Occurrence, Risk Assessment and Removal of Emerging Contaminants in Aquatic Environment

Occurrence, Risk Assessment and Removal of Emerging Contaminants in Aquatic Environment

Guest Editors

Xiaohu Lin
Binbin Shao
Jingcheng Xu

MDPI

Basel • Beijing • Wuhan • Barcelona • Belgrade • Novi Sad • Cluj • Manchester

Guest Editors

Xiaohu Lin
Hangzhou Institute of Ecological and Environmental Sciences
Hangzhou
China

Binbin Shao
College of Civil Engineering
Zhejiang University of Technology
Hangzhou
China

Jingcheng Xu
College of Environmental Science and Engineering
Tongji University
Shanghai
China

Editorial Office
MDPI AG
Grosspeteranlage 5
4052 Basel, Switzerland

This is a reprint of the Special Issue, published open access by the journal *Water* (ISSN 2073-4441), freely accessible at: https://www.mdpi.com/journal/water/special_issues/K56T336473.

For citation purposes, cite each article independently as indicated on the article page online and as indicated below:

Lastname, A.A.; Lastname, B.B. Article Title. *Journal Name* **Year**, *Volume Number*, Page Range.

ISBN 978-3-7258-5137-9 (Hbk)
ISBN 978-3-7258-5138-6 (PDF)
https://doi.org/10.3390/books978-3-7258-5138-6

Cover image courtesy of Xiaohu Lin

Contents

About the Editors

Xiaohu Lin

Xiaohu Lin is a Senior Engineer at the Hangzhou Institute of Ecological and Environmental Sciences, where he focuses on the application of artificial intelligence in ecological and environmental fields, "dual carbon" initiatives, and water environment treatment. He received his bachelor's and doctoral degrees from Tongji University, and was a joint Ph.D. student at the University of California, Santa Barbara. He also conducted postdoctoral research in collaboration with PowerChina Huadong Engineering Corporation Limited and the College of Environmental Science and Engineering at Tongji University. His primary research interests include the applications of AI in environmental science, the carbon footprints of products, green and low-carbon communities, integrated water environment governance, emerging contaminants, and the reuse of reclaimed water. Dr. Lin has published over 20 academic papers, including in SCI journals, has applied for more than 10 patents, and is the chief editor of one monograph.

Binbin Shao

Binbin Shao is a Research Associate Professor and master's supervisor whose research focuses on water pollution control technology. His work explores the mechanisms of pollutant purification and environmental remediation driven by non-radical oxidants, the reaction mechanisms of advanced oxidation processes such as Fenton-like systems and activated persulfate, and catalytic oxidation for the advanced treatment of metal complexes. He has published over 10 papers in authoritative academic journals, including *Environmental Science & Technology* and *Water Research*, and has led or participated in three national-level scientific research projects. He teaches undergraduate courses in Fluid Mechanics and graduate courses in Urban Water Conservation Theory and Technology, as well as Treatment Technologies and Engineering Cases for Recalcitrant Wastewater.

Jingcheng Xu

Jingcheng Xu is a Professor and Ph.D. supervisor at the College of Environmental Science and Engineering, Tongji University. He holds several key academic positions, including Vice Chairman and Secretary-General of the Shanghai Society for Environmental Sciences and Director of its Water Environment Professional Committee. His extensive career includes serving as Vice Dean and Deputy Party Secretary of his college. An esteemed educator recognized as a "Distinguished Teacher" at Tongji University, his research encompasses water pollution control and governance, advanced wastewater treatment and resource recovery, municipal drainage, and industrial process pollution control. Professor Xu has presided over more than 30 scientific research projects, has received over 30 national and provincial-level awards, has been the chief editor or co-editor of 13 textbooks and monographs, and has published over 100 academic papers.

Preface

The escalating diversity and quantity of synthetic chemicals entering our water systems represent one of the most pressing environmental challenges of the 21st century. These emerging contaminants (ECs)—a vast group that includes pharmaceuticals and industrial chemicals—are often present at trace concentrations, yet their persistence and biological activity raise profound concerns for the health of ecosystems and humans. Conventional treatment paradigms are frequently inadequate for their removal, necessitating urgent scientific innovation.

This Reprint, "Occurrence, Risk Assessment, and Removal of Emerging Contaminants in Aquatic Environments," was conceived to address this critical knowledge gap. Our aim was to assemble a comprehensive and diverse collection of high-quality research that captures the complexity of the EC problem. The scope of this work is intentionally broad, reflecting the multifaceted nature of the issue. It spans from fundamental investigations into the microbial mechanisms of co-metabolic degradation and the occurrence of specific pollutants in wastewater and drinking water, to the engineering of advanced materials like photocatalytic membranes and the implementation of intelligent control systems for treatment optimization.

This collection is addressed to the community of scientists, engineers, environmental managers, and policymakers who are at the forefront of protecting our aquatic ecosystems. It is our hope that the research presented in this Reprint will not only advance fundamental understanding, but also inspire the development and application of effective, sustainable, and scalable solutions to mitigate the threat of emerging contaminants, ensuring the safety and quality of water for generations to come.

Xiaohu Lin, Binbin Shao, and Jingcheng Xu
Guest Editors

water

Editorial

Occurrence, Risk Assessment, and Removal of Emerging Contaminants in Aquatic Environment

Xiaohu Lin [1,*], Binbin Shao [2] and Jingcheng Xu [3]

1 Hangzhou Institute of Ecological and Environmental Sciences, Hangzhou 310014, China
2 College of Civil Engineering, Zhejiang University of Technology, Hangzhou 310014, China; shaobb@zjut.edu.cn
3 College of Environmental Science and Engineering, Tongji University, Shanghai 200092, China; xujick@tongji.edu.cn
* Correspondence: tjhjxhlin@163.com

1. Introduction

The pervasive presence of emerging contaminants (ECs) in aquatic environments represents a significant and growing challenge for environmental science and public health in the 21st century [1–3]. Industrialization, agricultural intensification, and expanding urbanization have led to an explosive increase in the diversity and quantity of synthetic chemicals entering water systems [1,4]. These ECs encompass a wide range of substances, including pharmaceuticals and personal care products (PPCPs) [5,6], novel persistent organic pollutants (POPs) like per- and polyfluoroalkyl substances (PFASs) [7,8], endocrine-disrupting chemicals (EDCs) [9], disinfection by-products (DBPs) [10,11], engineered nanomaterials [12], microplastics [13], and flame retardants [14]. While often detected at trace concentrations (ng/L to µg/L levels), their continuous input into aquatic ecosystems, coupled with their potential persistence, bioaccumulation, and inherent biological activity, raises substantial concerns regarding long-term ecological impacts [15] and risks to human health [16].

Recent advancements in analytical chemistry have significantly improved our ability to detect and quantify these micropollutants in various environmental compartments, including wastewater [17,18], surface water [19], groundwater [20], and even drinking water [21]. However, significant knowledge gaps remain. The complex environmental fate, transport pathways, transformation products, and potential synergistic effects of EC mixtures are often poorly understood. Furthermore, conventional wastewater treatment plants (WWTPs) were not originally designed to remove these refractory compounds, often exhibiting limited and variable removal efficiencies, sometimes even acting as conduits for ECs and associated risks like antibiotic resistance genes (ARGs) into receiving waters. Consequently, there is an urgent need for research focusing on the comprehensive assessment of EC occurrence and risks, alongside the development and optimization of effective removal technologies and sustainable management strategies.

This Special Issue, "Occurrence, Risk Assessment, and Removal of Emerging Contaminants in Aquatic Environments", compiles ten original research articles and reviews that address these critical needs. The contributions herein explore the detection, fate, transport, and risk assessment of various ECs, evaluate conventional and advanced removal processes, and investigate novel management approaches, collectively advancing our understanding and offering potential solutions for safeguarding water quality.

https://doi.org/10.3390/w17111657

2. An Overview of Published Articles

This Special Issue compiles 10 insightful contributions covering a diverse range of topics central to the theme of emerging contaminants in aquatic systems.

Contributions 1, 2, and 5 delve into the biological treatment of specific recalcitrant organic pollutants, focusing on co-metabolism strategies. Wang et al. (Contribution 1) present a feasibility study utilizing excess sludge fermentation broth (FB) as an alternative, internal carbon source for the co-metabolic degradation of 2,4,6-trichlorophenol (2,4,6-TCP) in a sequencing batch reactor (SBR) system. Their findings demonstrate that this coupled system achieved stable and efficient 2,4,6-TCP removal (up to 240.13 mg/L) without external carbon sources, with the fermentation process yielding high concentrations of volatile fatty acids (VFAs), suggesting a cost-effective and sustainable approach. Wang and Li (Contribution 2) extended this work by exploring the degradation characteristics and underlying microbial mechanisms of using sludge FB. Through batch experiments and metagenomic analysis, they identified an optimal FB concentration range, pinpointed the inhibitory effects of specific VFAs (propionic acid), and revealed the enrichment of key chlorophenol degradation genes (e.g., PcpA, *chqB*, or *fadA*) and the associated bacterial genera like *Ralstonia* within the adapted sludge, providing deeper insights into the process's dynamics and genetic basis. Wang et al. (Contribution 5) further investigated the role of the carbon source by systematically comparing the effects of four common, easily degradable substrates (methanol, ethanol, sodium acetate, and sodium propionate) on 2,4,6-TCP degradation. Their results indicate that sodium acetate promoted the highest 2,4,6-TCP removal efficiency and stimulated the production of protective extracellular polymeric substances (EPSs), while different carbon sources led to distinct shifts in the microbial community structure and the abundance of functional metabolic genes, highlighting the significant influence of co-substrate choice on treatment performance and microbial ecology.

Contribution 3 explores advanced oxidation processes, specifically photocatalysis, for antibiotic removal. Lin et al. present the development and evaluation of novel composite photocatalytic membranes. Utilizing electrospinning, they successfully immobilized TiO_2 and TiO_2-reduced graphene oxide (rGO) onto polyacrylonitrile (PAN) nanofibers. Characterization confirmed the successful integration of the photocatalysts. Under simulated solar light, these PAN-TiO_2 and PAN-rGTi membranes exhibited significantly enhanced degradation rates for sulfamethoxazole (SMX) and enrofloxacin (ENR) compared to unmodified PAN membranes, addressing the challenge of catalyst recovery associated with powder forms. Importantly, the membranes demonstrated good stability and recyclability over five operational cycles, suggesting their potential for practical water purification applications.

Wastewater and sludge management strategies relevant to contaminant control are addressed in Contributions 4 and 7. Yang et al. (Contribution 4) report on a comprehensive full-chain approach to reprocessing historically landfilled municipal sludge in Shanghai, a significant challenge in megacities. Their study details the process from sludge extraction under geomembrane cover, through chemical conditioning (using PFSS/PEA or PAS/PEA) and subsequent dewatering to ~60% moisture content, to the physio-chemical treatment of the high-strength leachate generated and the evaluation of resource utilization pathways via co-incineration in power plants and solidification/modification for use as construction backfill. This work provides valuable insights into managing legacy waste streams that can act as reservoirs for various pollutants and reclaiming valuable urban land. Lu et al. (Contribution 7) focused on optimizing a critical WWTP process—chemical phosphorus removal. They developed an intelligent chemical dosing system for polyaluminum chloride (PAC) based on a feedforward prediction model combined with an adaptive fuzzy neural network P feedback controller. Pilot-scale experiments validated the optimal dosage, and subsequent implementation in a full-scale plant resulted in precise dosing control, achieving

100% effluent TP compliance and a 67% improvement in stability. Such process optimization enhances overall plant performance, potentially benefiting downstream EC removal, and reduces chemical consumption and sludge production, aligning with sustainability and low-carbon goals.

The occurrence, fate, and risks of specific EC classes are examined in Contributions 6 and 10. Liu et al. (Contribution 6) investigated 12 common organophosphate flame retardants (OPFRs) in a municipal WWTP in Hunan Province, China. Their analysis revealed that OPFRs were predominantly in the dissolved phase, with Tributoxyethyl phosphate (TBOEP) and tris(2-chloroethyl) phosphate (TCEP) being the most abundant. The overall removal efficiency was low (mean 39.1%), particularly for halogenated OPFRs which showed negative removal, indicating potential formation or release within the plant. Mass balance analysis indicated that a significant fraction (60.9%) was discharged via effluent, while adsorption to sludge (11.2%) and losses during treatment (biodegradation/biotransformation) accounted for the rest. The study highlights the inefficiency of conventional WWTPs in removing OPFRs and the associated ecological risks. Hernández et al. (Contribution 10) address disinfection by-products (DBPs) by determining the occurrence of chloroform ($CHCl_3$), a major trihalomethane (THM), in the drinking water supply of Cuenca, Ecuador. Sampling across three water treatment systems and their distribution networks over five months, they measured physicochemical parameters and $CHCl_3$ levels. While free chlorine residuals decreased along the distribution networks, $CHCl_3$ concentrations (ranging from 11.75 to 21.88 μg/L) remained below the Ecuadorian regulatory limit. No consistent correlation was found between $CHCl_3$ and the measured parameters, suggesting complex formation dynamics influenced by various factors, reinforcing the need for DBP monitoring in drinking water systems.

Finally, Contributions 8 and 9 provide valuable reviews synthesizing current knowledge. Wu et al. (Contribution 8) offer a comprehensive review of surfactant-enhanced remediation (SER) for non-aqueous phase liquid (NAPL)-contaminated soil and groundwater. The review details the mechanisms of surfactant action (mobilization, solubilization, and emulsification) and discusses the synergistic application of SER with various remediation techniques, including chemical oxidation, biodegradation, soil vapor extraction, electrokinetics, and thermal desorption. It also critically assesses the associated risks, such as residual surfactant toxicity, and explores the potential of more environmentally friendly biosurfactants. Zhu et al. (Contribution 9) present a broad review specifically focused on antibiotics within urban wastewater treatment systems. This review synthesizes information on the sources, occurrence, and potential ecological and human health risks of antibiotics and associated ARGs emanating from WWTPs. It covers the spectrum of detection methods, from enrichment techniques and immunoassays to advanced instrumental analysis and sensor technologies, and categorizes removal strategies including physical (membrane separation, adsorption), chemical (AOPs), and biological (activated sludge, MBRs) approaches, highlighting current limitations and challenges in effective antibiotic management in wastewater.

3. Conclusions and Future Directions

This Special Issue offers a multifaceted perspective on the pressing challenges posed by emerging contaminants in aquatic environments. The curated collection of ten articles spans a significant breadth of research, encompassing the investigation of specific contaminant classes such as chlorophenols, antibiotics, flame retardants, and disinfection by-products, alongside explorations into innovative remediation technologies and management strategies. Methodologically, the contributions showcase a diverse range of approaches, from detailed laboratory and pilot-scale experiments and field monitoring campaigns to advanced analytical techniques like metagenomics, comprehensive mass balance analyses, the development of intelligent control systems, and critical literature reviews.

Collectively, the research presented herein significantly advances our understanding of ECs. Studies like those by Wang et al. (Contributions 1 and 2) provide valuable insights into optimizing biological degradation pathways, demonstrating the potential of utilizing waste streams like sludge fermentate as sustainable co-substrates, and elucidating the complex interplay between carbon sources and microbial functional gene abundance. The work by Lin et al. (Contribution 3) highlights the promise of advanced materials, showing that electrospun photocatalytic membranes can effectively degrade antibiotics while overcoming the practical limitations of catalyst recovery. Investigations by Liu et al. (Contribution 6) and Hernández et al. (Contribution 10) underscore the limitations of existing treatment infrastructure in removing persistent compounds like OPFRs and managing DBP formation, respectively, providing crucial occurrence data and risk context. Furthermore, the studies by Yang et al. (Contribution 4) and Lu et al. (Contribution 7) demonstrate innovative approaches to managing legacy pollution (landfilled sludge) and optimizing existing treatment processes in ways that indirectly benefit overall contaminant control and resource management within WWTPs. The comprehensive reviews by Wu et al. (Contribution 8) and Zhu et al. (Contribution 9) synthesize the state-of-the-art in SER technologies and antibiotic management in wastewater systems, respectively, identifying key challenges and future research needs.

Despite the progress highlighted in this Special Issue, the field of emerging contaminants continues to face substantial hurdles, necessitating focused future research efforts. A critical area remains the development and scaling-up of efficient and cost-effective removal technologies. While novel materials like the photocatalytic membranes studied by Lin et al. (Contribution 3) show promise, transitioning these from lab-scale success to robust, full-scale application requires overcoming challenges related to long-term stability, fouling resistance, and economic viability. Further research into advanced oxidation processes, selective adsorbents, and optimizing biological processes, perhaps by harnessing specific microbial consortia or enzymes, is warranted. The synergistic combination of different treatment modalities, such as integrating physical pre-treatment with AOPs and biological polishing, deserves greater exploration.

Understanding the long-term ecological and health risks associated with chronic, low-level exposure to complex mixtures of ECs and their transformation products remains a paramount challenge. The work by Liu et al. (Contribution 6) on OPFR risk assessment exemplifies the need for such studies across a broader range of contaminants. Particular attention should be paid to the fate and transfer of antibiotic resistance genes through wastewater systems, a risk highlighted by Zhu et al. (Contribution 9), and the potential endocrine-disrupting effects of various ECs.

Continuous improvement in analytical methodologies is essential for accurate monitoring and risk assessment. Detecting ultra-trace concentrations of diverse ECs and their metabolites in complex matrices like wastewater and sludge requires ongoing innovation in sample preparation (enrichment/extraction) and instrumental analysis, possibly through the advanced sensor technologies discussed by Zhu et al.(Contribution 9) Developing rapid, cost-effective, and field-deployable monitoring tools would greatly enhance regulatory efforts and plant operational control.

Finally, bridging the gap between scientific understanding and effective management requires a holistic approach. This includes stronger source control measures, as emphasized by Zhu et al. (Contribution 9), optimizing existing infrastructure through approaches like the intelligent control systems developed by Lu et al. (Contribution 7), exploring sustainable solutions like biosurfactants for remediation (Contribution 8), and developing integrated assessment frameworks that consider the entire lifecycle of contaminants and treatment processes. The management of waste streams like landfilled sludge, addressed by Yang et al. (Contribution 4), is also a crucial component of preventing long-term environmental liabilities.

The research presented in this Special Issue provides valuable contributions to addressing the multifaceted challenge of emerging contaminants in aquatic environments. It is hoped that these articles will stimulate further investigation and innovation, ultimately leading to more effective strategies for protecting water resources and public health.

Acknowledgments: We extend our gratitude to all contributors and reviewers for their dedication to advancing this critical field. Their work collectively reinforces the urgency of addressing emerging contaminants through science-driven, sustainable approaches.

Conflicts of Interest: The authors declare no conflicts of interest.

List of Contributions:

1. Wang, J.; Sun, Z.; Li, J. Feasibility Study of Using Excess Sludge Fermentation Broth as a Co-Metabolic Carbon Source for 2,4,6-Trichlorophenol Degradation. *Water* **2023**, *15*, 4008. https://doi.org/10.3390/w15224008.
2. Wang, J.; Li, S. Exploring 2,4,6-Trichlorophenol Degradation Characteristics and Functional Metabolic Gene Abundance Using Sludge Fermentation Broth as the Carbon Source. *Water* **2023**, *15*, 4279. https://doi.org/10.3390/w15244279.
3. Liu, X.; Fang, H.; Wang, L.; Sun, D.; Zhao, G.; Xu, J. Photocatalytic Degradation of Sulfamethoxazole and Enrofloxacin in Water Using Electrospun Composite Photocatalytic Membrane. *Water* **2024**, *16*, 218. https://doi.org/10.3390/w16020218.
4. Yang, Y.; Luan, J.; Nie, J.; Zhang, X.; Du, J.; Zhao, G.; Dong, L.; Fan, Y.; Cui, H.; Li, Y. Reprocessing and Resource Utilization of Landfill Sludge—A Case Study in a Chinese Megacity. *Water* **2024**, *16*, 468. https://doi.org/10.3390/w16030468.
5. Wang, J.; Fang, H.; Li, S.; Yu, H. Delving into the Impacts of Different Easily Degradable Carbon Sources on the Degradation Characteristics of 2,4,6-Trichlorophenol and Microbial Community Properties. *Water* **2024**, *16*, 974. https://doi.org/10.3390/w16070974.
6. Liu, Y.; Song, Y.; Li, H.; Yang, Z. Occurrence, Fate, and Mass Balance Analysis of Organophosphate Flame Retardants in a Municipal Wastewater Treatment Plant in Hunan Province, China. *Water* **2024**, *16*, 1462. https://doi.org/10.3390/w16111462.
7. Lu, X.; Huang, S.; Liu, H.; Yang, F.; Zhang, T.; Wan, X. Research on Intelligent Chemical Dosing System for Phosphorus Removal in Wastewater Treatment Plants. *Water* **2024**, *16*, 1623. https://doi.org/10.3390/w16111623.
8. Wu, L.; Zhang, J.; Chen, F.; Li, J.; Wang, W.; Li, S.; He, L. Review of Surfactant-Enhanced Remediation Technology for NAPL Pollution in Soil and Groundwater. *Water* **2024**, *16*, 2093. https://doi.org/10.3390/w16152093.
9. Zhu, L.; Lin, X.; Di, Z.; Cheng, F.; Xu, J. Occurrence, Risks, and Removal Methods of Antibiotics in Urban Wastewater Treatment Systems: A Review. *Water* **2024**, *16*, 3428. https://doi.org/10.3390/w16233428.
10. Hernández, B.; Duque-Sarango, P.; Tonón, M.D.; Abril-González, M.; Pinos-Vélez, V.; García-Sánchez, C.R.; Rodríguez, M.J. Determination of the Occurrence of Trihalomethanes in the Drinking Water Supply of the City of Cuenca, Ecuador. *Water* **2025**, *17*, 591. https://doi.org/10.3390/w17040591.

References

1. Puri, M.; Gandhi, K.; Kumar, M.S. Emerging environmental contaminants: A global perspective on policies and regulations. *J. Environ. Manag.* **2023**, *332*, 117344. [CrossRef] [PubMed]
2. Rathi, B.S.; Kumar, P.S.; Show, P.L. A review on effective removal of emerging contaminants from aquatic systems: Current trends and scope for further research. *J. Hazard. Mater.* **2021**, *409*, 124413. [CrossRef] [PubMed]

3. Tong, X.E.; You, L.H.; Zhang, J.J.; Chen, H.T.; Nguyen, V.T.; He, Y.L.; Gin, K.Y.H. A comprehensive modelling approach to understanding the fate, transport and potential risks of emerging contaminants in a tropical reservoir. *Water Res.* **2021**, *200*, 117298. [CrossRef]
4. Kundu, P.; Dutta, N.; Bhattacharya, S. Application of microalgae in wastewater treatment with special reference to emerging contaminants: A step towards sustainability. *Front. Anal. Sci.* **2024**, *4*, 1513153. [CrossRef]
5. Reyes, N.; Geronimo, F.K.F.; Yano, K.A.V.; Guerra, H.B.; Kim, L.H. Pharmaceutical and Personal Care Products in Different Matrices: Occurrence, Pathways, and Treatment Processes. *Water* **2021**, *13*, 1159. [CrossRef]
6. Lu, S.; Wang, J.; Wang, B.D.; Xin, M.; Lin, C.Y.; Gu, X.; Lian, M.S.; Li, Y. Comprehensive profiling of the distribution, risks and priority of pharmaceuticals and personal care products: A large-scale study from rivers to coastal seas. *Water Res.* **2023**, *230*, 119591. [CrossRef]
7. Byrne, P.; Mayes, W.M.; James, A.L.; Comber, S.; Biles, E.; Riley, A.L.; Runkel, R.L. PFAS River Export Analysis Highlights the Urgent Need for Catchment-Scale Mass Loading Data. *Environ. Sci. Technol. Lett.* **2024**, *11*, 266–272. [CrossRef]
8. Pétré, M.A.; Salk, K.R.; Stapleton, H.M.; Ferguson, P.L.; Tait, G.; Obenour, D.R.; Knappe, D.R.U.; Genereux, D.P. Per- and polyfluoroalkyl substances (PFAS) in river discharge: Modeling loads upstream and downstream of a PFAS manufacturing plant in the Cape Fear watershed, North Carolina. *Sci. Total Environ.* **2022**, *831*, 154763. [CrossRef]
9. Liao, Z.; Jian, Y.; Lu, J.; Liu, Y.L.; Li, Q.Y.; Deng, X.Z.; Xu, Y.; Wang, Q.P.; Yang, Y.; Luo, Z.F. Distribution, migration patterns, and food chain human health risks of endocrine-disrupting chemicals in water, sediments, and fish in the Xiangjiang River. *Sci. Total Environ.* **2024**, *930*, 172484. [CrossRef]
10. Sanchis, J.; Redondo-Hasselerharm, P.E.; Villanueva, C.M.; Farre, M.J. Non targeted screening of nitrogen containing disinfection by-products in formation potential tests of river water and subsequent monitoring in tap water samples. *Chemosphere* **2022**, *303*, 135087. [CrossRef]
11. Wu, S.N.; Dong, H.Y.; Zhang, L.P.; Qiang, Z.M. Formation Characteristics and Risk Assessment of Disinfection By-Products in Drinking Water in Two of China's Largest Basins: Yangtze River Basin Versus Yellow River Basin. *ACS EST Water* **2023**, *4*, 79–90. [CrossRef]
12. Saharia, A.M.; Zhu, Z.; Aich, N.; Baalousha, M.; Atkinson, J.F. Modeling the transport of titanium dioxide nanomaterials from combined sewer overflows in an urban river. *Sci. Total Environ.* **2019**, *696*, 133904. [CrossRef]
13. Bian, P.Y.; Liu, Y.X.; Zhao, K.H.; Hu, Y.; Zhang, J.; Kang, L.; Shen, W.B. Spatial variability of microplastic pollution on surface of rivers in a mountain-plain transitional area: A case study in the Chin Ling-Wei River Plain, China. *Ecotoxicol. Environ. Saf.* **2022**, *232*, 113298. [CrossRef] [PubMed]
14. Chen, P.; Ma, S.T.; Yang, Y.; Qi, Z.H.; Wang, Y.J.; Li, G.Y.; Tang, J.H.; Yu, Y.X. Organophosphate flame retardants, tetrabromo-bisphenol A, and their transformation products in sediment of e-waste dismantling areas and the flame-retardant production base. *Ecotoxicol. Environ. Saf.* **2021**, *225*, 112717. [CrossRef]
15. Zhu, Q.H.; Li, X.D.; Song, F.H. Emerging Contaminants in Natural and Engineered Water Environments: Environmental Behavior, Ecological Effects and Control Strategies. *Water* **2025**, *17*, 1329. [CrossRef]
16. Yang, J.Y.; Zhang, X.; Liu, Z.S.; Yang, C.X.; Li, S.; Zhou, H.Y.; Gao, Z.X. The impact of emerging contaminants exposure on human health effects: A review of organoid assessment models. *Chem. Eng. J.* **2024**, *498*, 155882. [CrossRef]
17. Boro, D.; Chirania, M.; Verma, A.K.; Chettri, D.; Verma, A.K. Comprehensive approaches to managing emerging contaminants in wastewater: Identification, sources, monitoring and remediation. *Environ. Monit. Assess.* **2025**, *197*, 456. [CrossRef]
18. Ferreira, S.L.C.; Azevedo, R.S.A.; da Silva, J.D., Jr.; Teixeira, L.S.G.; dos Santos, I.F.; dos Santos, W.N.L.; Queiroz, A.F.S.; de Oliveira, O.M.C.; Guarieiro, L.L.N.; dos Anjos, J.P.; et al. Emerging contaminants—General aspects: Sources, substances involved, and quantification. *Appl. Spectrosc. Rev.* **2024**, *59*, 632–651. [CrossRef]
19. Zhang, Y.H.; Li, J.X.; Jiao, S.P.; Li, Y.; Zhou, Y.; Zhang, X.; Maryam, B.; Liu, X.H. Microfluidic sensors for the detection of emerging contaminants in water: A review. *Sci. Total Environ.* **2024**, *929*, 172734. [CrossRef]
20. Auersperger, P.; Korosa, A.; Mali, N.; Jamnik, B. Passive Sampling with Active Carbon Fibres in the Determination of Organic Pollutants in Groundwater. *Water* **2022**, *14*, 585. [CrossRef]
21. Paszkiewicz, M.; Godlewska, K.; Lis, H.; Caban, M.; Bia, A.; Stepnowski, P. Advances in suspect screening and non-target analysis of polar emerging contaminants in the environmental monitoring. *TrAC Trends Anal. Chem.* **2022**, *154*, 116671. [CrossRef]

water

MDPI

Article

Feasibility Study of Using Excess Sludge Fermentation Broth as a Co-Metabolic Carbon Source for 2,4,6-Trichlorophenol Degradation

Jianguang Wang [1,2,*], Zhirong Sun [1,*] and Jun Li [1]

1 National Engineering Laboratory for Advanced Municipal Wastewater Treatment and Reuse Technology, Beijing University of Technology, Beijing 100124, China
2 PowerChina Huadong Engineering Corporation Limited, Hangzhou 311122, China
* Correspondence: wjg909090@163.com (J.W.); zrsun@bjut.edu.cn (Z.S.)

Abstract: Excess sludge fermentation is a commonly employed method for carbon sources in wastewater treatment plants, but its use as a carbon source for chlorophenol removal has been relatively underexplored. In this study, a laboratory-scale sludge fermentation SBR (FSBR) was integrated with a 2,4,6-trichlorophenol (2,4,6-TCP) degradation SBR (DSBR), resulting in a stable removal of 2,4,6-TCP without the need for external carbon sources. In this coupled system, the concentrations of volatile fatty acids in FSBR remained constant, with acetic acid, propionic acid, butyric acid, and valeric acid concentrations reaching 322.04 mg COD/L, 225.98 mg COD/L, 274.76 mg COD/L, and 149.58 mg COD/L, respectively, and the acid production efficiency increased to 88.40%. Throughout the 110-day operational period, the activated sludge concentration in the DSBR was consistently maintained at 3021 ± 110 mg/L, and the sludge SVI remained stable at 70 mL/g. The maximum amount of 2,4,6-TCP removed reached 240.13 mg/L within a 12 h operating cycle. The use of excess sludge fermentation can completely replace commercial carbon sources for 2,4,6-TCP removal, leading to cost savings in chlorophenol treatment and broadening the applicability of this technology.

Keywords: 2,4,6-trichlorophenol; co-metabolism; excess sludge fermentation; carbon source; coupling process

1. Introduction

2,4,6-Trichlorophenol (2,4,6-TCP)-containing wastewater is a common form of organic effluent originating from the paper, printing, and dyeing industries. This wastewater is highly hazardous and accumulative, necessitating stringent treatment before discharge into the environment. Failure to do so could lead to substantial harm to aquatic ecosystems [1,2]. Currently, advanced oxidation techniques, including the Fenton method, ozone-catalyzed oxidation, and electrochemical catalytic oxidation, are employed to address persistent organic contaminants in wastewater [3–5]. Nevertheless, the widespread application of advanced oxidation methods is constrained by their rigorous treatment conditions, limited capacity, and substantial energy consumption. 2,4,6-TCP wastewater is categorized as a persistent contaminant due to its low five-day biochemical oxygen demand (BOD_5) to chemical oxygen demand (COD) ratio, which is less than 0.3 [6]. Additionally, the pronounced toxicity of 2,4,6-TCP exacerbates the challenges associated with its biological treatment. Consequently, the concept of biological co-metabolism was introduced by Stirling, D.I. et al. [7]: the addition of readily degradable organic compounds can stimulate the microbial degradation of recalcitrant organic compounds that cannot directly serve as carbon and energy sources. From an enzymatic metabolism perspective, the presence of easily degradable substrates induces the production of a broad-spectrum non-specific enzyme by microorganisms, which can facilitate the metabolism of recalcitrant organic compounds [8,9]. As a result, readily degradable carbon sources have been extensively investigated, as they play a pivotal role in influencing the effectiveness of biological co-metabolic treatment.

Previous research has revealed that readily degradable carbon sources offer more significant benefits compared to refractory carbon sources in enhancing the removal of 2,4,6-TCP [10]. Commonly employed biodegradable carbon sources, such as sodium acetate, glucose, and sucrose, have proven to be effective in removing various chlorophenol compounds, including trichlorophenol, dichlorophenol, and monochlorophenol [11–14]. Nevertheless, these readily degradable organic substances are typically obtained through artificial extraction or synthesis, making them expensive for large-scale applications in treating chlorophenol wastewater. Furthermore, various degradation devices used in chlorophenol treatment, such as Sequencing Batch Reactors (SBR) and Upflow Anaerobic Sludge Blanket reactors, still rely heavily on external carbon sources to enhance the biochemical characteristics of phenol-containing wastewater. Hence, the challenge remains to reduce treatment costs and enhance treatment sustainability when utilizing readily degradable organic compounds as the carbon source in biological co-metabolism processes.

The anaerobic digestion of excess sludge is a widely adopted approach for reducing sludge volume and harnessing resources in wastewater treatment plants (WWTP) [15,16]. By controlling the digestion process, it is possible to steer it toward the acidogenic phase, resulting in the production of short-chain fatty acids (SCFAs), including acetic acid, propionic acid, butyric acid, and valeric acid [17,18]. SCFAs, as high-quality carbon sources, have found application in municipal WWTP to address the shortage of carbon sources in managing domestic sewage [19]. Currently, research on sludge fermentation primarily focuses on the impact of the fermentation liquid as a carbon source on denitrification and phosphorus removal efficiency, as well as the study of fermentation conditions' influence [20,21]. Hu, C. et al. [22] investigated the impact of hydrolyzed acidification liquids from various residual sludges as carbon sources on denitrification. They found that the removal efficiency of nitrate nitrogen reached over 99% at the optimal hydraulic retention time (HRT). Specifically, the utilization rate of VFAs reached 90.6% at an HRT of 4 h, indicating that VFAs outperformed other hydrolyzed liquid components. Chen, Y. et al. [23] investigated the influence of surfactants (sodium dodecylbenzene sulfonate, SDBS) and alkaline conditions on VFA (volatile fatty acid) production. The results revealed that, at a hydraulic retention time of 10 h and under pH 10, VFAs production reached its peak at 2056 mg COD/L. However, there is limited research that explores the use of digestion products as a carbon source for co-metabolizing toxic pollutants.

The removal efficiency of the target pollutant is influenced by the type and addition level of the carbon source [24]. Anaerobic digestion products serve as mixed carbon sources, primarily composed of SCFAs, ethanol, butanol, and a variety of other organic materials [25]. SCFAs, being readily biodegradable, play a beneficial role in enhancing the removal rate of chlorophenols. To improve the removal rate of chlorophenols, it is essential to control fermentation conditions, thereby increasing the SCFAs level in the FB. Furthermore, the concentration of the carbon source also impacts co-metabolism efficiency and the growth of functional microbes [24,26]. The feasibility of substituting the single organic source with a complex FB as the co-metabolism carbon source warrants further investigation in the field of wastewater treatment.

In light of the background and the challenges identified, this study's primary objectives are as follows: to investigate the viability of utilizing excess sludge FB as the co-metabolism carbon source for the removal of 2,4,6-TCP, and to establish a coupled system integrating excess sludge FB and co-metabolism to achieve the prolonged, stable, and efficient removal of 2,4,6-TCP. This experiment marks the pioneering introduction of sludge FB into the co-metabolic system, holding significant implications for the sustained and cost-effective operation of biological co-metabolism processes. Moreover, the stability of the integrated system offers a novel avenue for the resource utilization of excess sludge in wastewater treatment. These findings have the potential to drive advancements in both wastewater treatment technology and the responsible management of excess sludge resources.

2. Materials and Methods

2.1. System Setup and the Reactor Operation

The operation system employed in this study consisted of two sequencing batch reactors (SBR), each with a working volume of 3 L, as illustrated in Figure 1. The Fermentation SBR (FSBR) served as the dedicated fermentation reactor, while the Degradation SBR (DSBR) was utilized as the co-metabolism reactor for the degradation of 2,4,6-TCP. Both the FSBR and DSBR were meticulously controlled through automated timers to ensure the coupling of these reactors and enable their prolonged and stable operation.

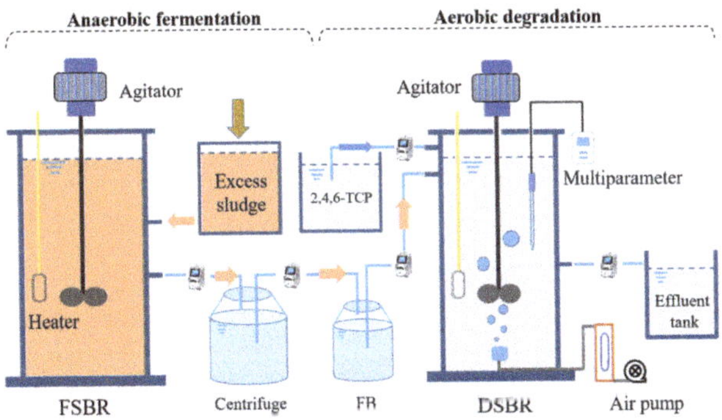

Figure 1. The schematic diagram of the experimental setup for this study is presented.

2.1.1. Long-Term Operation of FSBR

During the 180-day operation of the FSBR, as shown in Figure 2b, the FSBR operated for 24 h per cycle for the initial 110 days of operation, as depicted in Figure 2a. Each typical operation cycle was divided into three stages, comprising a 15 min discharge of FB, 15 min feeding of excess sludge, and a 23.5 h period of anaerobic fermentation. Throughout the entire cycle, a mechanical stirrer maintained a constant mixing rate of 200 revolutions per minute (rpm). The FSBR was held at a consistent temperature of 30 °C through the use of a heater. In each cycle, 300 mL of mixed FB was extracted from the reactor using a peristaltic pump to maintain a solid residence time (SRT) of 10 days. Subsequently, an equivalent volume of excess sludge was introduced into the reactor. Material exchange was carried out through the peristaltic pump to preserve an anaerobic environment within the FSBR. The Mixed Liquor Suspended Solids (MLSS) was consistently maintained at a level of 10,000 mg/L throughout the entire operation.

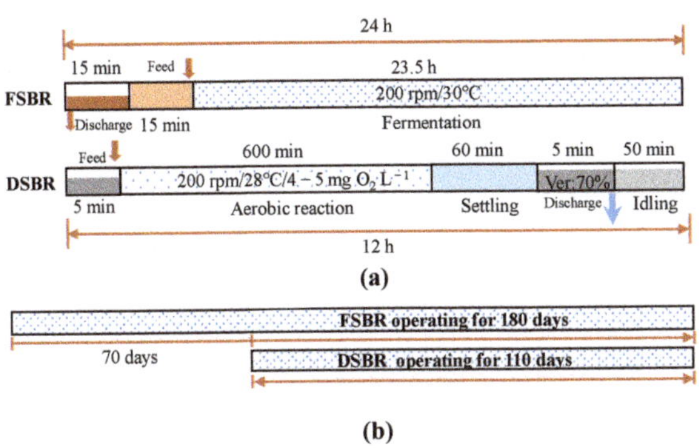

Figure 2. The typical operation of the system: (**a**) the operating mode of FSBR and DSBR, (**b**) the operation timeline of the FSBR-DSBR coupling process.

2.1.2. Long-Term Operation of DSBR

The DSBR was operated for a total of 110 days. DSBR was initiated after the FSBR had been in operation for 70 days and had reached a point where it could consistently produce a constant concentration of FB. The FB from FSBR was utilized as the co-catabolic carbon source and was introduced into DSBR along with the 2,4,6-TCP. DSBR operated with a cycle duration of 12 h, and a typical cycle, as illustrated in Figure 2a, included five stages (Figure 2a): a 5 min period for feeding synthetic wastewater; a 600 min period of aerobic reaction, maintaining an oxygen concentration of 4–5 mgO_2/L; a 60 min settling phase; a 5 min discharge phase with a volumetric exchange ratio of 70%; and a 50 min idling phase. The hydraulic retention time was consistently held at 24 h, and the SRT was maintained at 120 days by discharging 25 mL of mixed sludge per day. An agitator was used to thoroughly mix the activated sludge at a stirring speed of 200 rpm. Throughout the entire operation, the temperature was maintained at 28 °C using a constant heater. In our previous research, it has already been demonstrated that under conditions without the addition of a carbon source, activated sludge cannot attain a high concentration 2,4,6-TCP degradation capacity [24].

2.2. *Seeding Sludge and Influent Wastewater Composition*

The inoculum used in this study was derived from aerobic activated sludge collected from the aeration tank of the Xiaohongmen municipal WWTP located in Beijing, China. It is important to note that this activated sludge primarily serves in the treatment of municipal domestic wastewater and does not possess the capability to degrade 2,4,6-TCP. Before inoculation, the freshly acquired sludge underwent a washing process with tap water to eliminate impurities and contaminants. Subsequently, the initial concentration of this inoculum, amounting to 3000 mg/L, was introduced into both the FSBR and the DSBR for the study.

The feed for the FSBR comprised pre-treated excess activated sludge, sourced from the WWTP at Xiaohongmen, Beijing, along with the sludge discharged from the DSBR. The excess sludge had undergone hydrothermal treatment at 100 °C. This treatment is aimed at disintegrating the sludge cells, releasing extracellular polymeric substances, and making intracellular organic matter more accessible. This results in the generation of abundant substrates to support the anaerobic fermentation process. The treated sludge utilized in the FSBR had a concentration of 10,000 mg/L. The specific compositions and details of this treated sludge are outlined in Table 1.

Table 1. Compositions of added excess sludge and effluent fermentation broth (mg/L).

Components	TCOD	SCOD	SS	Proteins	Polysaccharide	VFAs (mg COD/L)	NH_4^+	PO_4^{3-}	NO_3^-
Influent	11,770	4984	10,830	1130	155	-	75.7	23.6	-
Effluent	1223.5	1120.2	-	-	-	974.5	634.4	193.4	5.2

Note: "-" represents values falling below the detection limit.

The influent of the DSBR included centrifugal-fermentation broth, 2,4,6-TCP within the concentration range of 0–200 mg/L, and trace elements. The composition of the trace elements is shown in Table S1 of the Supplementary Material. The centrifugal-fermentation broth was used as the co-metabolism carbon source in this experiment (Table 1).

2.3. *The Batch Experiment*

2.3.1. Mineralization and Chlorine Ion Removal Experiments of 2,4,6-TCP

The influent concentration of 2,4,6-TCP was set at 100 mg/L, and to eliminate any interference from chlorine ions in the influent, ultrapure water was used for preparation. The influent concentration of the FB was the same as that of DSBR, which is 150 mg COD/L. Dissolved oxygen was maintained at 4–5 mg/L. The experiment lasted for 10 h, with sampling intervals of 60 min. Mixed sludge samples were centrifuged, passed through a

0.22 μm filter membrane, and the clear liquid was analyzed for chloride ions, 2,4,6-TCP, and Total Organic Carbon (TOC) values.

2.3.2. Ammonia Nitrogen Concentration Influence Experiment

The experiment commenced with the addition of 100 mg/L of 2,4,6-TCP, and the influent concentration of the FB was maintained at 150 mg COD/L. In order to assess the influence of ammonia nitrogen (NH_4^+-N) concentrations, levels of 40 mg/L, 200 mg/L, 400 mg/L, 800 mg/L, and 1200 mg/L were tested. The experiment lasted for 10 h, maintaining the same sampling intervals and sample processing procedures as described in the previous test. The focus was on measuring the concentration of 2,4,6-TCP.

2.4. Analytical Methods

In this study, a comprehensive set of parameters was analyzed, including Total Chemical Oxygen Demand (TCOD), Soluble Chemical Oxygen Demand (SCOD), Ammonium Nitrogen (NH_4^+-N), Nitrate Nitrogen (NO_3^--N), Phosphate (PO_4^{3-}), Suspended Solids (SV), Sludge Volume Index (SVI), and Mixed Liquor Suspended Solids (MLSS). These measurements were conducted following the standard procedures outlined in the standard method [27].

The quantification of 2,4,6-TCP and SCFAs was carried out using high-performance liquid chromatography (HPLC, Waters 1525, Milford, MA, USA) and gas chromatography (Agilent 7890A, Santa Clara, CA, USA), respectively. The specific testing conditions were based on the methodology described by Wang, J. et al. [24] and Wang, B. et al. [18].

2.5. Calculation

The calculation of COD_{SCFAs} (mg/L) and the efficiency of SCFAs production (%) was performed using Equations (1) and (2):

$$COD_{SCFAs}\ (mg/L) = C_{SCFAs} \times n_x \tag{1}$$

$$\text{SCFAs production efficiency}\ (\%) = COD_{SCFAs}/COD_{Eff} \times 100\% \tag{2}$$

C_{SCFAs} (mg/L) represents the concentration of SCFAs as determined through liquid chromatography testing. The conversion factor, denoted as "n_x", was defined based on the methodology described by Wang, B. et al. [18]; COD_{Eff} stands for the COD of the effluent FB.

3. Results and Discussion

3.1. The Performance of FSBR in the Long-Term Operation

The stable acid production process in FSBR plays a crucial role in facilitating the efficient degradation of 2,4,6-TCP in DSBR. Overall, anaerobic sludge fermentation comprises four distinct stages: particulate organic matter dissolution and release, hydrolysis of soluble organic matter, acidogenesis, and methane production. Of these stages, converting particulate organic matter into soluble organic matter is a crucial step in anaerobic acidogenesis [28]. Consequently, several researchers have aimed to improve the solubilization of particulate organic matter by implementing various techniques including ultrasound, microwave treatment, heat treatment, the supplementation of surfactants, and alkaline treatment, as evidenced by previous studies [29–33].

The primary objective was to investigate the feasibility of utilizing sludge fermentation byproducts for the co-metabolic degradation of 2,4,6-TCP. To achieve this aim, sludge fermentation was conducted under optimal conditions with the intention of obtaining stable fermentation byproducts. Additionally, a thermal treatment method involving heating at 100 °C for 3 h was employed as a pretreatment for the residual sludge. A comparison of the sludge composition before and after pretreatment revealed a significant increase in the concentration of soluble organic substances in the mixed liquor, as shown in Table 1.

As shown in Figure 3, during the initial 10 days of the first run, VFAs production was low. In the subsequent period, from day 10 to day 30, the production of acetic acid and propionic acid initially increased, reaching 256.93 mg COD/L and 160.38 mg COD/L, respectively. However, at this point, the production of butyric acid and valeric acid remained low, resulting in an overall acid production efficiency of 55.95%. During days 30 to 70, VFAs gradually increased and stabilized, with concentrations of acetic acid, propionic acid, butyric acid, and valeric acid reaching 322.04 mg COD/L, 225.98 mg COD/L, 274.76 mg COD/L, and 149.58 mg COD/L, respectively. The acid production efficiency increased to 88.40%, which is significantly higher than the average acid production efficiency reported in the literature (55 ± 10.3%) [34]. After day 70, VFAs production remained stable.

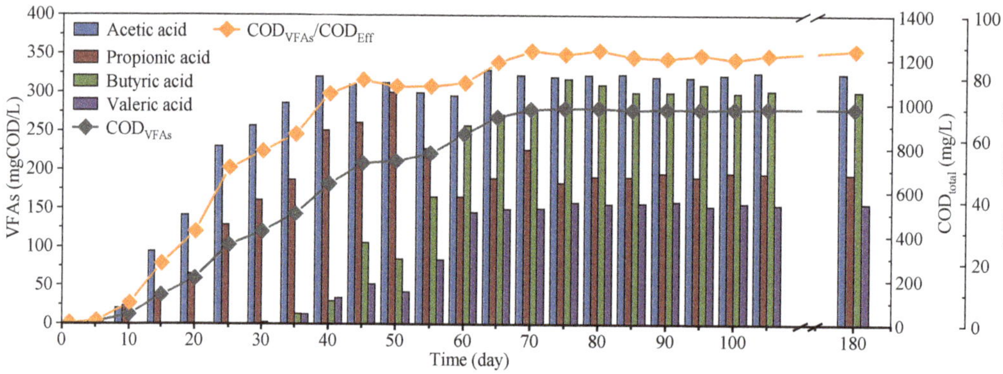

Figure 3. Long-term variation in VFA production in FSBR.

3.2. DSBR Performance in Long-Term Acclimation

3.2.1. 2,4,6-TCP Degradation Performance

The influent sludge fermentation liquid in the DSBR was consistently maintained at 150 mg COD/L, utilizing the activated sludge control method with a constant sludge concentration as described in Wang, J. et al. [24]. As shown in Figure 4a, a gradient increment approach was used for adding 2,4,6-TCP with influent ranging from 10 to 250 mg/L. The effluent 2,4,6-TCP was carefully monitored during each additional concentration. If a notable quantity of 2,4,6-TCP was detected in the effluent, the influent concentration was reduced or maintained to avoid impeding the activated sludge metabolism with excess inhibition from the 2,4,6-TCP. Over a lengthy operational period and with adjustments to the reactor, beneficial bacteria in the activated sludge were steadily enriched, enabling the decomposition of elevated 2,4,6-TCP concentrations. After a 110-day acclimation period, the influent 2,4,6-TCP was maintained at 250 mg/L, while the effluent 2,4,6-TCP remained consistently at 9.87 mg/L. This indicates that the functional bacteria achieved the maximum degradation concentration of 2,4,6-TCP, which is 240.13 mg/L.

Wang, J. et al. [35] used domestic wastewater as a substitute for commercial carbon sources and achieved a maximum degradation concentration of 2,4,6-TCP at 208 mg/L. When using glucose, sucrose, or starch as single carbon sources, they obtained 2,4,6-TCP degradation concentrations of 65 mg/L [10]. In this study, the obtained 2,4,6-TCP degradation concentration of 240.13 mg/L was significantly higher than the scenarios mentioned in the literature. The primary components of sludge fermentation liquid were volatile fatty acids (VFAs), and the FSBR achieved an acid production efficiency of 88.40%. VFAs were more easily biodegraded and utilized by microorganisms compared to domestic wastewater or single carbon sources. This may have explained why using sludge fermentation liquid as a carbon source yielded superior results compared to other carbon sources.

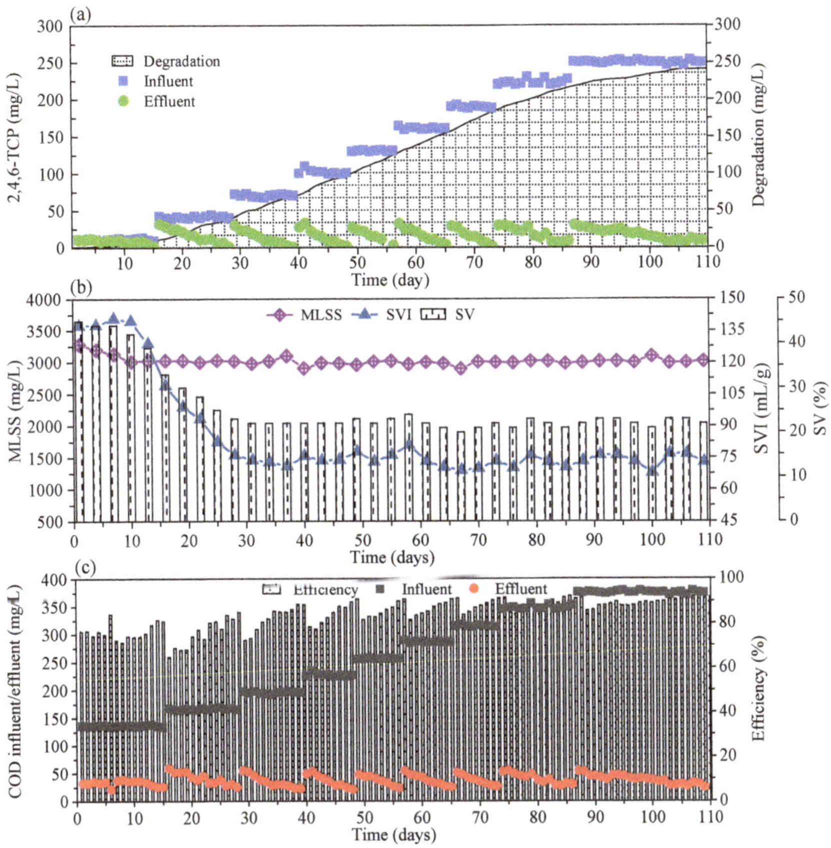

Figure 4. Operating characteristics of the DSBR during 110-day domestication: (**a**) the variation characteristics of influent and effluent of 2,4,6-TCP and degradable concentration; (**b**) the variations in activated sludge operating characteristics; (**c**) COD influent and effluent concentrations and removal efficiency.

3.2.2. COD Removal Performance

The influent and effluent COD, as well as the removal efficiency during the long-term operation of the DSBR, are depicted in Figure 4c. During the operation, COD was primarily contributed by the fermentation liquid and 2,4,6-TCP. It can be observed that the influent COD was correlated with 2,4,6-TCP, showing a gradient increase. Throughout the long-term operation of the reactor, maintaining effluent COD consistently below 50 mg/L signifies the stability of sludge properties and the absence of significant toxic inhibition.

However, the COD removal efficiency was relatively low during the early acclimation phase, ranging from 70% to 80%. In the stable operational phase, the removal efficiency can exceed 90%. Therefore, throughout the entire acclimation period, the DSBR demonstrates a substantial capability for COD degradation.

3.2.3. Sludge Characteristics

Before the start of the DSBR operation, the inoculated sludge concentration was 3280 ± 100 mg/L. After 110 days of operation, the sludge concentration slightly decreased but was maintained at 3021 ± 110 mg/L, with no significant fluctuations during this period. This indicates that a sludge fermenter with a concentration of 150 mg COD/L can sustain the carbon source metabolism of activated sludge and maintain a constant sludge concentration.

Furthermore, the sedimentation performance of the sludge during DSBR operation can be reflected by calculating the SVI value, and a good sedimentation performance helps to reduce the loss of activated sludge during the DSBR drainage phase. In the initial 0–10 days, the sludge's SVI value was relatively high, averaging 137 mL/g, indicating slight expansion [36]. From day 10 to day 30, it rapidly decreased to a stable level of 70 mL/g. These results indicate that an influent concentration of 150 mg COD/L can maintain the normal metabolism of activated sludge and ensure the proper operation of the reactor.

3.3. Mineralization

The absence of 2,4,6-TCP in the long-term experiment effluent does not necessarily indicate complete microbial metabolism. Only when complete dechlorination and mineralization were achieved could it be confirmed that 2,4,6-TCP was thoroughly metabolized by microorganisms. Therefore, a batch test was established to demonstrate that the microorganisms in the DSBR possess the capability to completely degrade 2,4,6-TCP. The 2,4,6-TCP dechlorination was confirmed by comparing the Cl^{-1} in the effluent to its theoretical Cl^{-1} based on its molecular formula. Complete 2,4,6-TCP mineralization was indicated by the total organic carbon (TOC) value in the effluent.

The influent 2,4,6-TCP was set at 100 mg/L, and the fermentation liquid was added at the same concentration as in the long-term DSBR process, which was 150 mg COD/L. As shown in Figure 5, the 2,4,6-TCP at 100 mg/L was completely degraded within 300 min, achieving a removal rate of 100%. In the reaction solution, the Cl^{-1} concentration reached its highest point at 360 min, measuring 53.90 mg/L, which was consistent with the theoretical value for 2,4,6-trichlorophenol. This indicates that 2,4,6-TCP achieved nearly 100% dechlorination. The delay of 60 min in reaching the maximum Cl^{-1} concentration in the solution was attributed to the fact that 2,4,6-TCP initially underwent degradation into intermediate products bearing Cl^{-1}. The initial TOC was 69.20 mg/L, and this value was contributed by 2,4,6-TCP, sludge fermentation liquid, and some of the membrane-bound bacteria. At 360 min, the TOC decreased to 10.67 mg/L and remained constant until the end of the reaction, resulting in a removal rate of 84.58%. The lowest TOC and the highest Cl^{-1} content both occurred at 360 min, indicating that 2,4,6-TCP achieved simultaneous mineralization and dechlorination.

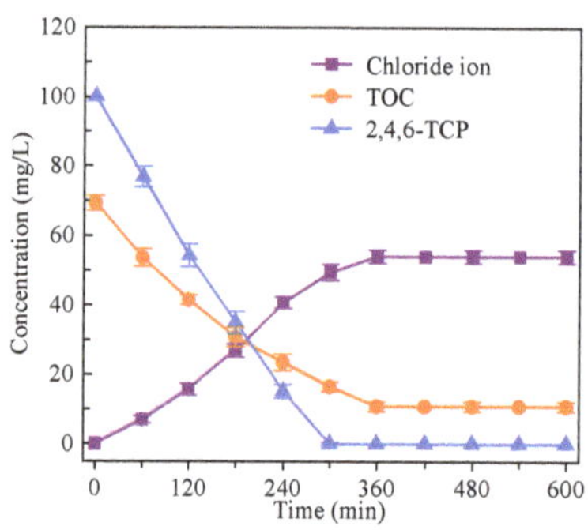

Figure 5. Mineralization characteristics of 2,4,6-TCP using fermentation broth as the carbon source.

3.4. The Impact of Ammonia Nitrogen Influent Concentration on the Degradation of 2,4,6-TCPl

High concentrations of NH_4^+-N are a significant characteristic of sludge fermentation. In this study, a heat pretreatment method was employed to process the influent sludge of the FSBR, which accelerated the release of nitrogen-containing compounds generated from extracellular polymeric substances and cell lysis. As a result, the NH_4^+-N content in the FB produced by FSBR reached as high as 634.4 mg/L. This concentration is notably higher than the 144.7 mg/L NH_4^+-N content produced using alkaline sludge fermentation methods, as reported in the literature [37]. When using sludge FB as a carbon source in denitrification processes, to mitigate the impact of high NH_4^+-N levels, it is common to employ a chemical method for NH_4^+-N and phosphorus removal [38]. In this study, no pretreatment of the FB precipitate was conducted. Therefore, it is necessary to investigate the influence of different influent NH_4^+-N concentrations on the metabolism of 2,4,6-TCP. Batch tests were conducted with a 2,4,6-TCP concentration set at 100 mg/L and influent NH_4^+-N concentrations of 40 mg/L, 170 mg/L, 340 mg/L, 680 mg/L, and 1360 mg/L.

As depicted in Figure 6, NH_4^+-N concentrations ranging from 0 to 680 mg/L exhibited no significant impact on the metabolism of 2,4,6-TCP. However, when the influent NH_4^+-N was raised to 1360 mg/L, there was a noticeable inhibition of 2,4,6-TCP metabolism. Changes in sludge fermentation conditions can lead to fluctuations in effluent NH_4^+-N, subsequently affecting the metabolism of 2,4,6-TCP. Therefore, when NH_4^+-N levels are excessively high in the FB, it is essential to employ necessary pretreatment methods to reduce the influent NH_4^+-N concentration. This is performed to prevent the inhibition of 2,4,6-TCP metabolism.

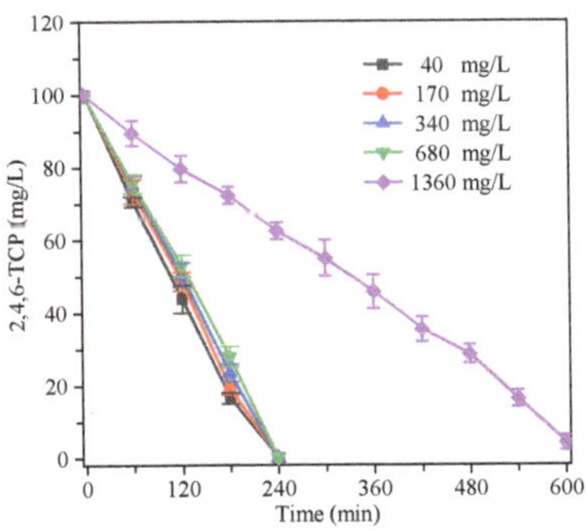

Figure 6. Degradation characteristics of 2,4,6-trichlorophenol under different ammonia nitrogen influent concentrations.

3.5. *Novel Strategy for Degrading 2,4,6-TCP in a Pilot-Scale Application*

2,4,6-TCP wastewater, characterized by its high toxicity, stands apart from general wastewater such as domestic sewage, imposing more stringent requirements on treatment methods. However, practicality and cost-effectiveness are paramount in engineering applications. Currently, microbial co-metabolism methods predominantly rely on artificially extracted or synthesized single organic compounds as carbon sources, thus incurring a substantial economic burden in practical operations.

This study presents groundbreaking evidence that sludge fermentation liquor not only finds application in biological nitrogen and phosphorus removal processes, but also serves as an exceptional mixed carbon source for microbial co-metabolism. Furthermore, sludge fermentation contributes to the consumption of surplus sludge from wastewater treatment plants, reducing the residual sludge generated during the treatment of chlorophenol wastewater. Figure 7 depicts the pilot-scale application for degrading 2,4,6-TCP using sludge fermentation liquid as a carbon source.

During the pilot-scale operation, considering that the pre-treatment method of thermal hydrolysis for residual sludge may lack operational feasibility, it is advisable to replace the residual sludge fermentation with alkaline fermentation to enhance practical applicability. Alkaline fermentation is a more mature fermentation method, where the fermentation sludge can achieve higher acid production efficiency without the need for special treatment [34,39].

In practical applications, it is essential to determine the dosage of sludge fermentation liquid to ensure that its introduction does not lead to competition with the metabolism of 2,4,6-TCP. The control strategy employed can be achieved by maintaining a constant sludge concentration.

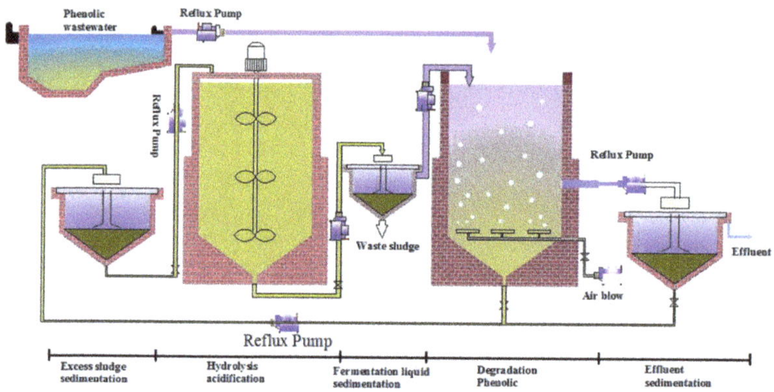

Figure 7. The schematic diagram of the pilot-scale conceptual apparatus for degrading 2,4,6-TCP using sludge fermentation liquid as a carbon source.

In the pilot-scale operation, the pre-treatment of sludge fermentation liquid will involve natural sedimentation, which differs from the centrifugation method used in small-scale studies. Sludge fermentation liquid's settling performance is poor, and natural settling will inevitably introduce fermentation bacteria into the DSBR. Therefore, the pilot-scale operation requires further research into the acclimatization of 2,4,6-TCP degradation bacteria and operational parameters under the conditions of mixed fermentation liquid addition. The sludge retention time in the degradation unit was maintained at 120 days, and the resulting residual sludge was recirculated back to the fermentation unit as a fermentation substrate.

4. Conclusions

The utilization of sludge fermentation liquid as a carbon source for the degradation of 2,4,6-TCP presents a viable strategy to tackle the problem of exorbitant treatment expenses linked to the incorporation of external carbon sources. Throughout the 180-day operational period, the concentrations of VFAs in FSBR remained constant, with acetic acid, propionic acid, butyric acid, and valeric acid concentrations reaching 322.04 mg COD/L, 225.98 mg COD/L, 274.76 mg COD/L, and 149.58 mg COD/L, respectively. The acid production efficiency peaked at 88.40%, further substantiating the significant improvement in acid production rates in sludge fermentation through the application of thermal pretreatment. The maximum removal of 2,4,6-TCP reached 240.13 mg/L within a 12 h operating cycle, significantly outperforming the use of single commodity carbon sources or other mixed carbon sources. However, the composition and dosage of sludge fermentation liquid will directly affect the removal of 2,4,6-TCP, which remains an aspect to be explored in future research.

Supplementary Materials: The following supporting information can be downloaded at: https://www.mdpi.com/article/10.3390/w15224008/s1, Table S1: The DSBR Influent Trace Elements Concentrations.

Author Contributions: Conceptualization, J.W.; data curation, J.W.; formal analysis, J.W.; writing—original draft, J.W.; writing—review and editing, J.W., Z.S. and J.L. All authors have read and agreed to the published version of the manuscript.

Funding: This research was supported by the scientific program of PowerChina Huadong Engineering Corporation Limited (KY2022-HS-02-20).

Data Availability Statement: Data are contained within the article and Supplementary Materials.

Conflicts of Interest: Author Jianguang Wang was employed by the company PowerChina Huadong Engineering Corporation Limited. The remaining authors declare that the research was conducted in the absence of any commercial or financial relationships that could be construed as a potential conflict of interest.

References

1. Eker, S.; Kargi, F. COD, 2,4,6-trichlorophenol (TCP) and toxicity removal from synthetic wastewater in a rotating perforated-tubes biofilm reactor. *J. Hazard. Mater.* **2008**, *159*, 306–312. [CrossRef] [PubMed]
2. Gaya, U.I.; Abdullah, A.H.; Hussein, M.Z.; Zainal, Z. Photocatalytic removal of 2,4,6-trichlorophenol from water exploiting commercial ZnO powder. *Desalination* **2010**, *263*, 176–182. [CrossRef]
3. Chanikya, P.; Nidheesh, P.V.; Syam Babu, D.; Gopinath, A.; Suresh Kumar, M. Treatment of dyeing wastewater by combined sulfate radical based electrochemical advanced oxidation and electrocoagulation processes. *Sep. Purif. Technol.* **2021**, *254*, 117570. [CrossRef]
4. Liu, Y.; Zhao, Y.; Wang, J. Fenton/Fenton-like processes with in-situ production of hydrogen peroxide/hydroxyl radical for degradation of emerging contaminants: Advances and prospects. *J. Hazard. Mater.* **2021**, *404*, 124191. [CrossRef] [PubMed]
5. Ouali, S.; Loulergue, P.; Biard, P.; Nasrallah, N.; Szymczyk, A. Ozone compatibility with polymer nanofiltration membranes. *J. Membr. Sci.* **2021**, *618*, 118656. [CrossRef]
6. Correa, J. Aerobic degradation of 2,4,6-TCP content in ECF bleached effluent. *Environ. Int.* **2003**, *29*, 459–465. [CrossRef] [PubMed]
7. Stirling, D.I.; Dalton, H. The fortuitous oxidation and cometabolism of various carbon compounds by whole-cell suspensions of Methylococcus capsulatus (Bath). *FEMS Microbiol. Lett.* **1979**, *5*, 315–318. [CrossRef]
8. Alvarez-Cohen, L.; Speitel, G.E., Jr. Kinetics of aerobic cometabolism of chlorinated solvents. *Biodegradation* **2001**, *12*, 105–126. [CrossRef]
9. Goltz, M.N.; Bouwer, E.J.; Huang, J. Transport issues and bioremediation modeling for the in situ aerobic co-metabolism of chlorinated solvents. *Biodegradation* **2001**, *12*, 127–140. [CrossRef]
10. Wang, J.; Sun, Z. Effects of different carbon sources on 2,4,6-trichlorophenol degradation in the activated sludge process. *Bioprocess Biosyst. Eng.* **2020**, *43*, 2143–2152. [CrossRef]
11. Majumder, P.S.; Gupta, S.K. Effect of carbon sources and shock loading on the removal of chlorophenols in sequential anaerobic-aerobic reactors. *Bioresour. Technol.* **2008**, *99*, 2930–2937. [CrossRef]
12. Mun, C.H.; Ng, W.J.; He, J. Aclidogenic sequencing batch reactor start-up procedures for induction of 2,4,6-trichlorophenol dechlorination. *Water Res.* **2008**, *42*, 1675–1683. [CrossRef] [PubMed]
13. Quan, X.C.; Shi, H.C.; Liu, H.; Wang, J.L.; Qian, Y. Removal of 2,4-dichlorophenol in a conventional activated sludge system through bioaugmentation. *Process Biochem.* **2004**, *39*, 1701–1707. [CrossRef]
14. Ziagova, M.; Kyriakou, G.; Liakopoulou-Kyriakides, M. Co-metabolism of 2,4-dichlorophenol and 4-Cl-m-cresol in the presence of glucose as an easily assimilated carbon source by Staphylococcus xylosus. *J. Hazard. Mater.* **2009**, *163*, 383–390. [CrossRef]
15. Shin, J.; Rhee, C.; Shin, J.; Jang, H.M.; Shin, S.G.; Kim, Y.M. Determining the composition of bacterial community and relative abundance of specific antibiotics resistance genes via thermophilic anaerobic digestion of sewage sludge. *Bioresour. Technol.* **2020**, *311*, 123510. [CrossRef]
16. Zhang, M.; Wang, Y. Effects of Fe-Mn-modified biochar addition on anaerobic digestion of sewage sludge: Biomethane production, heavy metal speciation and performance stability. *Bioresour. Technol.* **2020**, *313*, 123695. [CrossRef]
17. Lee, W.S.; Chua, A.S.M.; Yeoh, H.K.; Ngoh, G.C. A review of the production and applications of waste-derived volatile fatty acids. *Chem. Eng. J.* **2014**, *235*, 83–99. [CrossRef]
18. Wang, B.; Wang, S.; Li, B.; Peng, C.; Peng, Y. Integrating waste activated sludge (WAS) acidification with denitrification by adding nitrite (NO_2^-). *Biomass Bioenergy* **2014**, *67*, 460–465. [CrossRef]
19. Gao, Y.; Guo, L.; Shao, M.; Hu, F.; Wang, G.; Zhao, Y.; Gao, M.; Jin, C.; She, Z. Denitrification performance evaluation and kinetics analysis with mariculture solid wastes (MSW) derived carbon source in marine recirculating aquaculture systems (RAS). *Bioresour. Technol.* **2020**, *313*, 123649. [CrossRef] [PubMed]
20. Ucisik, A.S.; Henze, M. Biological hydrolysis and acidification of sludge under anaerobic conditions: The effect of sludge type and origin on the production and composition of volatile fatty acids. *Water Res.* **2008**, *42*, 3729–3738. [CrossRef]
21. Zhang, P.; Chen, Y.; Zhou, Q. Waste activated sludge hydrolysis and short-chain fatty acids accumulation under mesophilic and thermophilic conditions: Effect of pH. *Water Res.* **2009**, *43*, 3735–3742. [CrossRef]
22. Hu, C.; Guo, Y.; Guo, L.; Zhao, Y.; Jin, C.; She, Z.; Gao, M. Comparation of thermophilic bacteria (TB) pretreated primary and secondary waste sludge carbon sources on denitrification performance at different HRTs. *Bioresour. Technol.* **2020**, *297*, 122438. [CrossRef] [PubMed]
23. Chen, Y.; Liu, K.; Su, Y.; Zheng, X.; Wang, Q. Continuous bioproduction of short-chain fatty acids from sludge enhanced by the combined use of surfactant and alkaline pH. *Bioresour. Technol.* **2013**, *140*, 97–102. [CrossRef] [PubMed]
24. Wang, J.; Sun, Z. Exploring the effects of carbon source level on the degradation of 2,4,6-trichlorophenol in the co-metabolism process. *J. Hazard. Mater.* **2020**, *392*, 122293. [CrossRef] [PubMed]

25. Qi, W.; Chen, T.; Wang, L.; Wu, M.; Zhao, Q.; Wei, W. High-strength fermentable wastewater reclamation through a sequential process of anaerobic fermentation followed by microalgae cultivation. *Bioresour. Technol.* **2017**, *227*, 317–323. [CrossRef] [PubMed]
26. Hori, K.; Mii, J.; Morono, Y.; Tanji, Y.; Unno, H. Kinetic analyses of trichloroethylene cometabolism by toluene-degrading bacteria harboring a tod homologous gene. *Biochem. Eng.* **2005**, *26*, 59–64. [CrossRef]
27. Apha. *Standard Methods for the Examination of Water and Wastewater*, 12th ed.; United Book Press: Washington, DC, USA, 1998.
28. Feng, L.; Yan, Y.; Chen, Y. Kinetic analysis of waste activated sludge hydrolysis and short-chain fatty acids production at pH 10. *J. Environ. Sci.* **2009**, *21*, 589–594. [CrossRef] [PubMed]
29. Jiang, S.; Chen, Y.; Zhou, Q.; Gu, G. Biological short-chain fatty acids (SCFAs) production from waste-activated sludge affected by surfactant. *Water Res.* **2007**, *41*, 3112–3120. [CrossRef]
30. Yan, Y.; Feng, L.; Zhang, C.; Wisniewski, C.; Zhou, Q. Ultrasonic enhancement of waste activated sludge hydrolysis and volatile fatty acids accumulation at pH 10.0. *Water Res.* **2010**, *44*, 3329–3336. [CrossRef]
31. Liao, P.H.; Lo, K.V.; Chan, W.I.; Wong, W.T. Sludge reduction and volatile fatty acid recovery using microwave advanced oxidation process. *J. Environ. Sci. Health Part A-Toxic/Hazard. Subst. Environ. Eng.* **2007**, *42*, 633–639. [CrossRef]
32. Yang, Q.; Luo, K.; Li, X.; Wang, D.; Zheng, W.; Zeng, G.; Liu, J. Enhanced efficiency of biological excess sludge hydrolysis under anaerobic digestion by additional enzymes. *Bioresour. Technol.* **2010**, *101*, 2924–2930. [CrossRef] [PubMed]
33. Uma Rani, R.; Kaliappan, S.; Adish Kumar, S.; Rajesh Banu, J. Combined treatment of alkaline and disperser for improving solubilization and anaerobic biodegradability of dairy waste activated sludge. *Bioresour. Technol.* **2012**, *126*, 107–116. [CrossRef] [PubMed]
34. Yuan, Y.; Wang, S.; Liu, Y.; Li, B.; Wang, B.; Peng, Y. Long-term effect of pH on short-chain fatty acids accumulation and microbial community in sludge fermentation systems. *Bioresour. Technol.* **2015**, *197*, 56–63. [CrossRef] [PubMed]
35. Wang, J.; Sun, Z. Successful application of municipal domestic wastewater as a co-substrate in 2,4,6-trichlorophenol degradation. *Chemosphere* **2021**, *280*, 130707. [CrossRef]
36. Mesquita, D.P.; Amaral, A.L.; Ferreira, E.C. Identifying different types of bulking in an activated sludge system through quantitative image analysis. *Chemosphere* **2011**, *85*, 643–652. [CrossRef]
37. Yuan, Y.; Liu, J.; Ma, B.; Liu, Y.; Wang, B.; Peng, Y. Improving municipal wastewater nitrogen and phosphorous removal by feeding sludge fermentation products to sequencing batch reactor (SBR). *Bioresour. Technol.* **2016**, *222*, 326–334. [CrossRef]
38. Karakashev, D.; Schmidt, J.E.; Angelidaki, I. Innovative process scheme for removal of organic matter, phosphorus and nitrogen from pig manure. *Water Res.* **2008**, *42*, 4083–4090. [CrossRef]
39. Yuan, Y.; Peng, Y.; Liu, Y.; Jin, B.; Wang, B.; Wang, S. Change of pH during excess sludge fermentation under alkaline, acidic and neutral conditions. *Bioresour. Technol.* **2014**, *174*, 1–5. [CrossRef]

water

MDPI

Article

Exploring 2,4,6-Trichlorophenol Degradation Characteristics and Functional Metabolic Gene Abundance Using Sludge Fermentation Broth as the Carbon Source

Jianguang Wang [1,2,3,*] and Shiyi Li [1,3]

1 PowerChina Huadong Engineering Corporation Limited, Hangzhou 311122, China
2 National Engineering Laboratory for Advanced Municipal Wastewater Treatment and Reuse Technology, Beijing University of Technology, Beijing 100124, China
3 Huadong Eco-Environmental Engineering Research Institute of Zhejiang Province, Hangzhou 311122, China
* Correspondence: wjg909090@163.com

Abstract: The use of sludge fermentation broth (FB) as a co-metabolic carbon source for treating 2,4,6-trichlorophenol (2,4,6-TCP) wastewater is a novel strategy. The key to the feasibility of this strategy is whether the FB can promote the growth of functional microorganisms that are capable of degrading 2,4,6-TCP. This study focused on long-term acclimatized sludge and investigated the impact of key operating parameters such as the sludge FB concentration and the influent concentration of 2,4,6-TCP on the removal efficiency of chlorophenol. The research findings revealed that when the influent concentration of sludge FB exceeded 300 mg COD/L, it significantly inhibited the degradation of 2,4,6-TCP. Simulation experiments using individual VFA components as influent carbon sources showed that excessive propionic acid addition can inhibit the degradation of 2,4,6-TCP, indicating the need to control the concentration of propionic acid in the fermentation conditions. Metagenomic analysis further showed that sludge FB can promote the enrichment of microbial chlorophenol degradation genes, including *PcpA*, *pcaF*, *pcaI*, *Mal-r*, *chqB*, and *fadA*. The abundances of these six chlorophenol degradation genes were as follows: 1152 hits (*PcpA*), 112 hits (*pcaF*), 10,144 hits (*pcaI*), 12,552 hits (*Mal-r*), 8022 hits (*chqB*), and 20,122 hits (*fadA*). Compared with other types of carbon sources, sludge FB demonstrates distinct advantages in terms of leading to the highest chlorophenol degradation concentration and the abundance of functional microbial communities. This study has successfully demonstrated the feasibility of using sludge FB as a co-metabolic carbon source for the degradation of 2,4,6-TCP.

Keywords: 2,4,6-trichlorophenol; functional gene; microbial community; co-metabolism

1. Introduction

2,4,6-Trichlorophenol (2,4,6-TCP) is a persistent organic compound. Its molecular formula features three chlorine substituents, which significantly increase its biotoxicity compared with mono- and dichlorophenols [1,2]. Its remarkable chemical stability has led to a wider range of applications [3] than other chlorophenols, resulting in higher environmental concentrations of 2,4,6-TCP [4]. Consequently, many researchers have focused on developing techniques for removing 2,4,6-TCP, including biological co-metabolism [5], and bio-electrochemical methods [1,6–8]. The bio-co-metabolism technique involved enhancing the biodegradability of 2,4,6-TCP wastewater by adding readily degradable carbon sources [2]. Over time, the technique has evolved from using commercial carbon sources like sucrose and glucose to employing other organic wastewater streams as co-metabolic carbon sources [9]. This shift has significantly reduced the application cost of the co-metabolic technique, thereby increasing its practicality. A crucial aspect of this progress has been the enrichment and cultivation of 2,4,6-TCP functional microbial communities.

Research on the co-metabolism of biological processes can employ mixed microbial cultures. Wang, J et al. [5] investigated the degradation of 2,4,6-TCP using sucrose as a co-metabolic carbon source. They utilized mixed cultures from a wastewater treatment plant as the inoculum sludge and identified Norank_p_Saccharibacteria as the predominant taxa after domestication. Additionally, they observed varying abundances of these taxa with different sucrose concentrations. Similarly, Zhao, J et al. [10] used sludge from a wastewater treatment plant as inoculum and studied the degradation mechanism of 4-chlorophenol with starch and sodium acetate as carbon sources. The microbial communities utilizing starch and sodium acetate both had Proteobacteria as the dominant phylum, with abundances of 32.15% and 43.43%, respectively.

In contrast, other researchers employed single strains to investigate the degradation mechanisms of 2,4,6-TCP. *Cupriavidus necator JMP134* was frequently employed as an aerobic co-metabolism bacterium with strong 2,4,6-TCP degradation capabilities. It was often utilized to investigate the functional genes that are involved in the aerobic metabolism pathway of 2,4,6-TCP. *Cupriavidus necator JMP134* contained all the tcp degradation genes, enabling the efficient synthesis of metabolic enzymes not only for 2,4,6-TCP but also for its different metabolic by-products, resulting in the complete degradation of 2,4,6-TCP [11,12]. The degradation process by *Cupriavidus necator JMP134* did not lead to the accumulation of metabolic intermediates, thus greatly enhancing the mineralization efficiency of 2,4,6-TCP. *Ralstonia pickettii DTP0602* is another extensively tested strain, sharing the same phenol degradation pathway as *Cupriavidus necator JMP134*. However, the functional genes that were responsible for metabolism were entirely different [13]. Wang, C C et al. [14] isolated pure strains that are capable of utilizing 2,4,6-TCP from a mixed microbial community grown on substrates containing chlorophenolic compounds: *Pseudomonas spp. strain 01* and *Pseudomonas spp. strain 02*. These two aerobic bacteria individually exhibited low removal rates for 2,4,6-TCP. When 200~400 mg/L of phenol was added as a co-metabolic substrate, the removal rates for 2,4,6-TCP could be increased to 65% and 48%, respectively. However, further evidence is needed to confirm whether the 2,4,6-TCP degradation active sludge, adapted by adding a mixed carbon source, contains the aforementioned microbial communities.

Research on 2,4,6-TCP-degrading bacteria has primarily concentrated on changes in the microbial community [15,16]. However, there has been limited investigation into the expression of functional genes. The continuous introduction of mixed wastewater into the co-metabolic system could potentially alter the functional bacterial community due to the presence of numerous suspended microorganisms. This could, in turn, impact the degradation efficiency of 2,4,6-TCP. Metagenomic technology, a technique that is capable of analyzing microbial abundance at the gene level [17], presents a viable solution to this issue. It facilitates the examination of microorganisms that are involved in carbon source metabolism and 2,4,6-TCP degradation within the reactor. Importantly, this method allows for the exploration of the potential relationship between the bacteria introduced through mixed wastewater and the original bacterial community. This approach not only enhances our understanding of the degradation process but also provides valuable insights into the impact of introduced bacteria on the functional bacterial community.

In our previous research, the feasibility of utilizing sludge fermentation liquid as a carbon source to domesticate bacteria that are capable of degrading 2,4,6-TCP has been meticulously demonstrated [18]. Based on the above research background, this study focuses on 2,4,6-TCP-degrading bacteria cultivated using sludge fermentation broth as a carbon source. Batch experiments are conducted to validate the influence of different reactor operating conditions on the degradation properties of the microbial community. Simultaneously, both high-throughput and metagenomic analysis techniques were employed to examine the original sludge, fermentation sludge, and chlorophenol-degrading bacteria. This approach allowed us to understand the impact of sludge fermentation broth on the abundance of 2,4,6-TCP degradation genes.

2. Materials and Methods

2.1. Seeding Sludge

Three types of activated sludge were employed in this research. The excess sludge (CS) was collected from the secondary clarifier of a wastewater treatment plant. The degradation sludge (DS), which was acclimated from the CS and had the ability to degrade 2,4,6-TCP, was used with sludge fermentation liquid as the carbon source. The fermentation sludge (FS) was used to provide the sludge fermentation liquid.

CS does not possess the capability to degrade 2,4,6-TCP or ferment acid. The DS demonstrated a maximum degradation concentration of 240 mg/L for 2,4,6-TCP. The FS exhibited an acid production rate of 80.40%, with a peak acid concentration of 974.5 mgCOD/L.

2.2. The Batch Experiment

Batch experiments were conducted within a small-scale sequential batch reactor (SBR), as illustrated in Figure 1. The effective volume of this reactor was 750 mL. The operating conditions for the batch experiments were as follows: the temperature was set at 28 °C, dissolved oxygen was maintained at 4–5 mgO_2/L, and the sludge operational stirring speed was set at 200 rpm. During the operation of the batch experiments, sampling was conducted using a syringe, with each sampling event collecting 10 mL. The pretreatment conditions for batch experiment samples involved centrifugation at 4000 rpm and membrane filtration (0.22 μm). Subsequently, various water quality parameters were further analyzed.

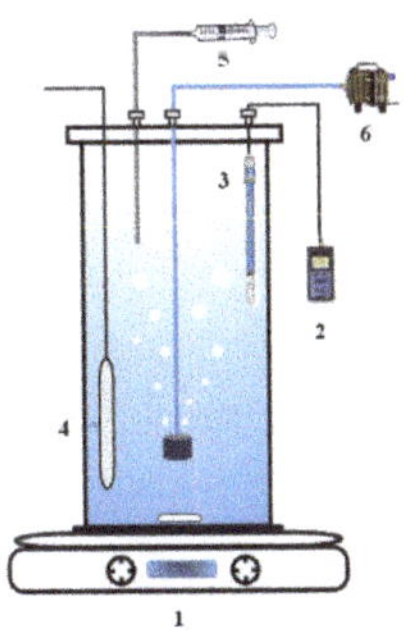

Figure 1. The schematic diagram of batch test SBR (1. magnetic stirrer; 2. WTW water quality monitor; 3. dissolved oxygen and temperature probes; 4. constant temperature heater; 5. sampling syringe; 6. air pump).

2.2.1. Test 1: Studying the Impact of the Dosage of Sludge Fermentation Liquid on the Degradation of 2,4,6-TCP

The influent concentration of the fermentation liquid was calculated in terms of COD equivalents, with concentrations set at 0, 150, 300, and 600 mg COD/L. Sampling intervals ranged from 10 to 30 min. The influent concentration of 2,4,6-TCP was 70 mg/L.

2.2.2. Test 2: Exploring the Influence of the Fermentation Liquid Composition on the Degradation of 2,4,6-TCP

The primary components of the sludge fermentation liquid are VFAs, with the major constituents being acetic acid, propionic acid, butyric acid, valeric acid, and other volatile fatty acids, along with a small portion of lipids and proteins [19]. Given the difficulty in purifying volatile components, sodium acetate, sodium propionate, sodium butyrate, and sodium valerate were used to simulate the VFAs' composition. The alteration of the solution pH induced by sodium acetate, sodium propionate, sodium butyrate, and sodium valerate was rectified by adjusting the pH to neutral using hydrochloric acid. The influent concentration was calculated in terms of COD and was set at 150 mg COD/L for each of these components. The influent includes a simulated carbon source at 150 mg COD/L and 2,4,6-TCP at 100 mg/L. Sampling intervals were set at 60 min.

2.2.3. Test 3: The Impact of Varying Concentrations of 2,4,6-TCP on the Degradation Characteristics of Sludge

The dosage of sludge fermentation liquid was set at 150 mg COD/L. The influent concentrations of 2,4,6-TCP were established at 50 mg/L, 100 mg/L, 150 mg/L, 200 mg/L, 230 mg/L, and 250 mg/L, respectively. Sampling intervals were set at 60 min.

2.2.4. Test 4: Investigating the Influence of Chloride Ion Concentration on the Degradation Characteristics of Sludge

2,4,6-TCP contains three chlorine atoms within its molecular structure. As the reaction progresses, 2,4,6-TCP is continuously oxidized, releasing chlorine ions into the reaction solution. Therefore, it is essential to investigate the influence of the accumulating chlorine ion concentration on the metabolism of 2,4,6-TCP. Sodium chloride served as the primary compound providing chlorine ions, and the impact of chloride ion concentration on the degradation of 2,4,6-TCP in sludge was examined. Batch experiments were conducted under the same conditions as the long-term operation of the SBR, with chloride ion concentrations set in the range of 1000 mg/L, 2000 mg/L, 3000 mg/L, and 5400 mg/L. Sampling intervals were set at 60 min. The influent concentration of 2,4,6-TCP was 100 mg/L.

2.2.5. Test 5: The Effect of Temperature on 2,4,6-TCP Degradation

Prior to the commencement of the reaction, the influent concentration of 2,4,6-TCP was 100 mg/L, while the influent concentration of sludge fermentation liquid was 150 mg COD/L. The investigation was carried out at temperatures of 10 °C, 20 °C, 28 °C, and 40 °C. The experiment lasted for 10 h, with sampling intervals of 60 min.

2.3. Analytical Methods

2.3.1. Standard Parameters

2,4,6-TCP was detected using liquid chromatography, chloride ions were detected using ion chromatography, and volatile fatty acids were detected using gas chromatography. Specific testing conditions for these three parameters are detailed in the attached document.

2.3.2. Sludge Microbial Community and Genetic Analysis

In this study, a total of three types of sludge samples were tested. The activated sludge from the secondary sedimentation tank of the wastewater treatment plant, when used as the original biological sample, was named excess sludge (ES). The active sludge sample, stabilized through the utilization of sludge fermentation liquid as a carbon source for the degradation of 2,4,6-TCP, was named degradation sludge (DS). The fermentation active sludge remaining within the sludge fermentation reactor was named fermentation sludge (FS).

High-throughput methods and metagenomics were employed for the analysis of microbial community and gene abundance. Detailed analytical procedures are available in the Supplementary Materials. The raw data from the metagenomic analysis have been deposited in the NCBI database under accession number PRJNA707137.

3. Results and Discussion

3.1. The Impact of Sludge Fermentation Liquid Dosage

Degradable organic compounds were found to enhance the degradation of 2,4,6-TCP, and this enhancing effect was intensified with an increase in the concentration of the carbon source [5]. It was also demonstrated that 2,4,6-TCP was not adversely affected in the short term when mixed carbon sources containing recalcitrant components were present [9]. In this study, FB served as a typical mixed carbon source with a VFA content reaching 88.4%. Therefore, it was imperative to investigate the impact of adding FB on the degradation of 2,4,6-TCP.

As shown in Figure 2a, there was no significant difference in the degradation of 2,4,6-TCP when the influent FB was either 0 or 150 mgCOD/L. In both cases, complete degradation was achieved within 300 min. However, when the influent FB concentrations were increased to 300 mgCOD/L and 600 mgCOD/L, the degradation times for 2,4,6-TCP extended to 420 min and 540 min, respectively.

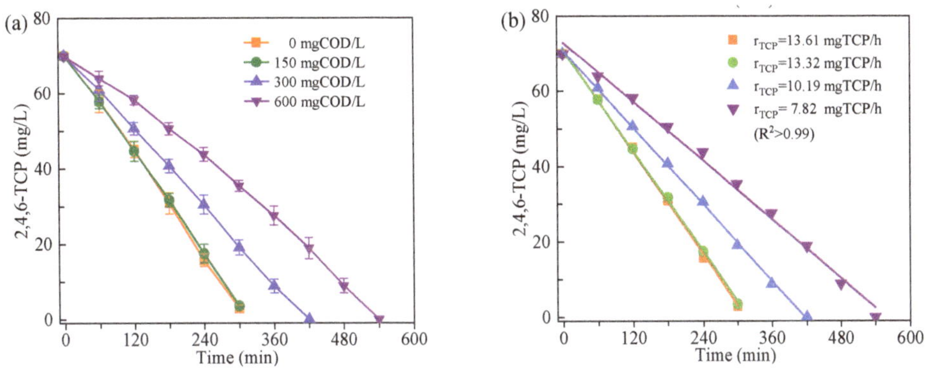

Figure 2. (**a**) The effects of adding different fermentation broth levels on 2,4,6-TCP degradation, (**b**) average degradation rate.

As depicted in Figure 2b, calculations through fitting provided the average degradation rates of 2,4,6-TCP at different FB levels, which were 13.61 mgTCP/h, 13.32 mgTCP/h, 10.19 mgTCP/h, and 7.82 mgTCP/h. It can be observed that there is a competitive metabolic phenomenon between FB and 2,4,6-TCP. This differs from the case when sodium acetate and sodium propionate are used. The reason for this phenomenon may be the interference caused by other organic compounds that are present in the FB on the degradation of 2,4,6-TCP. In the short term, not adding FB can achieve the best removal efficiency of 2,4,6-TCP. However, this is not suitable for the long-term stable operation of the reactor [5]. An FB concentration of 150 mgCOD/L can maintain a stable sludge concentration and has a relatively minor inhibitory effect on 2,4,6-TCP degradation.

3.2. *Effect of VFA Compositions on 2,4,6-TCP Degradation*

It remains to be further demonstrated which specific component among VFAs, including acetic acid, propionic acid, butyric acid, and valeric acid, may be inhibited in the degradation of 2,4,6-TCP when added in excessive amounts. To explore the impact of the addition of these components, the simulation of the above four VFA components was achieved using different fatty acid salts, and the effect of their concentration on the degradation of 2,4,6-TCP was investigated. The influent concentration of 2,4,6-TCP was set at 100 mg/L, while the influent concentration of fatty acid salts was uniformly set at 150 mgCOD/L.

As shown in Figure 3, when sodium acetate, sodium butyrate, and sodium valerate were used as carbon sources, 2,4,6-TCP was completely degraded within 240 min, with average degradation rates of 24.93 mgTCP/h, 24.98 mgTCP/h, and 24.94 mgTCP/h, respectively, and there were no significant differences. However, when sodium propionate was used as a carbon source, 2,4,6-TCP could only be completely degraded by the 300th minute, with an average degradation rate of 20.19 mgTCP/h, which is significantly lower than the other three carbon sources. These results indicate that among the VFAs, acetic acid, butyric acid, and valeric acid can enhance the removal of 2,4,6-TCP, while propionic acid has a certain degree of inhibition on the degradation of 2,4,6-TCP. Based on these observations, by adjusting the sludge fermentation conditions, it is possible to increase the content of acetic acid, butyric acid, and valeric acid in the total VFAs, thereby enhancing the removal efficiency of 2,4,6-TCP.

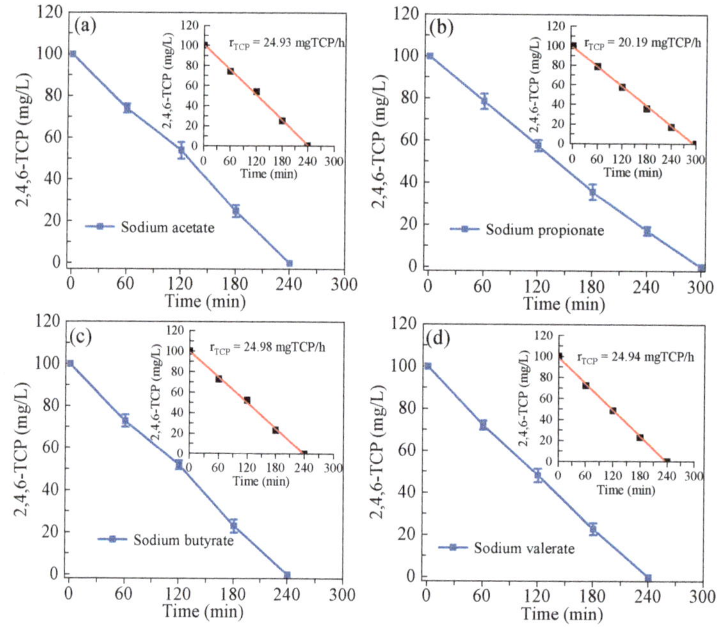

Figure 3. The effects of different VFA components on 2,4,6-TCP degradation, (**a**) sodium acetate, (**b**) sodium propionate, (**c**) sodium butyrate, and (**d**) sodium valerate.

3.3. The Impact of Influent 2,4,6-TCP on Its Degradation

As shown in Figure 4, the specific degradation rates at different 2,4,6-TCP concentrations were investigated. It can be observed that at influent concentrations of 50 mg/L, 100 mg/L, and 150 mg/L of 2,4,6-TCP, the corresponding specific degradation rates were 8.28 mgTCP/g·VSS·h, 8.34 mgTCP/g·VSS·h, and 8.37 mgTCP/g·VSS·h, respectively. When the influent concentration of 2,4,6-TCP was raised to 200 mg/L and 230 mg/L, the specific degradation rates increased to 9.48 mgTCP/g·VSS·h and 9.63 mgTCP/g·VSS·h, respectively. However, when the concentration of 2,4,6-TCP was further increased to 250 mg/L, the specific degradation rate rapidly decreased to 8.32 mgTCP/g·VSS·h.

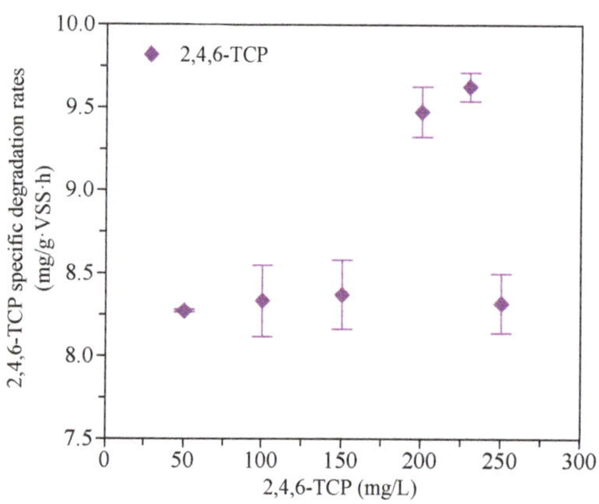

Figure 4. Variation in specific degradation rates of 2,4,6-TCP with its initial concentration (all values are means (n = 3)).

These results indicate that, at a certain influent concentration of 2,4,6-TCP, the specific degradation rate increases with the increase in influent concentration. However, due to the toxicity of 2,4,6-TCP, even with long-term acclimation of the activated sludge, excessively high influent concentrations can still inhibit the microbial degradation activity. The floccular sludge used in this study exhibited significantly higher degradation efficiency for 2,4,6-TCP compared with the use of granular sludge [20].

3.4. Effect of Chloride Ion on 2,4,6-TCP Degradation

Dechlorination is an important indicator for the environmentally friendly treatment of 2,4,6-TCP, and whether the removal of chloride ions will affect the further degradation of 2,4,6-TCP needs further investigation. Using sodium chloride to simulate the concentration of chloride ions released by 2,4,6-TCP, the influence of its influent concentration on the degradation of 2,4,6-TCP was studied. As shown in Figure 5a, when the influent chloride ion concentration ranged from 1 to 3 g/L, 2,4,6-TCP was completely removed within 240 min. However, when the chloride ion concentration was increased to 5.4 g/L, the degradation of 2,4,6-TCP was significantly inhibited. The tolerance threshold of activated sludge to chloride ions was below 5.4 g/L. Furthermore, the chloride ion concentration varied with the influent 2,4,6-TCP and the reactor's operational mode.

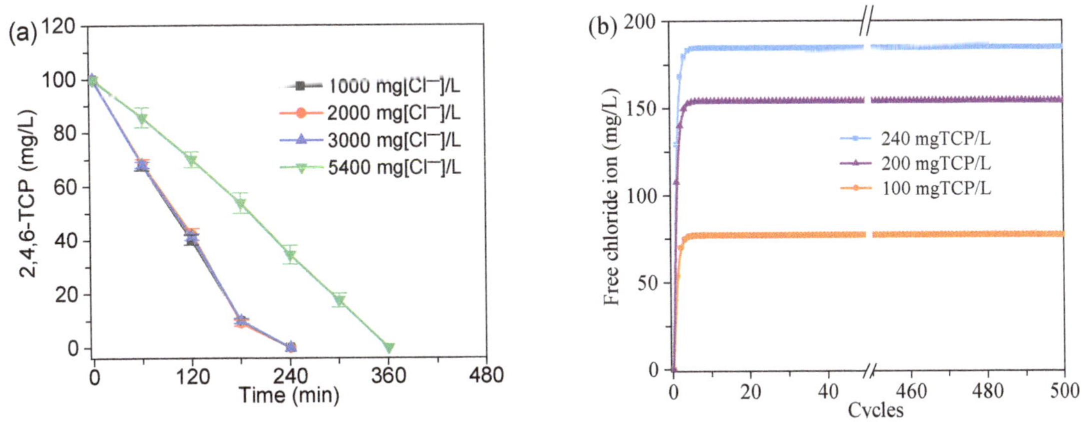

Figure 5. (**a**) The effect of different chloride ion concentrations on 2,4,6-TCP degradation; (**b**) the relationship between the release of chloride ions and the operating cycle with the addition of different 2,4,6-TCP (SBR drainage ratio of 0.7).

In Figure 5b, under the conditions of different influent 2,4,6-TCP (100 mg/L, 200 mg/L, and 240 mg/L) and an SBR effluent ratio of 0.7, the relationship between Cl^{-1} in the reaction liquid and the SBR operational cycles was calculated. It can be observed that within the first four operational cycles, the Cl^{-1} increased rapidly. However, starting from the fifth cycle, the production and discharge of Cl^{-1} reached equilibrium. The final equilibriums of Cl^{-1} were 184.77 mg/L, 153.89 mg/L, and 76.95 mg/L, respectively. Therefore, under a constant SBR effluent ratio, the Cl^{-1} generated by the dechlorination of 2,4,6-TCP reached an equilibrium. In this study, the maximum degradation concentration of 2,4,6-TCP was 240 mg/L, with an SBR effluent ratio of 0.7, resulting in Cl^{-1} below 185 mg/L, while the highest Cl^{-1} tolerance of the activated sludge was below 5.4 g/L. Consequently, the Cl^{-1} generated by the dechlorination of 2,4,6-TCP will not have a long-term impact on the reactor's operation.

3.5. Effect of Temperature on 2,4,6-TCP Metabolism

At different temperatures, the degradation characteristics of 2,4,6-TCP are illustrated in Figure 6. At 28 °C, which was the long-term acclimation temperature for the activated sludge, it was observed that the sludge exhibited the highest degradation activity for 2,4,6-TCP. It could remove 100 mg/L of 2,4,6-TCP within 300 min. However, when the temperature was raised to 40 °C, the initial degradation rate of 2,4,6-TCP was faster, but the degradation significantly slowed down in the later stages. This may have been due to the higher external temperature accelerating the metabolic rate of the carbon source, leading to a lack of necessary carbon source supply in the later stages of operation. When the temperature was lowered to 10 °C and 20 °C, at the end of the cycle, 2,4,6-TCP still remained incompletely degraded.

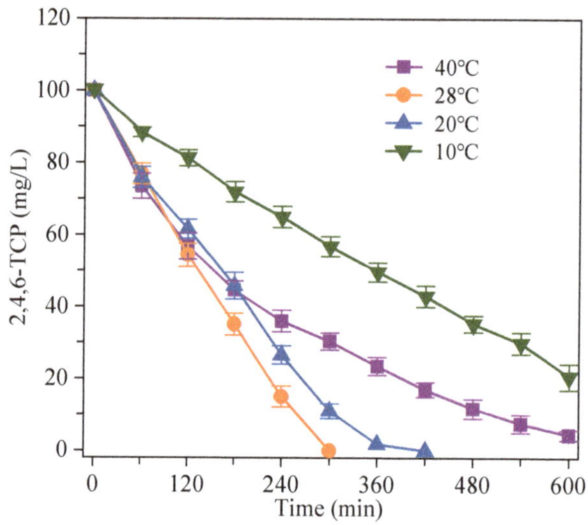

Figure 6. Degradation characteristics of 2,4,6-TCP at different operating temperatures.

3.6. Analysis of FSBR-DSBR Process Bacterial Community

The active sludge tested in this experiment includes three types: residual sludge, which serves as the feedstock for the FSBR; fermentative sludge; and sludge capable of degrading 2,4,6-TCP. Residual sludge acts as the substrate for fermentation, and the sludge FB serves as the carbon source for 2,4,6-TCP degradation. Therefore, it is possible that both residual sludge and the FB may have a certain impact on the microbial community within the target unit.

3.6.1. Analysis of Functional Microbial Community

As shown in Figure 7, at the phylum level of anaerobic digestion, there are a total of 12 dominant bacterial phyla among the three sludge samples. Among these, *Proteobacteria* is the predominant phylum in the residual sludge, accounting for 31.61% of the total abundance. In contrast, *Firmicutes* dominates in the fermentative sludge, representing a substantial proportion at 55.56%. *Firmicutes* is a commonly observed phylum in sludge fermentation [21–25]. The higher abundance of *Firmicutes* observed in this study aligns with the effective acid production during FSBR. Other phyla with relatively high abundances include *Proteobacteria* (29.31%) and *Actinobacteria* (2.73%).

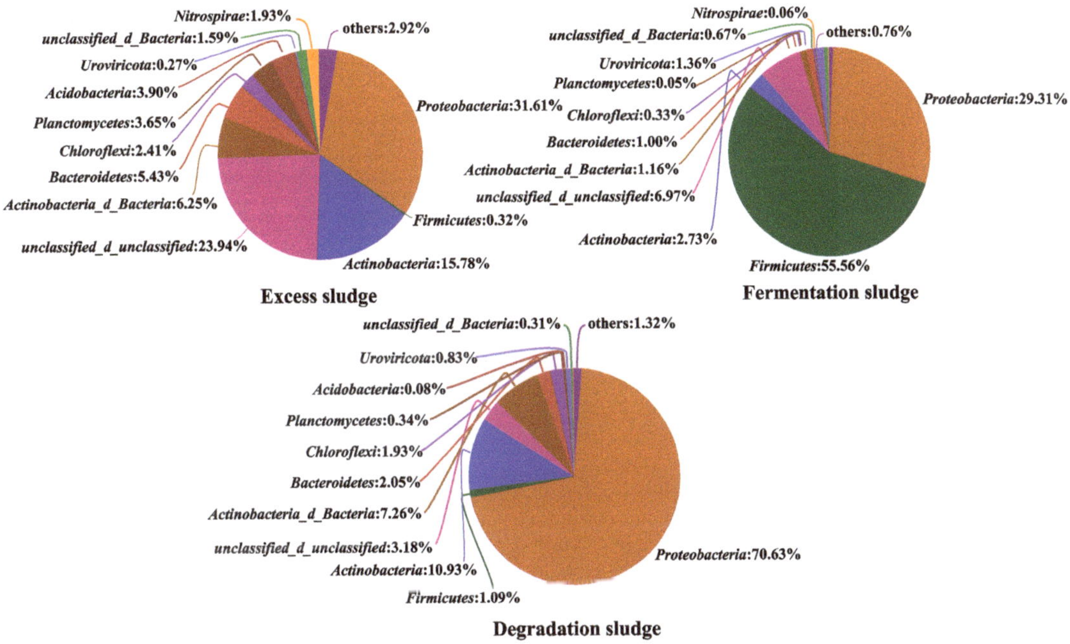

Figure 7. Bacterial community evolution of residual sludge, fermented sludge, and 2,4,6-TCP-degraded sludge at phylum level.

In the sludge that is capable of degrading 2,4,6-TCP, the dominant bacterial phylum is *Proteobacteria*, representing a high proportion of 70.63%. *Proteobacteria* is a key phylum and is associated with the metabolism of 2,4,6-TCP [26], and this finding aligns with the efficient 2,4,6-TCP degradation observed in DSBR. Furthermore, in residual sludge, *Proteobacteria* (31.61%) is the dominant phylum, while fermentative sludge is dominated by *Firmicutes* (55.56%). This suggests that the use of residual sludge as a feedstock substrate did not significantly affect the microbial community structure in the fermentative sludge. This is likely because the heat treatment of residual sludge, its use as the fermentation substrate in FSBR, and the anaerobic fermentation environment favored the dominance of *Firmicutes*. Simultaneously, the suspended sludge in the sludge FB did not significantly impact the microbial community in DSBR.

As shown in Figure 8, at the genus level, *Lactobacillus* was detected in the fermentation sludge, representing 54.06% of the total, and many studies have reported it as a dominant genus in anaerobic activated sludge and acid-producing fermentation processes [27–29]. Therefore, the presence of the *Lactobacillus* genus is favorable for the acid production in sludge fermentation, resulting in an acid production rate of over 88.4%. Additionally, 3.49% of the *Dechloromonas* genus was detected, which plays a significant role in the hydrolysis and acidification of organic matter under anaerobic conditions [22,30,31]. In this experiment, heat-treated residual sludge was used as the feedstock sludge, which contained a substantial amount of polysaccharides and protein components. *Dechloromonas* genus can effectively hydrolyze these organic substances and promote hydrolytic acidification, accelerating acid production.

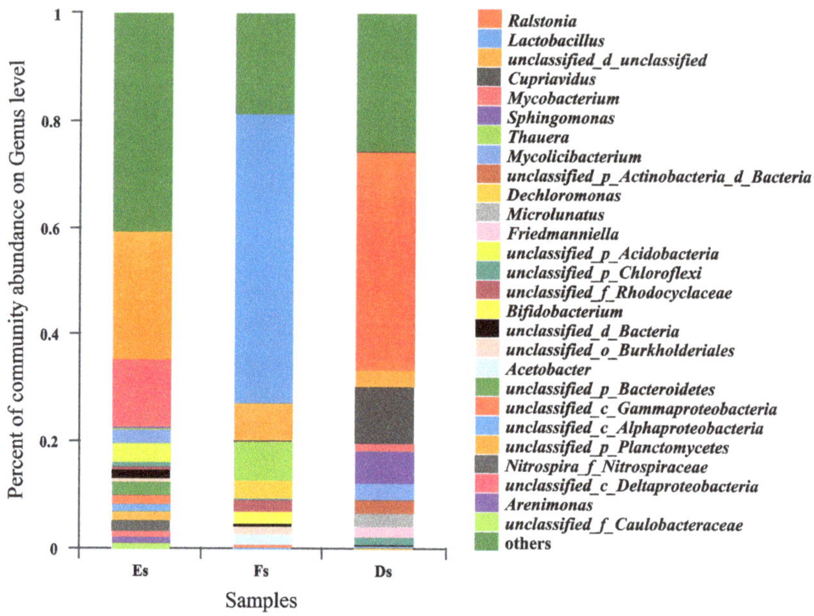

Figure 8. Bacterial community evolution of residual sludge, fermented sludge, and 2,4,6-TCP-degraded sludge at genus level (Es: excess sludge; Fs: fermentation sludge; Ds: degradation sludge).

Through high-throughput analysis of the sludge involved in the degradation of 2,4,6-trichlorophenol, it was discovered that the *Ralstonia* genus was the most abundant genus in the reactor, accounting for as much as 40.89%. Many studies have found a close metabolic relationship between the *Ralstonia* genus and phenol, pentachlorophenol, 4-chlorophenol, and 2,4,6-trichlorophenol [13,32–35]. Other genera with abundances exceeding 1% include *Cupriavidus* (10.52%), *Sphingomonas* (6.18%), *Mycolicibacterium* (2.97%), *Microlunatus* (2.39%), *Friedmanniella* (1.94%), and *Mycobacterium* (1.35%). Among these, the *Cupriavidus genus* [36–39], the *Sphingomonas* genus [40–42], and the *Mycobacterium* genus [43–45] are known to possess the ability to degrade phenol, 4-chlorophenol, 2,4,6-trichlorophenol, 2,3,4,5-tetrachlorophenol, and pentachlorophenol.

Compared with other organic carbon sources, the use of sludge fermentation liquid as a carbon source significantly promoted the enrichment of these chlorophenol-degrading bacteria, particularly the *Ralstonia genus*, which reached a high proportion of 40.89%. The enrichment of these chlorophenol-degrading bacteria is consistent with the removal efficiency of 2,4,6-trichlorophenol.

3.6.2. Analysis of 2,4,6-TCP Functional Gene Abundance and Distribution

In Figure 9, the abundance of functional genes and their distribution proportions among different genera are depicted. At the genetic level, there were a total of six functional genes that were associated with 2,4,6-trichlorophenol metabolism, namely, *PcpA*, *pcaF*, *pcaI*, *Mal-r*, *chqB*, and *fadA*, which was consistent with previous research [9]. The abundance of functional genes in the sludge samples was 52,104 hits, significantly higher than when domestic wastewater was used as a carbon source [9]. This difference in gene abundance may have explained why the highest 2,4,6-trichlorophenol degradation concentration was achieved using sludge fermentation liquid rather than domestic wastewater as the carbon source.

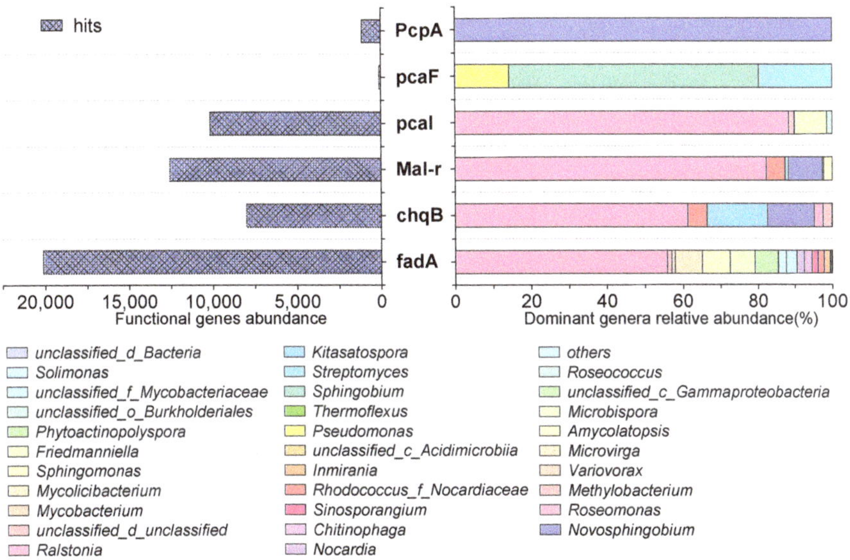

Figure 9. Abundance of 2,4,6-TCP functional genes and the contribution of dominant genera to functional genes.

The individual gene abundances were as follows: 1152 hits (*PcpA*), 112 hits (*pcaF*), 10,144 hits (*pcaI*), 12,552 hits (*Mal-r*), 8022 hits (*chqB*), and 20,122 hits (*fadA*). Although *pcaF* had a relatively low abundance of only 112 hits, it is worth noting that *pcaF* is positioned at the end of the 2,4,6-trichlorophenol metabolic pathway and is responsible for degrading less toxic by-products. This lower abundance of *pcaF* did not impact the overall effectiveness of 2,4,6-trichlorophenol degradation. In contrast, the functional genes at the metabolic front end had relatively high abundances.

PcpA was exclusively contributed by the *Novosphingobium* genus, and the content of *Novosphingobium* had a direct relationship with the removal efficiency of 2,4,6-trichlorophenol. *PcaF* was contributed by the *Pseudomonas* (contribution ratio: 14.29%), *Sphingobium* (66.07%), and *Streptomyces* (19.64%) genera. Multiple genera contributed to *pcaI*, *Mal-r*, *chqB*, and *fadA*, with *Ralstonia* being the most prominent contributor for each, with contribution ratios of 87.54%, 82.12%, 60.91%, and 52.64%, respectively. *Ralstonia* was also the most abundant genus in the sludge used for 2,4,6-trichlorophenol degradation. Therefore, the abundance of *Novosphingobium*, *Pseudomonas*, *Sphingobium*, *Streptomyces*, and *Ralstonia* genera directly influences the metabolic characteristics of 2,4,6-trichlorophenol when using sludge fermentation liquid as a co-metabolic carbon source.

4. Conclusions

Compared with the carbon sources documented in the literature, sludge fermentation broth has demonstrated the ability to enhance the proliferation of functional microorganisms and facilitate the degradation of 2,4,6-TCP. The fermentation liquid derived from sludge exhibits the potential to completely replace other commercially available carbon sources, thereby resulting in a significant reduction in operational investments for practical wastewater treatment. However, the presence of propionic acid components in sludge fermentation broth can partially inhibit the degradation of 2,4,6-TCP. Therefore, during the operation of the coupled fermentation and acid production process, it is necessary to control the level of propionic acid at a lower concentration. Pilot-scale experiments have confirmed that metabolic competition still exists, and the addition of fermentation broth at excessively high concentrations can inhibit the metabolism of 2,4,6-TCP. The analysis of the metabolic genes of functional bacterial strains revealed the presence of six chlorophenol degradation genes, with the following abundances: 1152 hits (*PcpA*), 112 hits (*pcaF*), 10,144 hits (*pcaI*), 12,552 hits (*Mal-r*), 8022 hits (*chqB*), and 20,122 hits (*fadA*). This study has successfully demonstrated the feasibility of using sludge fermentation broth as a co-metabolic carbon source for the degradation of 2,4,6-TCP.

Supplementary Materials: The following supporting information can be downloaded at https://www.mdpi.com/article/10.3390/w15244279/s1: Figure S1: 2-4 Liquid chromatographic peak of 2,4,6-TCP; Figure S2: General process of high-throughput sequencing. References [19,46–48] are cited in the Supplementary Materials.

Author Contributions: Conceptualization, J.W.; data curation, J.W.; formal analysis, S.L., J.W.; writing—original draft, J.W.; writing—review and editing, J.W. All authors have read and agreed to the published version of the manuscript.

Funding: This research was supported by the scientific program of PowerChina Huadong Engineering Corporation Limited (KY2022-HS-02-20).

Data Availability Statement: Data are contained within the article and Supplementary Materials.

Conflicts of Interest: Authors Jianguang Wang was employed by the company PowerChina Huadong Engineering Corporation Limited. The remaining authors declare that the research was conducted in the absence of any commercial or financial relationships that could be construed as a potential conflict of interest.

References

1. Xu, H.; Tong, N.; Huang, S.; Zhou, S.; Li, S.; Li, J.; Zhang, Y. Degradation of 2,4,6-trichlorophenol and determination of bacterial community structure by micro-electrical stimulation with or without external organic carbon source. *Bioresour. Technol.* **2018**, *263*, 266–272. [CrossRef] [PubMed]
2. Wang, J.; Sun, Z. Effects of different carbon sources on 2,4,6-trichlorophenol degradation in the activated sludge process. *Bioprocess Biosyst. Eng.* **2020**, *43*, 2143–2152. [CrossRef] [PubMed]
3. Chen, W.; Lee, T.; Chen, C. Polypyrrole-induced active-edge-S and high-valence-Mo reinforced composites with boosted electrochemical performance for the determination of 2,4,6-trichlorophenol in the aquatic environment. *Chemosphere* **2023**, *335*, 139003. [CrossRef] [PubMed]
4. Gao, J.; Liu, L.; Liu, X.; Zhou, H.; Huang, S.; Wang, Z. Levels and spatial distribution of chlorophenols –2,4-Dichlorophenol, 2,4,6-trichlorophenol, and pentachlorophenol in surface water of China. *Chemosphere* **2008**, *71*, 1181–1187. [CrossRef] [PubMed]
5. Wang, J.; Sun, Z. Exploring the effects of carbon source level on the degradation of 2,4,6-trichlorophenol in the co-metabolism process. *J. Hazard. Mater.* **2020**, *392*, 122293. [CrossRef] [PubMed]
6. Lin, X.; Li, Z.; Liang, B.; Zhai, H.; Cai, W.; Nan, J.; Wang, A. Accelerated microbial reductive dechlorination of 2,4,6-trichlorophenol by weak electrical stimulation. *Water Res.* **2019**, *162*, 236–245. [CrossRef]
7. Zou, C.; Wang, M.; Chen, Y.; Qin, Y.; Zhao, Y.; Qiao, L.; Zhu, S.; Chen, T.; Yuan, Y. Effects of different cathodic potentials on performance, microbial community structure and function for bioelectrochemical-stimulated dechlorination of 2,4,6-trichlorophenol in sediments. *Environ. Res.* **2023**, *216*, 114477. [CrossRef] [PubMed]
8. Khan, N.; Khan, M.D.; Ansari, M.Y.; Ahmad, A.; Khan, M.Z. Bio-electrodegradation of 2,4,6-Trichlorophenol by mixed microbial culture in dual chambered microbial fuel cells. *J. Biosci. Bioeng.* **2019**, *127*, 353–359. [CrossRef]
9. Wang, J.; Sun, Z. Successful application of municipal domestic wastewater as a co-substrate in 2,4,6-trichlorophenol degradation. *Chemosphere* **2021**, *280*, 130707. [CrossRef]
10. Zhao, J.; Li, Y.; Chen, X.; Li, Y. Effects of carbon sources on sludge performance and microbial community for 4-chlorophenol wastewater treatment in sequencing batch reactors. *Bioresour. Technol.* **2018**, *255*, 22–28. [CrossRef]
11. Hayes, R.P.; Webb, B.N.; Subramanian, A.K.; Nissen, M.; Popchock, A.; Xun, L.; Kang, C. Structural and Catalytic Differences between Two FADH2-Dependent Monooxygenases: 2,4,5-TCP 4-Monooxygenase (TftD) from *Burkholderia cepacia* AC1100 and 2,4,6-TCP 4-Monooxygenase (TcpA) from *Cupriavidus necator* JMP134. *Int. J. Mol. Sci.* **2012**, *13*, 9769–9784. [CrossRef] [PubMed]
12. Belchik, S.M.; Schaeffer, S.M.; Hasenoehrl, S.; Xun, L. A β-barrel outer membrane protein facilitates cellular uptake of polychlorophenols in *Cupriavidus necator*. *Biodegradation* **2010**, *21*, 431–439. [CrossRef] [PubMed]
13. Hatta, T.; Fujii, E.; Takizawa, N. Analysis of two gene clusters involved in 2,4,6-trichlorophenol degradation by *Ralstonia pickettii* DTP0602. *Biosci. Biotechnol. Biochem.* **2012**, *76*, 892–899. [CrossRef]
14. Wang, C.C.; Lee, C.M.; Lu, C.J.; Chuang, M.S.; Huang, C.Z. Biodegradation of 2,4,6-trichlorophenol in the presence of primary substrate by immobilized pure culture bacteria. *Chemosphere* **2000**, *41*, 1873–1879. [CrossRef]

15. Tong, N.; Yuan, J.; Xu, H.; Huang, S.; Sun, C.; Wen, X.; Zhang, Y. Effects of 2,4,6-trichlorophenol on simultaneous nitrification and denitrification: Performance, possible degradation pathway and bacterial community structure. *Bioresour. Technol.* **2019**, *290*, 121757. [CrossRef]
16. Huang, L.; Shi, Y.; Wang, N.; Dong, Y. Anaerobic/aerobic conditions and biostimulation for enhanced chlorophenols degradation in biocathode microbial fuel cells. *Biodegradation* **2014**, *25*, 615–632. [CrossRef] [PubMed]
17. Jadeja, N.B.; Purohit, H.J.; Kapley, A. Decoding microbial community intelligence through metagenomics for efficient wastewater treatment. *Funct. Integr. Genom.* **2019**, *19*, 839–851. [CrossRef]
18. Wang, J.; Sun, Z.; Li, J. Feasibility Study of Using Excess Sludge Fermentation Broth as a Co-Metabolic Carbon Source for 2,4,6-Trichlorophenol Degradation. *Water* **2023**, *15*, 4008. [CrossRef]
19. Wang, B.; Wang, S.; Li, B.; Peng, C.; Peng, Y. Integrating waste activated sludge (WAS) acidification with denitrification by adding nitrite (NO_2^-). *Biomass Bioenergy* **2014**, *67*, 460–465. [CrossRef]
20. Ma, J.; Quan, X.; Yang, Z.; Li, A. Biodegradation of a mixture of 2,4-dichlorophenoxyacetic acid and multiple chlorophenols by aerobic granules cultivated through plasmid pJP4 mediated bioaugmentation. *Chem. Eng. J.* **2012**, *181*, 144–151. [CrossRef]
21. Yuan, Y.; Wang, S.; Liu, Y.; Li, B.; Wang, B.; Peng, Y. Long-term effect of pH on short-chain fatty acids accumulation and microbial community in sludge fermentation systems. *Bioresour. Technol.* **2015**, *197*, 56–63. [CrossRef] [PubMed]
22. Yuan, Y.; Liu, J.; Ma, B.; Liu, Y.; Wang, B.; Peng, Y. Improving municipal wastewater nitrogen and phosphorous removal by feeding sludge fermentation products to sequencing batch reactor (SBR). *Bioresour. Technol.* **2016**, *222*, 326–334. [CrossRef] [PubMed]
23. Karakashev, D.; Schmidt, J.E.; Angelidaki, I. Innovative process scheme for removal of organic matter, phosphorus and nitrogen from pig manure. *Water Res.* **2008**, *42*, 4083–4090. [CrossRef] [PubMed]
24. Nelson, M.C.; Morrison, M.; Yu, Z. A meta-analysis of the microbial diversity observed in anaerobic digesters. *Bioresour. Technol.* **2011**, *102*, 3730–3739. [CrossRef] [PubMed]
25. Zheng, X.; Su, Y.; Li, X.; Xiao, N.; Wang, D.; Chen, Y. Pyrosequencing reveals the key microorganisms involved in sludge alkaline fermentation for efficient short-chain fatty acids production. *Environ. Sci. Technol.* **2013**, *47*, 4262–4268. [CrossRef]
26. Gómez-Acata, S.; Vital-Jácome, M.; Pérez-Sandoval, M.V.; Navarro-Noya, Y.E.; Thalasso, F.; Luna-Guido, M.; Conde-Barajas, E.; Dendooven, L. Microbial community structure in aerobic and fluffy granules formed in a sequencing batch reactor supplied with 4-chlorophenol at different settling times. *J. Hazard. Mater.* **2018**, *342*, 606–616. [CrossRef]
27. Tamis, J.; Joosse, B.; Leeuw, K.; Kleerebezem, R. High-rate ethanol production at low pH using the anaerobic granular sludge process. *Biotechnol. Bioeng.* **2021**, *118*, 1943–1950. [CrossRef]
28. Lian, T.; Zhang, W.; Cao, Q.; Wang, S.; Dong, H. Enhanced lactic acid production from the anaerobic co-digestion of swine manure with apple or potato waste via ratio adjustment. *Bioresour. Technol.* **2020**, *318*, 124237. [CrossRef]
29. Wang, P.; Qiao, Z.; Li, X.; Su, Y.; Xie, B. Functional characteristic of microbial communities in large-scale biotreatment systems of food waste. *Sci. Total Environ.* **2020**, *746*, 141086. [CrossRef]
30. Shi, L.; Du, R.; Peng, Y.; Li, Y. Successful establishment of partial denitrification by introducing hydrolytic acidification of slowly biodegradable organic matter. *Bioresour. Technol.* **2020**, *315*, 123887. [CrossRef]
31. Shi, L.; Du, R.; Peng, Y.; Li, Y. Simultaneous carbon reutilization for primary sludge and stable nitrite production in a hydrolytic acidification coupled with partial denitrification system to treat nitrate contaminant. *Bioresour. Technol.* **2020**, *318*, 124062. [CrossRef] [PubMed]
32. Laemmli, C.M.; Johan, H.J.L.; Alexander, J.B.Z.; Jan, R.V.D.M. Characterization of a econd tfd gene cluster for chlorophenol and chlorocatechol metabolism on Plasmid pJP4 in *Ralstonia eutropha* JMP134(pJP4). *J. Bacteriol.* **2000**, *182*, 4165–4172. [CrossRef] [PubMed]
33. Moormann, H.; Kuschk, P.; Stottmeister, U. The effect of rhizodeposition from helophytes on bacterial degradation of phenolic compounds. *Acta Biotechnol.* **2002**, *22*, 107–112. [CrossRef]
34. Torii, H.; Hirofumi, H.; Yabe, T.; Takizawa, N.; Hatta, T. A unique transcriptional regulator HadR Involved in 2,4,6-trichlorophenol degradation in *Ralstonia pickettii* DTP0602. *J. Biotechnol.* **2010**, *150*, 250. [CrossRef]
35. Wang, W.; Wang, S.; Zhang, J.; Hu, Z.; Zhang, X.; Muñoz Sierra, J. Degradation kinetics of pentachlorophenol and changes in anaerobic microbial community with different dosing modes of co-substrate and zero-valent iron. *Int. Biodeterior. Biodegrad.* **2016**, *113*, 126–133. [CrossRef]
36. Sanchez, M.A.; Gonzalez, B. Genetic characterization of 2,4,6-trichlorophenol degradation in *Cupriavidus necator* JMP134. *Appl. Environ. Microbiol.* **2007**, *73*, 2769–2776. [CrossRef] [PubMed]
37. Fang, L.; Qin, H.; Shi, T.; Wu, X.; Li, Q.X.; Hua, R. Ortho and para oxydehalogenation of dihalophenols catalyzed by the monooxygenase TcpA and NAD(P)H:FAD reductase Fre. *J. Hazard. Mater.* **2020**, *388*, 121787. [CrossRef]
38. Ledger, T.; Pieper, D.H.; Gonzalez, B. Chlorophenol hydroxylase encoded by plasmid pJP4 differentially contribute to chlorophenoxyacetic acid degradation. *Appl. Environ. Microbiol.* **2006**, *72*, 2783. [CrossRef]
39. Ying, X. Chemotaxis of *Cupriavidus necator* JMP134 towards aromatic compounds. *Res. J. Chem. Environ.* **2013**, *17*, 10–15.
40. Kim, Y.; Murugesan, K.; Schmidt, S.; Bokare, V.; Jeon, J.; Kim, E.; Chang, Y. Triclosan susceptibility and co-metabolism-a comparison for three aerobic pollutant-degrading bacteria. *Bioresour. Technol.* **2011**, *102*, 2206–2212. [CrossRef]

41. Mannisto, M.K.; Tiirola, M.A.; Puhakka, J.A. Degradation of 2,3,4,6-tetrachlorophenol at low temperature and low dioxygen concentrations by phylogenetically different groundwater and bioreactor bacteria. *Biodegradation* **2001**, *12*, 291–301. [CrossRef] [PubMed]
42. Rutgers, M.; Breure, A.M.; van Andel, J.G.; Duetz, W.A. Growth yield coefficients of *Sphingomonas* sp. strain P5 on various chlorophenols in chemostat culture. *Appl. Microbiol. Biotechnol.* **1997**, *48*, 656–661. [CrossRef]
43. Burback, B.L.; Perry, J.J. Biodegradation and biotransformation of groundwater pollutant mixtures by *Mycobacterium vaccae*. *Appl. Environ. Microbiol.* **1993**, *59*, 1025–1029. [CrossRef] [PubMed]
44. Burback, B.L.; Perry, J.J.; Rudd, L.E. Effect of environmental-pollutants and their metabolites on a soil mycobacterium. *Appl. Microbiol. Biotechnol.* **1994**, *41*, 134–136. [CrossRef]
45. Mannisto, M.K.; Salkinoja-Salonen, M.S.; Puhakka, J.A. In situ polychlorophenol bioremediation potential of the indigenous bacterial community of boreal groundwater. *Water Res.* **2001**, *35*, 2496–2504. [CrossRef]
46. Bardi, M.J.; Oliaee, M.A. Impacts of different operational temperatures and organic loads in anaerobic co-digestion of food waste and sewage sludge on the fate of SARS-CoV-2. *Process Saf. Environ. Prot.* **2021**, *146*, 464–472. [CrossRef]
47. Czaplicka, M. Sources and transformations of chlorophenols in the natural environment. *Sci. Total Environ.* **2004**, *322*, 21–39. [CrossRef]
48. Cui, B.; Yang, Q.; Liu, X.; Wu, W.; Liu, Z.; Gu, P. Achieving partial denitrification-anammox in biofilter for advanced wastewater treatment. *Environ. Int.* **2020**, *138*, 105612. [CrossRef]

water

MDPI

Article

Photocatalytic Degradation of Sulfamethoxazole and Enrofloxacin in Water Using Electrospun Composite Photocatalytic Membrane

Xiaohu Lin [1,2,3,*], Haifeng Fang [1,3], Libing Wang [1,3], Danyan Sun [2], Gang Zhao [2,4] and Jingcheng Xu [2,*]

1 PowerChina Huadong Engineering Corporation Limited, Hangzhou 311122, China
2 College of Environmental Science and Engineering, Tongji University, Shanghai 200092, China
3 Huadong Eco-Environmental Engineering Research Institute of Zhejiang Province, Hangzhou 311122, China
4 Shanghai Urban Construction Design & Research Institute (Group) Co., Ltd., Shanghai 200125, China
* Correspondence: tjhjxhlin@tongji.edu.cn (X.L.); jcxutj@126.com (J.X.); Tel.: +86-0571-56613288 (X.L.); +86-021-65982010 (J.X.)

Abstract: Photocatalysis has emerged as a promising technology for the removal of emerging contaminants such as antibiotics from water. Fixing photocatalytic materials on polymers to prepare applicable membranes is a feasible method for applying photocatalysis. This study explored the preparation of composite PAN-TiO_2 and PAN-TiO_2-rGO (PAN-rGTi) photocatalytic membranes by combining TiO_2, TiO_2-reduced graphene oxide (rGO) and polyacrylonitrile (PAN) using electrospinning. Characterization through SEM and EDS analysis confirms the composite membrane's microstructure and elemental composition. The electrospun PAN-TiO_2 and PAN-rGTi composite membranes exhibit a stable and efficient photocatalytic performance in degrading sulfamethoxazole (SMX) and enrofloxacin (ENR), two typical antibiotics commonly found in water bodies. Photocatalytic degradation experiments under simulated solar light reveal the superior performance of the composite photocatalytic membranes compared to PAN alone, with a notable increase in the reaction rate constants of PAN-TiO_2 (1.8 to 2.2 times for SMX and 3.2 to 4.0 times for ENR) and even higher enhancements for PAN-rGTi (2.8 to 3.0 times for SMX and 5.4 to 6.5 times for ENR) compared to PAN alone. Despite minor decreases (from 97.6% to 90.4%) in activity over five cycles, the photocatalytic composite membranes remain effective, showcasing their stability and recyclability. This study highlights the potential application of PAN-TiO_2 and PAN-rGTi composite membranes as sustainable and effective materials for removing emerging contaminants from water. Further exploration should focus on optimizing materials for specific emerging contaminants and improving their application feasibility for wastewater and water treatment and water purification in water bodies.

Keywords: photocatalytic degradation; sulfamethoxazole; enrofloxacin; polyacrylonitrile; composite membrane

1. Introduction

In recent years, emerging contaminants, mainly including antibiotics, endocrine-disrupting chemicals (EDCs) and microplastics, have attracted increasing attention and concern due to the high detection frequency in aquatic environments [1–4] and the associated risks to ecosystems and public health. To mitigate the risks from emerging contaminants, various technologies, including adsorption [5], advanced oxidation [6,7], and biological treatment [8], have been studied and developed in recent years. Among these technologies, photocatalytic oxidation has shown high efficiency and promising potential in removing various emerging contaminants, thanks to its advantages of high removal efficiency, a simple process, easy operation, and no secondary pollution [9,10]. Marvelous studies on photocatalytic materials, especially semiconductor materials, have been conducted and reported. Common photocatalytic materials, such as TiO_2, ZnO, SiO_2, SnO_2,

WO_3, Fe_2O_3, InO_3, ZnS, CdS, etc. [11,12], exhibit excellent photocatalytic performance in removing emerging contaminants from water. Moreover, by harnessing the exceptional photocatalytic properties of materials like TiO_2 and ZnO and combining them with carbon materials such as graphene oxide (GO) [13], carbon nanotubes [14], C_3N_4 [15], mesoporous carbon materials [16], etc., the specific surface area and conductivity of carbon materials are fully exploited, enhancing the photocatalytic activity and application potential of the materials. Existing research has demonstrated the significant advantages of these composite materials in removing emerging contaminants in water. However, current photocatalytic materials are usually studied and applied in the form of powder or particles. Powdered or particulate materials disperse readily in water, allowing for enhanced interaction with contaminants in water, thereby demonstrating excellent photocatalytic performance [17,18]. Nevertheless, powdered or granular photocatalytic materials face challenges in applications, such as being easy to agglomerate in the preparation process and difficult to recycle from water [9,19,20], limiting their usability and engineering application.

To address the limitations of conventional photocatalytic materials, researchers have explored innovative approaches for immobilizing photocatalytic materials [21–23], enhancing their stability and reusability. One promising strategy involves the development of photocatalytic nanocomposites, where photocatalytic materials are incorporated into a stable matrix or support material. Polymer-based carriers offer a viable solution for stabilizing photocatalytic materials and facilitating their separation from treated water [24–26]. In numerous studies, the removal efficiency of pollutants in dyes such as methyl orange and rhodamine B through photocatalytic degradation has been reported to reach 70–100% [25,27]. Polymers like polyethylene (PE), polytetrafluoroethylene (PTFE), polypropylene (PP), polyacrylonitrile (PAN), polyaniline (PANI), polyethersulfone (PES) and polydimethylsiloxane (PDMS) have also drawn attention as common polymer matrices for photocatalysts [28–30]. Among various methods for immobilizing photocatalysts in polymers, electrospinning, recognized for its effectiveness and versatility, has gained substantial attention in wastewater treatment. This is due to its capability to produce nanofibers with high surface area and porosity, as well as its convenience for separation, recovery, and reuse operations [31,32]. Recent studies have demonstrated successful applications of electrospun nanofibers as carriers for photocatalysts [31,33].

Despite the progress made in using polymer-based carriers for fixed-bed photocatalytic systems, there are still some challenges that need to be addressed. Existing studies predominantly focused on a limited range of pollutants or polymer materials, necessitating further exploration of more composite materials and their applicability to a broader spectrum of contaminants. While many studies confirm the efficacy of these photocatalytic composite membranes in degrading pollutants like dyes [34,35], further investigation into emerging contaminants, such as antibiotics, remains inadequate. Additionally, careful consideration is required in the selection and design of suitable polymer materials and photocatalysts as specific contaminants require careful consideration to achieve optimal removal efficiency. Furthermore, the stability and reusability of polymer-based carriers and immobilized photocatalysts warrant further investigation.

Consequently, this study aims to develop PAN-TiO_2 and PAN-TiO_2-rGO (PAN-rGTi) composite photocatalytic membranes by combining TiO_2, TiO_2-reduced graphene oxide (rGO) and polyacrylonitrile (PAN) using electrospinning. The objective is to evaluate their performance in degrading sulfamethoxazole (SMX) and enrofloxacin (ENR) in water. The key innovations of this research include: (1) the use of electrospinning to immobilize TiO_2 nanoparticles and TiO_2-rGO on PAN nanofibers, creating a stable and efficient photocatalytic membrane; (2) investigating the recyclability and stability of the composite membrane over multiple cycles of SMX and ENR degradation, effectively addressing emerging contaminants in wastewater treatment and water reclamation in wastewater treatment plants and water purification in rivers and lakes.

2. Methods and Materials

2.1. Materials and Regents

SMX (analytic standard) and ENR (analytic standard) were purchased from Sigma-Aldrich. Acetonitrile, methanol, and ethyl acetate of at least HPLC grade were obtained from Sigma-Aldrich (St. Louis, MO, USA). PAN (Mw = 150,000) was acquired from Shanghai Aladdin Biochemical Technology Co., Ltd. (Shanghai, China). *N,N*-dimethylformamide (DMF, analytical reagent, 99.5%) and ethanol absolute were supplied by Sinopharm Chemical Reagent Co., Ltd. (Shanghai, China). Moreover, 3-Methacryloxypropyltrimethoxysilane (MEMO, analytic regent) was procured from Tianjin BaiMa Technology Co., Ltd. (Tianjin, China). Graphene oxide (GO) powder (lateral size of 0.5–5 μm and thickness of 1–3 nm) was synthesized using the Hummers method and provided by Nanjing XFNANO Materials Tech Co., Ltd. (Nanjing, China). The Chemical Abstracts Service (CAS) numbers of the major chemicals are listed in Table S1. Ultrapure water (resistivity 18.2 $M\Omega \cdot cm^{-1}$ at 25 °C) was produced by a Merck Millipore water purification system (Darmstadt, Germany) and was used in related experiments.

2.2. Preparation of PAN Membrane and Composite Membrane

The PAN membrane and composite membrane were prepared using an electrospinning machine (TL-Pro-BM, Tongli Tech, Shenzhen, China), similar to in our previous study [36]. A 6% PAN solution was prepared by dissolving 1.8 g PAN in 30 mL DMF and stirred by magnetic stirring overnight before electrospinning. Additionally, 0.5 g P25 TiO_2 was weighed and added into a beaker containing 40 mL methanol and 10 mL ethanol, with the addition of 0.1 mL of MEMO reagent. The mixture was stirred by magnetic stirring overnight.

Two injection pumps were installed on the same side of the drum collector, and the injection tube was fixed on the same mobile platform. The PAN solution and TiO_2 dispersion were loaded into two 10 mL syringes, respectively. The speed of the mobile platform was maintained at 50 mm/s, with the scanning starting point at 30 mm and the scanning endpoint at 300 mm. Both the PAN solution and TiO_2 dispersion were fed at a constant rate through a 20# stainless steel needle (inner diameter 0.99 mm). The voltage set on the needle was 13 kV, the voltage set on the drum was −2 kV, and the distance from the tip of the needle to the collector was 15 cm. The drum speed was set to 500 rpm/min and the collection time was 10 h. During this process, the electrospun PAN nanofibers and the electro-sprayed TiO_2 nanoparticles were simultaneously collected on the drum collector to form a composite membrane of nanoparticles and fibers. Finally, the composite membrane was dried in a vacuum oven at 50 °C for 12 h to remove the residual solvent and then placed in a dry box for use.

The preparation of TiO_2-rGO (rGTi) material has been reported by some related studies [37–39]. Similarly, it was prepared by a hydrothermal method in this study. Initially, a certain amount of GO powder was dispersed in a 90 mL ultrapure water/ethanol solution (volume ratio of 2:1). The dispersion underwent ultrasonic treatment for 3 h in an ultrasonic bath to obtain a well-dispersed GO solution. Subsequently, 800 mg of P25 TiO_2 powder was added to the 90 mL GO dispersion, and the mixture was stirred at 500 rpm for 30 min. The resulting mixture was then transferred to a 150 mL Teflon-lined stainless-steel autoclave and subjected to hydrothermal treatment at 180 °C for 6 h, followed by cooling to room temperature. The reaction mixture was centrifuged at 3900 rpm for 15 min to obtain a centrifugal precipitate. The precipitate was washed several times with anhydrous ethanol and ultrapure water, and finally, it was dried in a vacuum oven at 60 °C for 8 h. In the synthesis of materials, the mass ratios of GO to P25 were set at 1% and 2%, denoted as rGTi-1 and rGTi-2, respectively. During the electrospinning stage, the main processes and parameters are essentially the same as those in the preparation method of the PAN-TiO_2 composite membrane.

2.3. Characteristics of PAN Membrane and Composite Membrane

A scanning electron microscope (SEM, ZEISS Gemini 300, Carl Zeiss, Jena, Germany) was used to analyze the surface microstructure and morphology, and the element mapping was carried out by an energy-dispersive X-ray spectrometer (EDS, Oxford Xplore , Oxford Instruments, Abingdon, UK) equipped with an SEM.

2.4. Photocatalytic Degradation of SMX and ENR Using Photocatalytic Membrane

The prepared PAN membrane and composite membrane were employed in the photocatalytic degradation of two common antibiotics in water. This study investigates the efficacy of PAN-TiO_2 and PAN-rGTi composite membranes in the photocatalytic degradation of typical antibiotics. Photodegradation experiments of SMX and ENR were conducted under simulated solar light provided by a photochemical reactor (Phchem III, NBeT, Beijing NBET Technology Co., Ltd., Beijing, China) equipped with a 500 W Xenon lamp, as stated in a previous study [40]. In the experiment, approximately 1.8 cm × 10 cm membranes were cut and placed in a quartz test tube. To support the morphology of the membrane in water, the metal mesh of the membrane collected during the spinning process was placed together with the membrane, ensuring a stable state in the test tube. The control group with just the PAN membrane was set to explore the difference in the photocatalytic degradation effect of the composite membrane loaded with TiO_2 and rGTi. At the same time, due to the introduction of metal mesh as a support structure, a blank control group with only metal mesh was set up in the experiment to eliminate the possible interference of metal mesh on the reaction. The experimental process included the dark adsorption stage (30 min) and photocatalytic reaction stage (60–180 min). In this group of experiments, the device used is the light reactor mentioned above. The light source used to simulate the solar light source was a 500 W xenon lamp light source, and the current was set to 8 A. The initial concentration of SMX or ENR was set as 5 mg/L, the samples were taken at certain time points during the reaction process, and the concentrations of SMX or ENR antibiotics were analyzed using high-performance liquid chromatography (HPLC) (Agilent HPLC 1200, Agilent Technologies, Santa Clara, CA, USA) using a variable wavelength detector (VWD) and a Shim-pack VP-ODS column (250 mm × 4.6 mm), with the analytic method similar to the previous study [40].

3. Results and Discussion

3.1. The Characteristics of PAN and Composite Membrane

The SEM images in Figure 1 depict the morphologies of the PAN, PAN-TiO_2 and PAN-rGTi membranes. The PAN membrane, fabricated through electrospinning without a photocatalyst, showcases a typical PAN nanofiber structure. Upon the introduction of the TiO_2 material, visible changes occur, with some TiO_2 nanoparticles sprayed onto the surface of PAN nanofibers. This process results in the creation of surface roughness and a defect structure, as shown in Figure 1e. It is noteworthy that not all TiO_2 nanoparticles were uniformly integrated with the PAN surface; some remained either loosely associated or were not loaded into the material. The resulting rough and defective structure of TiO_2 particles on the PAN nanofiber surface, along with the formation of a nanofiber structure composed of TiO_2 and PAN, plays a crucial role in enhancing the photocatalytic activity sites of the PAN membrane. This, in turn, allows the composite membrane to exhibit notable photocatalytic performance.

The element analysis of the PAN membrane and PAN-TiO_2 composite membrane was carried out by energy-dispersive spectrometer surface-scanning analysis mapping, and the corresponding elements were observed. As shown in Figure 2, the elemental surface sweeping results of the PAN-TiO_2 composite membrane offered the distribution of C, Ti, O, and N elements and the corresponding element weight ratios. The weight ratio of elements C, N, Ti, and O differs more from the theoretical value for PAN and less for TiO_2; thus, the accuracy of weight percentages may be lower for low-mass elements. The characterization of this elemental ratio primarily aims to confirm the combination of the two materials.

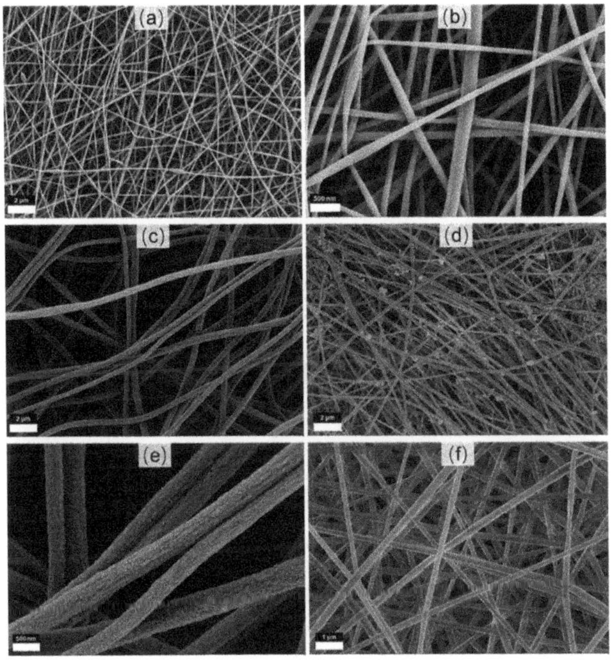

Figure 1. SEM images of PAN membrane under (**a**) 2 μm and (**b**) 500 nm scale, PAN-TiO_2 composite membrane under (**c**) 2 μm, (**d**) 2 μm and (**e**) 500 nm scale and PAN-rGTi composite membrane under (**f**) 1 μm scale.

3.2. Photocatalytic Degradation of SMX and ENR

The concentration variations of SMX and ENR during the reaction and corresponding kinetic fittings for the photocatalytic reaction stage are shown in Figures S1 and 3. A previous study [40] established that the degradation reactions of both SMX and ENR adhere to pseudo-first-order kinetics, a pattern consistent with the photocatalytic degradation stage in this study. Following the dark adsorption stage, the metal mesh has a small amount of adsorption (7.4%) for SMX in the reaction system, and the adsorption of SMX on the PAN membrane was more obvious (18.7%), which may account for a larger adsorption area. The PAN composite membrane loaded with TiO_2 had the largest adsorption capacity for SMX, with the PAN-TiO_2-2 composite membrane adsorbing 34.2% of SMX and the PAN-TiO_2-4 composite membrane adsorbing 37.3% of SMX. This indicated that the PAN membrane composed of a large number of fibers could adsorb and retain a certain number of pollutants in its structure, and after TiO_2 particles were loaded on the PAN fiber, the structural pores were smaller, which helped to increase the capacity of adsorption and retention of pollutants. Similar trends are observed in the dark adsorption and photocatalytic degradation phases of ENR. While the PAN membrane adsorbs more ENR than the group with just a metal mesh, both groups exhibit a comparable final total removal ratio for ENR by the end of the photochemical reaction phase. In the PAN-TiO_2-2 and PAN-TiO_2-4 systems, a noticeable photocatalytic degradation effect is evident compared to the PAN membrane and the metal mesh groups. The reaction rate constants during the photochemical reaction phase are increased by 3.2 to 4.0 times.

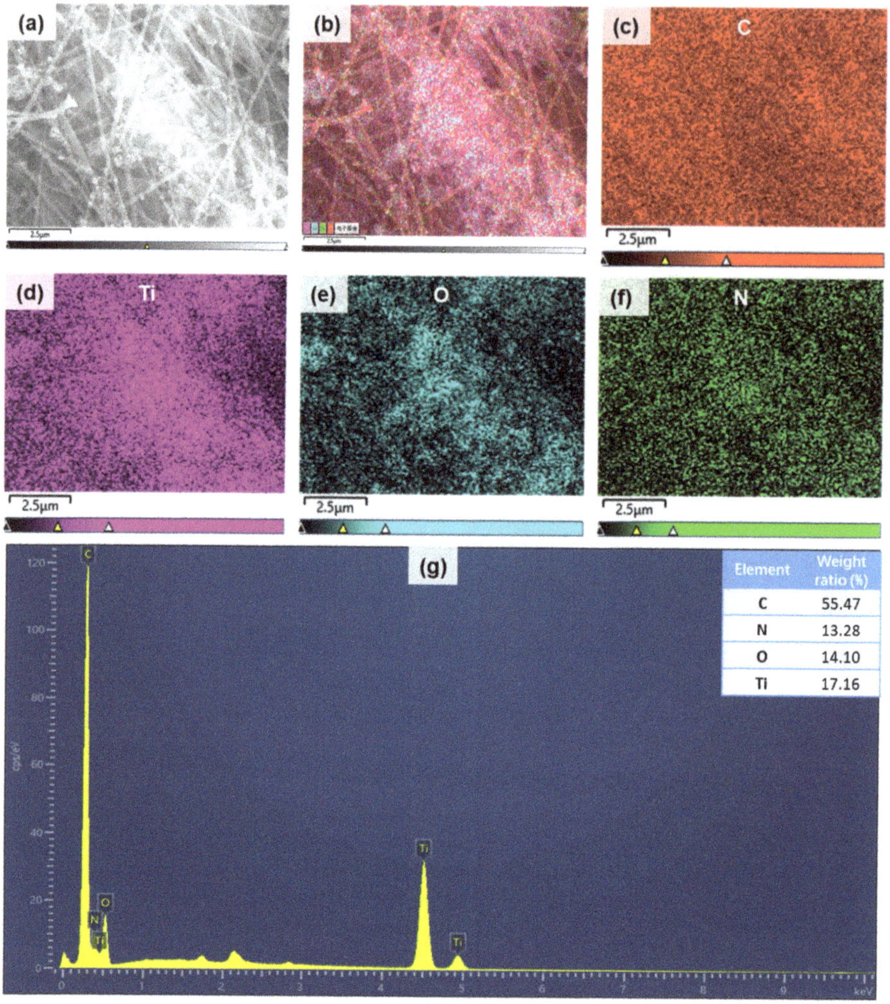

Figure 2. (**a**) SEM micrograph, (**b**) energy-dispersive X-ray spectroscopy (EDS) layered image, corresponding EDS elemental mapping for (**c**) C, (**d**) Ti, (**e**) O, (**f**) N, and (**g**) EDS pattern of of PAN-TiO_2 composite membrane.

In the photocatalytic reaction, although the PAN membrane adsorbs more SMX than the group with metal mesh alone, the total removal efficiencies of SMX in both groups were close, indicating that the PAN membrane had no significant catalytic effect on the photodegradation of SMX. Moreover, the photodegradation rate of SMX in the PAN membrane group was even slightly lower than that in the metal mesh group during the photocatalytic reaction stage. This may be attributed to the PAN membrane affecting the light transmission in the reaction system, thereby reducing the photodegradation rate of SMX and resulting in a lower total removal rate.

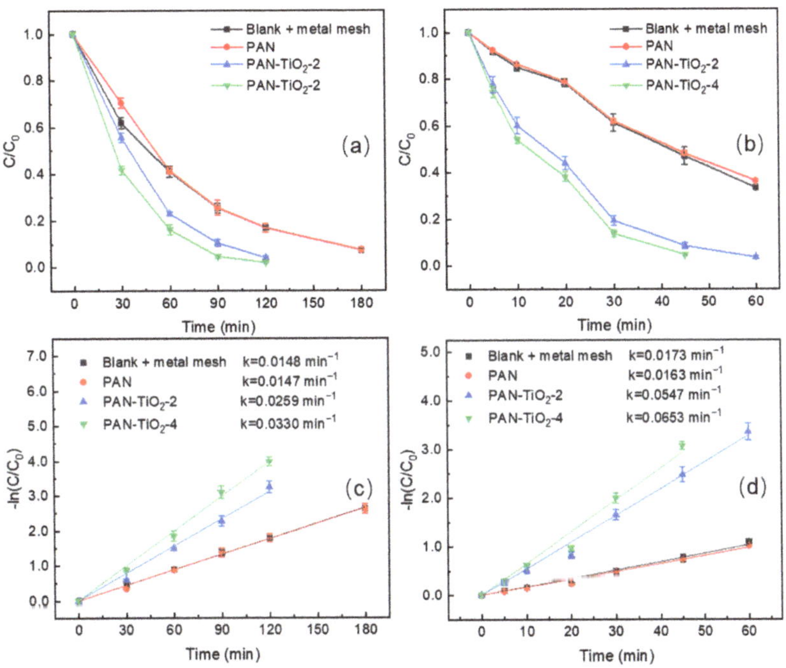

Figure 3. The concentrations of (**a**) SMX and (**b**) ENR in the photocatalytic degradation stage with PAN-TiO_2 composite membrane and the corresponding kinetic curves of (**c**) SMX and (**d**) ENR with the initial concentration of 5 mg/L and uncontrolled pH at room temperature (20 °C).

The PAN-TiO_2 composite membrane, with the addition of TiO_2, played a catalytic degradation role in the photoreaction process. The reaction constants of PAN-TiO_2-2 and PAN-TiO_2-4 relative to the PAN membrane and the blank group increased by 1.8–2.2 times. Su et al. [41] prepared TiO_2/PAN composite nanofiber membranes by electrospinning, demonstrating commendable air filtration performance and photocatalytic capabilities. Notably, as the mass ratio of TiO_2 to PAN increased, the efficiency of photocatalytic toluene removal exhibited a corresponding rise. The optimal performance was achieved at a TiO_2/PAN mass ratio of 4:1, yielding a toluene conversion rate of 97.9%. While the specific pollutants targeted differed, Su et al.'s findings showcased robust photocatalytic performance in the composite membrane, aligning with our study. Similarly, in the investigation conducted by Xu et al. [42] on PAN/TiO_2/PANI, it was observed that augmenting the TiO_2 ratio in the composite membrane led to an enhancement in photocatalytic performance.

A parallel investigation was conducted to assess the photocatalytic application of the PAN-rGTi composite membrane. A reaction tube with only a metal mesh served as the blank control group, while a tube with only a PAN membrane served as the control group. Tubes containing PAN-rGTi-1 and PAN-rGTi-2 were placed into separate test tubes, undergoing a dark adsorption stage followed by a photoreaction stage under xenon lamp illumination. The concentration changes and reaction constants for the photoreaction process of SMX and ENR are illustrated in Figure 4a–d. Following the dark adsorption stage, the PAN membrane adsorbed more pollutants compared to the metal mesh alone. However, during the photoreaction stage, the photocatalytic degradation rate of pollutants in tubes containing the PAN membrane was slightly lower than that of the group with only the metal mesh. In contrast, the PAN-rGTi composite membrane demonstrated excellent performance in both adsorption and photocatalytic properties. Analyzing the removal efficiency of SMX during the dark adsorption and photoreaction stages, as well as the reaction constants during the photoreaction stage for the PAN membrane, PAN-TiO_2 membrane, and PAN-rGTi composite membrane (Table 1), reveals that the adsorption performance of the PAN-TiO_2 composite membrane is improved compared to the PAN membrane, reaching 2.2 to 2.5 times. The adsorption capacity of PAN-rGTi is further enhanced, increasing to around three times. Comparing the experimental group with the PAN-TiO_2 composite membrane to the blank group and the photodegradation reaction rate constant of SMX and ENR in the PAN membrane, the PAN-TiO_2 composite membrane exhibited an increase of 1.8 to 2.2 times and 3.2 to 4.0 times during the photoreaction stage, respectively. The photocatalytic activity of the PAN-rGTi composite membrane was even higher, showing an enhancement of 2.8 to 3.0 times and 5.4 to 6.5 times. These results highlight the excellent photocatalytic performance of the photocatalytic composite membrane.

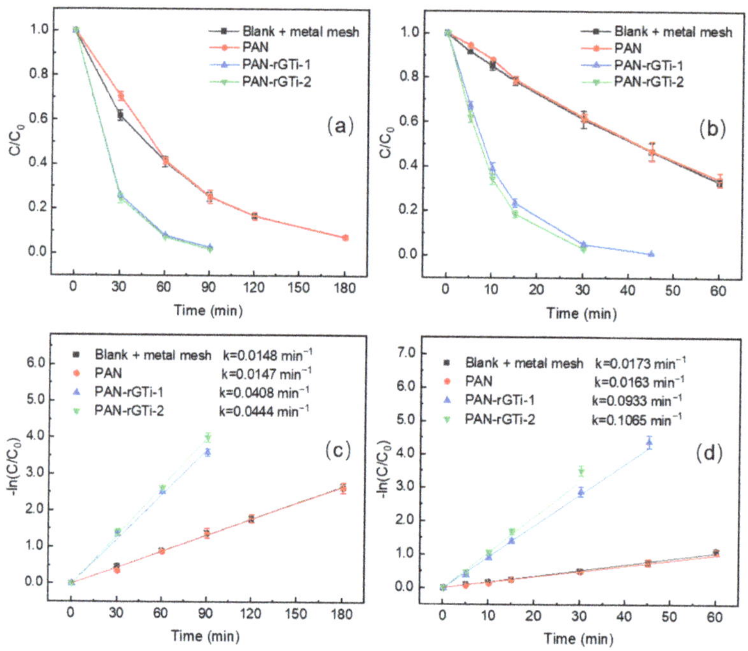

Figure 4. Adsorption and photocatalytic degradation of (**a**) SMX and (**b**) ENR with PAN-rGTi composite membrane and kinetic curves of (**c**) SMX and (**d**) ENR with the initial concentration of 5 mg/L and uncontrolled pH at room temperature (20 °C).

Table 1. The removal of SMX by PAN-TiO_2 and PAN-rGTi composite membrane in different reaction stage with the initial concentration of 5 mg/L and uncontrolled pH at room temperature (20 °C).

	Blank + Metal Mesh	PAN Membrane	PAN-TiO_2-2	PAN-TiO_2-4	PAN-rGTi-1	PAN-rGTi-2
Removal efficiency in adsorption stage	2.86%	16.82%	37.72%	42.61%	47.96%	50.85%
Removal efficiency in photocatalytic degradation stage	92.7%	92.6%	~100%	~100%	~100%	~100%
Total removal efficiency	92.9%	93.8%	~100%	~100%	~100%	~100%
Reaction constant in photocatalytic degradation stage (min^{-1})	0.148	0.147	0.259	0.330	0.408	0.444

3.3. Recyclability and Application Feasibility of Photocatalytic Composite Membrane

To assess the application potential of the prepared photocatalytic composite membrane, the feasibility of membrane reuse was investigated using ENR as the research target. The PAN-TiO_2 composite membrane underwent repeated application under nearly identical conditions for five cycles to evaluate its photocatalytic removal efficiency of ENR. After each adsorption and photoreaction stage, the membrane underwent thorough washing and ultrapure water soaking before being dried for the subsequent cycle. As shown in Figure 5, after five cycles, the removal efficiency of ENR by the PAN-TiO_2 composite membrane for photocatalytic degradation gradually decreased from 97.6% to 90.4%. Despite this reduction, the PAN-TiO_2 composite membrane maintained high photocatalytic activity. The reaction constant during the photocatalytic reaction process decreased from 0.064 min^{-1} in the first cycle to 0.039 min^{-1} in the fifth cycle, remaining more than twice as high as the experimental group without a photocatalytic composite membrane. This demonstrated the stability of the electrospun PAN-TiO_2 composite membrane, showcasing its ability to be reused multiple times. In the study of Su et al. [41], the removal efficiency of toluene by PAN-TiO_2 composite membrane was only slightly reduced when it was reused five times and still maintained a high removal efficiency. Shi et al. [43] also reused the PAN@TiO_2/Ag composite nanofiber membrane five times under visible light to remove methylene blue and found that the removal efficiency of photocatalytic degradation was slightly reduced from 99.0% to 93.0% after five cycles.

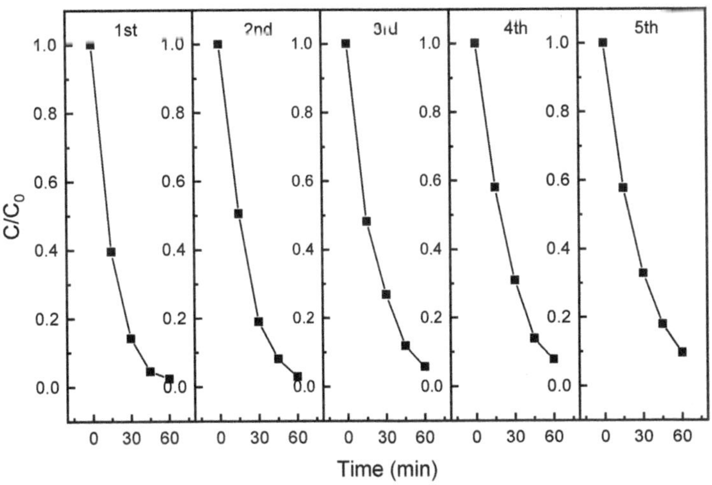

Figure 5. Five circling runs for photocatalytic degradation of ENR with PAN-TiO_2 membrane.

It is important to note that the vertical positioning of the membrane during experiments may lead to slight changes in the light contact area due to water flow disturbances and potential accidental damage. This could result in wrinkles or local defects, leading to a corresponding decrease in catalytic performance during subsequent uses. Similar observations by Sun et al. [44] also indicated that the prepared PAN/TiO_2 composite membrane still kept good stability after 10 cycles of reuse, but it suffered slight damage during deionized water cleaning. Due to the particularity of the preparation process, they also realized that the damaged membrane could be dissolved in DMF again and reshaped, and a new membrane could be prepared again, and the photocatalytic activity was not significantly reduced, which helped to further reduce the cost of photocatalytic materials and avoid the pollution caused by discarding material.

Cleaning and maintenance during the reuse process emerged as a critical factor influencing photocatalytic membrane performance. While pollutants in the aqueous phase were nearly completely removed during the photocatalytic reaction, the residual incomplete photodegradation of pollutants within the membrane and adsorbed products from the photodegradation stage could affect catalytic performance in subsequent reuse cycles. In comparison to photocatalytic powders, the photocatalytic composite membrane exhibited a slight reduction in catalytic reaction rates due to factors such as the contact area and degree between the catalyst and pollutants. However, it maintained excellent catalytic performance, making it more suitable for practical engineering applications due to advantages like easy recovery, reuse, flexible application forms, and stable performance.

Figure 6 presents the conceptual scenarios for the application of photocatalytic composite membranes in the engineering practice of reclaimed water reuse in rivers, including ultraviolet (UV) disinfection tanks in wastewater treatment plants and actual urban rivers. UV disinfection, as an essential disinfection process before reclaimed water replenishment into rivers, provides a UV light source that can be further utilized. With the deepening of subsequent research, photocatalytic composite membranes are expected to play an effective photocatalytic role in ultraviolet disinfection tanks, further removing emerging contaminants from reclaimed water [45]. In actual urban rivers, photocatalytic membranes can be fixed on the water surface, utilizing sunlight to catalyze reactions. When combined with various ecological restoration technologies such as biological filters and submerged plants in existing water bodies, they can further purify water quality, ensuring the safety of reclaimed water reuse and overall water body quality. Therefore, photocatalytic composite membranes have promising applications, and conducting more in-depth research is essential to advance their practical use.

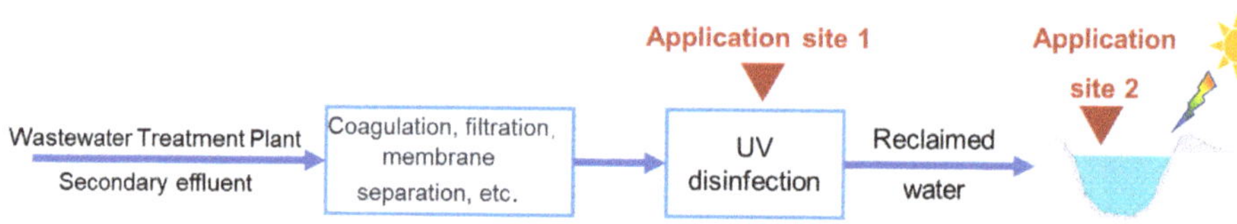

Figure 6. Proposed application sites for photocatalytic membranes.

4. Conclusions

The study investigated the preparation and application of PAN-TiO_2 and PAN-rGTi composite photocatalytic membranes prepared by electrospinning for the degradation of emerging contaminants: SMX and ENR. Electrospinning technology effectively immobilizes TiO_2 nanoparticles and rGTi onto PAN nanofibers, resulting in the preparation of a stable photocatalytic composite membrane. SEM and EDS images reveal the microstructure of the PAN-TiO_2 composite fiber membrane. After the electrostatic spraying of TiO_2, a multilayered TiO_2-coated coating forms on PAN nanofibers, exhibiting a well-defined defective structure. In the photocatalytic degradation of SMX and ENR, the reaction rate constants of PAN-TiO_2 increased by approximately 1.8 to 2.2 times and 3.2 to 4.0 times, respectively, compared to the PAN membrane system. PAN-rGTi demonstrated even better photocatalytic effects, with reaction rate constants increasing to approximately 2.8 to 3.0 times and 5.4 to 6.5 times, respectively, compared to the PAN membrane system. Cyclic experiments indicate that after five repeated uses, the catalytic performance of the photocatalytic composite membrane remains excellent. Taking ENR as an example, the removal efficiency of the PAN-TiO_2 composite membrane gradually decreased from 97.6% to 90.4%, maintaining high photocatalytic activity. The slight decrease in activity is attributed to minimal localized damage and wrinkles during repeated use, indicating that the composite membrane exhibits good catalytic activity and stability.

This research highlights the potential of PAN-TiO_2 and PAN-rGTi composite membranes as effective and sustainable materials for the removal of emerging contaminants from water. Further improvement can be achieved through additional research and an exploration of applications. Future research should focus on optimizing materials for a wider range of emerging contaminants and enhancing their feasibility for wastewater and water treatment in diverse environmental conditions. The developed membranes, with their stable photocatalytic activity and recyclability, hold promise for practical engineering applications in water purification and treatment. Additionally, this study envisions the application of these membranes in UV disinfection tanks and urban rivers, contributing to the overall improvement of water quality and the safety of reclaimed water reuse. The continued exploration and refinement of these innovative photocatalytic membranes, as well as the stability, reusability, scalability, and cost-effectiveness of this technology, are crucial for advancing their real-world applicability and addressing emerging water quality challenges.

Supplementary Materials: The following supporting information can be downloaded at: https://www.mdpi.com/article/10.3390/w16020218/s1, Figure S1: Adsorption and photocatalytic degradation of (a) SMX and (b) ENR with PAN-TiO_2 composite membrane with the initial concentration of 5 mg/L and uncontrolled pH at room temperature (20 °C); Table S1: Chemical Abstracts Service (CAS) Numbers of the major chemicals.

Author Contributions: Conceptualization, X.L.; methodology, X.L., D.S. and J.X.; software, X.L., D.S. and G.Z.; validation, X.L., G.Z. and J.X.; resources, H.F., L.W. and J.X.; data curation, X.L.; writing—original draft preparation, X.L.; writing—review and editing, X.L. and J.X.; visualization, X.L.; supervision, J.X.; project administration, H.F. and J.X.; funding acquisition, H.F., L.W. and J.X. All authors have read and agreed to the published version of the manuscript.

Funding: This research was supported by a scholarship from the China Scholarship Council (CSC) (Grant No. 201906260067) and the scientific program of PowerChina Huadong Engineering Corporation Limited (KY2018-SHJ-02).

Data Availability Statement: All relevant data are included in the paper or its Supplementary Materials.

Conflicts of Interest: Authors X.L., H.F. and L.W. are employed by the company PowerChina Huadong Engineering Corporation Limited, and author G.Z. is employed by the company Shanghai Urban Construction Design & Research Institute (Group) Co., Ltd. The remaining authors declare that the research was conducted in the absence of any commercial or financial relationships that could be construed as a potential conflict of interest.

References

1. Lin, X.H.; Xu, J.C.; Keller, A.A.; He, L.; Gu, Y.H.; Zheng, W.W.; Sun, D.Y.; Lu, Z.B.; Huang, J.W.; Huang, X.F.; et al. Occurrence and risk assessment of emerging contaminants in a water reclamation and ecological reuse project. *Sci. Total Environ.* **2020**, *744*, 11. [CrossRef] [PubMed]
2. Sabri, N.A.; Schmitt, H.; Van der Zaan, B.; Gerritsen, H.W.; Zuidema, T.; Rijnaarts, H.H.M.; Langenhoff, A.A.M. Prevalence of antibiotics and antibiotic resistance genes in a wastewater effluent-receiving river in The Netherlands. *J. Environ. Chem. Eng.* **2020**, *8*, 102245. [CrossRef]
3. Schmidt, C.; Kumar, R.; Yang, S.; Buettner, O. Microplastic particle emission from wastewater treatment plant effluents into river networks in Germany: Loads, spatial patterns of concentrations and potential toxicity. *Sci. Total Environ.* **2020**, *737*, 139544. [CrossRef] [PubMed]
4. Cundy, A.B.; Rowlands, F.M.; Lu, G.; Wang, W.X. A systematic review of emerging contaminants in the Greater Bay Area (GBA), China: Current baselines, knowledge gaps, and research and management priorities. *Environ. Sci. Policy* **2022**, *131*, 196–208. [CrossRef]
5. Rathi, B.S.; Kumar, P.S. Application of adsorption process for effective removal of emerging contaminants from water and wastewater. *Environ. Pollut.* **2021**, *280*, 116995. [CrossRef]
6. Wols, B.A.; Hofman-Caris, C.H.M. Review of photochemical reaction constants of organic micropollutants required for UV advanced oxidation processes in water. *Water Res.* **2012**, *46*, 2815–2827. [CrossRef]
7. Priyadarshini, M.; Das, I.; Ghangrekar, M.M.; Blaney, L. Advanced oxidation processes: Performance, advantages, and scale-up of emerging technologies. *J. Environ. Manag.* **2022**, *316*, 115295. [CrossRef]
8. Samal, K.; Bandyopadhyay, R.; Dash, R.R. Biological Treatment of Contaminants of Emerging Concern in Wastewater: A Review. *J. Hazard. Toxic Radioact. Waste* **2022**, *26*, 04022002. [CrossRef]
9. Deng, F.; Shi, H.; Guo, Y.; Luo, X.; Zhou, J. Engineering paths of sustainable and green photocatalytic degradation technology for pharmaceuticals and organic contaminants of emerging concern. *Curr. Opin. Green Sustain. Chem.* **2021**, *29*, 100465. [CrossRef]
10. Silvestri, S.; Fajardo, A.R.; Iglesias, B.A. Supported porphyrins for the photocatalytic degradation of organic contaminants in water: A review. *Environ. Chem. Lett.* **2022**, *20*, 731–771. [CrossRef]

11. Mirzaei, A.; Chen, Z.; Haghighat, F.; Yerushalmi, L. Removal of pharmaceuticals and endocrine disrupting compounds from water by zinc oxide-based photocatalytic degradation: A review. *Sustain. Cities Soc.* **2016**, *27*, 407–418. [CrossRef]
12. Feng, Y.; Rijnaarts, H.H.M.; Yntema, D.; Gong, Z.; Dionysiou, D.D.; Cao, Z.; Miao, S.; Chen, Y.; Ye, Y.; Wang, Y. Applications of anodized TiO_2 nanotube arrays on the removal of aqueous contaminants of emerging concern: A review. *Water Res.* **2020**, *186*, 116327. [CrossRef] [PubMed]
13. Shi, Y.; Yu, Z.; Li, Z.; Zhao, X.; Yuan, Y. In-Situ Synthesis of TiO_2@GO Nanosheets for Polymers Degradation in a Natural Environment. *Polymers* **2021**, *13*, 2158. [CrossRef] [PubMed]
14. Yoon, C.-J.; Lee, S.-H.; Kwon, Y.-B.; Kim, K.; Lee, K.-H.; Kim, S.M.; Kim, Y.-K. Fabrication of sustainable and multifunctional TiO_2@carbon nanotube nanocomposite fibers. *Appl. Surf. Sci.* **2021**, *541*, 148332. [CrossRef]
15. Li, Y.; Zhang, Q.; Lu, Y.; Song, Z.; Wang, C.; Li, D.; Tang, X.; Zhou, X. Surface hydroxylation of TiO_2/g-C_3N_4 photocatalyst for photo-Fenton degradation of tetracycline. *Ceram. Int.* **2022**, *48*, 1306–1313. [CrossRef]
16. Jansson, I.; Garcia-Garcia, F.J.; Sanchez, B.; Suarez, S. Key factors to develop hybrid photoactive materials based on mesoporous carbon/TiO_2 for removal of volatile organic compounds in air streams. *Appl. Catal. A Gen.* **2021**, *623*, 118281. [CrossRef]
17. Melinte, V.; Stroea, L.; Chibac-Scutaru, A.L. Polymer Nanocomposites for Photocatalytic Applications. *Catalysts* **2019**, *9*, 986. [CrossRef]
18. Epelle, E.I.; Okoye, P.U.; Roddy, S.; Gunes, B.; Okolie, J.A. Advances in the Applications of Nanomaterials for Wastewater Treatment. *Environments* **2022**, *9*, 141. [CrossRef]
19. Luna, M.; Gatica, J.M.; Vidal, H.; Mosquera, M.J. One-pot synthesis of Au/N-TiO_2 photocatalysts for environmental applications: Enhancement of dyes and NO_x photodegradation. *Powder Technol.* **2019**, *355*, 793–807. [CrossRef]
20. Chu, Y.; Fan, J.; Wang, R.; Liu, C.; Zheng, X. Preparation and immobilization of Bi_2WO_6/BiOI/g-C_3N_4 nanoparticles for the photocatalytic degradation of tetracycline and municipal waste transfer station leachate. *Sep. Purif. Technol.* **2022**, *300*, 121867. [CrossRef]
21. Oulhakem, O.; Zahdi, H.; Belaiche, M.; Laalioui, S.; Naimi, Z.; Ikken, B.; Sekkat, Z.; Alaoui, K.B. One-step immobilization of tungsten oxide on microporous silica surface as a photocatalyst for water pollutant removal. *Microporous Mesoporous Mater.* **2022**, *335*, 111784. [CrossRef]
22. Xue, Y.; Kamali, M.; Zhang, X.; Askari, N.; De Preter, C.; Appels, L.; Dewil, R. Immobilization of photocatalytic materials for (waste)water treatment using 3D printing technology-advances and challenges. *Environ. Pollut.* **2023**, *316*, 120549. [CrossRef] [PubMed]
23. Mansurov, R.R.; Safronov, A.P.; Lakiza, N.V.; Beketov, I.V. Photocatalytic Activity of Titanium Dioxide Nanoparticles Immobilized in the Polymer Network of Polyacrylamide Hydrogel. *Russ. J. Appl. Chem.* **2017**, *90*, 1712–1721. [CrossRef]
24. Hasnan, N.S.N.; Mohamed, M.A.; Anuar, N.A.; Sukur, M.F.A.; Yusoff, S.F.M.; Mokhtar, W.N.A.W.; Hir, Z.A.M.; Shohaimi, N.A.M.; Rafaie, H.A. Emerging polymeric-based material with photocatalytic functionality for sustainable technologies. *J. Ind. Eng. Chem.* **2022**, *113*, 32–71. [CrossRef]
25. Zhao, Y.; Wang, Y.; Xiao, G.; Su, H. Fabrication of biomaterial/TiO_2 composite photocatalysts for the selective removal of trace environmental pollutants. *Chin. J. Chem. Eng.* **2019**, *27*, 1416–1428. [CrossRef]
26. Zhao, Y.; Tao, C.; Xiao, G.; Su, H. Controlled synthesis and wastewater treatment of Ag_2O/TiO_2 modified chitosan-based photocatalytic film. *RSC Adv.* **2017**, *7*, 11211–11221. [CrossRef]
27. Enesca, A.; Cazan, C. Polymer Composite-Based Materials with Photocatalytic Applications in Wastewater Organic Pollutant Removal: A Mini Review. *Polymers* **2022**, *14*, 3291. [CrossRef] [PubMed]
28. Ahmad, N.; Anae, J.; Khan, M.Z.; Sabir, S.; Yang, X.J.; Thakur, V.K.; Campo, P.; Coulon, F. Visible light-conducting polymer nanocomposites as efficient photocatalysts for the treatment of organic pollutants in wastewater. *J. Environ. Manag.* **2021**, *295*, 113362. [CrossRef]
29. Zakria, H.S.; Othman, M.H.D.; Kamaludin, R.; Kadir, S.; Kurniawan, T.A.; Jilani, A. Immobilization techniques of a photocatalyst into and onto a polymer membrane for photocatalytic activity. *RSC Adv.* **2021**, *11*, 6985–7014. [CrossRef]
30. Lin, Q.; Zeng, G.; Yan, G.; Luo, J.; Cheng, X.; Zhao, Z.; Li, H. Self-cleaning photocatalytic MXene composite membrane for synergistically enhanced water treatment: Oil/water separation and dyes removal. *Chem. Eng. J.* **2022**, *427*, 131668. [CrossRef]
31. Zhou, X.; Shao, C.; Yang, S.; Li, X.; Guo, X.; Wang, X.; Li, X.; Liu, Y. Heterojunction of *g*-C3N4/BiOI Immobilized on Flexible Electrospun Polyacrylonitrile Nanofibers: Facile Preparation and Enhanced Visible Photocatalytic Activity for Floating Photocatalysis. *ACS Sustain. Chem. Eng.* **2018**, *6*, 2316–2323. [CrossRef]
32. Zhu, J.; Shao, C.; Li, X.; Han, C.; Yang, S.; Ma, J.; Li, X.; Liu, Y. Immobilization of ZnO/polyaniline heterojunction on electrospun polyacrylonitrile nanofibers and enhanced photocatalytic activity. *Mater. Chem. Phys.* **2018**, *214*, 507–515. [CrossRef]
33. Sun, F.; Xie, Y.; Xu, D.; Liu, F.; Qi, H.; Ma, Q.; Yang, Y.; Yu, H.; Yu, W.; Dong, X. Electrospun self-supporting double Z-scheme tricolor-typed microfiber oriented-heterostructure photocatalyst with highly effective hydrogen evolution and organic pollutants degradation. *J. Environ. Chem. Eng.* **2023**, *11*, 109169. [CrossRef]
34. Li, S.; Thiyagarajan, D.; Lee, B.-K. Efficient removal of methylene blue from aqueous solution by ZIF-8-decorated helicoidal electrospun polymer strips. *Chemosphere* **2023**, *333*, 138961. [CrossRef] [PubMed]
35. Sarkodie, B.; Amesimeku, J.; Frimpong, C.; Howard, E.K.; Feng, Q.; Xu, Z. Photocatalytic degradation of dyes by novel electrospun nanofibers: A review. *Chemosphere* **2023**, *313*, 137654. [CrossRef] [PubMed]

36. Zheng, W.W.; Xu, J.C.; Wang, L.Y.; Zhang, J.L.; Chu, W.H.; Liu, J.; Lu, L.J.; Cai, C.; Peng, K.M.; Huang, X.F. Electro-enhanced rapid separation of nanosized oil droplets from emulsions via the superhydrophilic micro-sized pore membrane. *Sep. Purif. Technol.* **2023**, *314*, 123453. [CrossRef]
37. Diamantopoulou, A.; Sakellis, E.; Romanos, G.E.; Gardelis, S.; Ioannidis, N.; Boukos, N.; Falaras, P.; Likodimos, V. Titania photonic crystal photocatalysts functionalized by graphene oxide nanocolloids. *Appl. Catal. B Environ.* **2019**, *240*, 277–290. [CrossRef]
38. Tolosana-Moranchel, A.; Casas, J.A.; Bahamonde, A.; Pascual, L.; Granone, L.I.; Schneider, J.; Dillert, R.; Bahnemann, D.W. Nature and photoreactivity of TiO_2-rGO nanocomposites in aqueous suspensions under UV-A irradiation. *Appl. Catal. B Environ.* **2019**, *241*, 375–384. [CrossRef]
39. Yu, L.; Tang, B. Photocatalytic Degradation of Phenolic Compounds from Wastewater Using Titanium dioxide@reduced Graphene Oxide (TiO_2@rGO) Nanocomposites. *Int. J. Electrochem. Sci.* **2021**, *16*, 210915. [CrossRef]
40. Lin, X.; Zhou, W.; Li, S.; Fang, H.; Fu, S.; Xu, J.; Huang, J. Photodegradation of Sulfamethoxazole and Enrofloxacin under UV and Simulated Solar Light Irradiation. *Water* **2023**, *15*, 517. [CrossRef]
41. Su, J.; Yang, G.; Cheng, C.; Huang, C.; Xu, H.; Ke, Q. Hierarchically structured TiO_2/PAN nanofibrous membranes for high-efficiency air filtration and toluene degradation. *J. Colloid Interface Sci.* **2017**, *507*, 386–396. [CrossRef] [PubMed]
42. Xu, B.; Wang, X.; Huang, Y.; Liu, J.; Wang, D.; Feng, S.; Huang, X.; Wang, H. Electrospinning preparation of PAN/TiO_2/PANI hybrid fiber membrane with highly selective adsorption and photocatalytic regeneration properties. *Chem. Eng. J.* **2020**, *399*, 125749. [CrossRef]
43. Shi, Y.; Yang, D.; Li, Y.; Qu, J.; Yu, Z.-Z. Fabrication of PAN@TiO_2/Ag nanofibrous membrane with high visible light response and satisfactory recyclability for dye photocatalytic degradation. *Appl. Surf. Sci.* **2017**, *426*, 622–629. [CrossRef]
44. Sun, X.-X.; Liu, G.; Li, R.; Meng, Y.; Wu, J. Polyporous PVDF/TiO_2 photocatalytic composites for photocatalyst fixation, recycle, and repair. *J. Am. Ceram. Soc.* **2021**, *104*, 6290–6298. [CrossRef]
45. Moreno-Andrés, J.; Rueda-Márquez, J.J.; Homola, T.; Vielma, J.; Moríñigo, M.A.; Mikola, A.; Sillanpää, M.; Acevedo-Merino, A.; Nebot, E.; Levchuk, I. A comparison of photolytic, photochemical and photocatalytic processes for disinfection of recirculation aquaculture systems (RAS) streams. *Water Res.* **2020**, *181*, 115928. [CrossRef]

water

MDPI

Article

Reprocessing and Resource Utilization of Landfill Sludge—A Case Study in a Chinese Megacity

Yifeng Yang [1], Jingshuai Luan [1], Jing Nie [2], Xin Zhang [1,*], Jiong Du [1], Gang Zhao [3], Lei Dong [1], Yong Fan [1], He Cui [1,*] and Yubo Li [1]

[1] Shanghai Municipal Engineering Design Institute (Group) Co., Ltd., Shanghai 200092, China; yangyifeng@smedi.com (Y.Y.); luanjingshuai@smedi.com (J.L.); dujiong@smedi.com (J.D.); donglei@smedi.com (L.D.); fanyongsmedi@163.com (Y.F.); liyubo@smedi.com (Y.L.)

[2] Shanghai Chengtou Water Engineering Project Management Co., Ltd., Shanghai 201103, China; niejingshct@126.com

[3] Shanghai Urban Construction Design & Research Institute Groups Co., Ltd., Shanghai 200125, China; zhaogang@sucdri.com

* Correspondence: zhangxin@smedi.com (X.Z.); cuihe@smedi.com (H.C.); Tel.: +86-136-7167-6724 (X.Z. & H.C.)

Abstract: In the past, due to improper sludge treatment technology and the absence of treatment standards, some municipal sludge was simply dewatered and then sent to landfills, occupying a significant amount of land and posing a serious threat of secondary pollution. To free up land in the landfill area for the expansion of a large-scale wastewater treatment plant (WWTP) in Shanghai, in this study, we conducted comprehensive pilot research on the entire chain of landfill sludge reprocessing and resource utilization. Both the combination of polyferric silicate sulfate (PFSS) and polyetheramine (PEA) and the combination of polyaluminum silicate (PAS) and polyetheramine (PEA) were used for sludge conditioning before dewatering, resulting in dewatered sludge with approximately 60% moisture content. The combined process involved coagulation and sedimentation, flocculation, and oxidation to treat the leachate generated during dewatering. The treatment process successfully met the specified water pollutant discharge concentration limits for the leachate, with the concentration of ammonia nitrogen in the effluent as low as 15.6 mg/L. Co-incineration in a power plant and modification were applied to stabilize and harmlessly dispose of the dewatered sludge. The coal-generating system ran stably, and no obvious problems were observed in the blending process. In the modification experiment, adding 5% to 7% of the solidifying agent increased the sludge bearing ratio by 53% and 57%, respectively. This process effectively reduced levels of fecal coliforms and heavy metals in the sludge but had a less noticeable effect on organic matter content. The modified sludge proved suitable for use as backfill material in construction areas without requirements for organic matter. The results of this study provide valuable insights for a completed full-scale landfill sludge reclamation and land resource release project.

Keywords: landfill sludge treatment; conditioning; dewatering; co-incineration; leachate treatment

1. Introduction

Municipal sludge is the byproduct of municipal wastewater treatment, consisting of complex materials such as organic matter, microbial biomass, protozoans, inorganic particles, and colloids [1]. The raw sludge is characterized by a high moisture content, high organic matter content, and strong smell. With the continuous increase in wastewater treatment during China's urbanization process, the generation of municipal sludge has also increased [2]. In the past few decades, landfilling has been the conventional method for municipal sludge treatment in China due to its simplicity and cost advantage in handling large quantities of sludge [3]. However, sludge that was directly dumped into landfills without proper pretreatment was not stabilized. Long-term storage of sludge with a high moisture content could easily lead to secondary pollution of the surrounding soil, water, and air [4,5].

Subsequent dumping of garbage in the landfill could cause compression of the sludge, excessive deformation, and insufficient strength, which might lead to landfill engineering accidents. Furthermore, in the context of increasingly limited urban construction land, landfill sites for sludge have occupied large areas and had a significant restraining effect on the development of surrounding areas [6]. Therefore, the removal and reprocessing of municipal sludge from landfill sites to mitigate the historical sludge accumulation has become a new direction in the field of municipal sludge treatment. Typically, to handle and recycle the landfill sludge, the sludge must be taken out from the landfill site first and then dewatered and disposed of properly. Moreover, the leachate generated during the dewatering process must be treated to meet the discharge standard. Co-incineration of sludge in power plants has been widely used as an alternative method to utilize sludge [7–9]. In China's megacities, like Shanghai, the use of dewatered sludge for co-treatment in coal-fired power plants is encouraged [10,11]. However, few studies have reported the co-treatment in power plants of sludge that has been landfilled and then dewatered. Leachate, as a byproduct of landfill sludge, is characterized by high concentrations of nitrogen and phosphorus. Comparatively, the concentration of nitrogen in sludge landfill leachate is typically even higher than that in traditional solid waste landfill leachate [12].

Some researchers have used chemical and biological technology to remove ammonium nitrogen from landfill sludge leachate [13–17]. It is worth noting that biological treatment methods, such as the activated sludge process, usually cost too much energy and occupy a large land area. On the other hand, only biological treatment of leachate can meet discharge standards due to the high concentrations of pollutants [18]. Therefore, the combination of physio-chemical technology for the simultaneous removal of nitrogen and phosphorus is becoming a promising method to handle high nitrogen concentrations in leachate.

The temporary sludge landfill site used in this study is located on the east side of a large-scale WWTP, adjacent to the Yangtze River, with a landfill area of approximately 25 ha. It was constructed in 2004 to address the issue of municipal sludge disposal. Starting in June 2010, to control the odor from the landfill site and its impact on the surrounding environment, the WWTP implemented capping and covering measures on the entire sludge landfill area. Currently, with limited available land for the Phase III expansion of the wastewater treatment plant, the urgency and necessity of releasing the land within the sludge temporary storage area have become apparent.

Through this study, we aim to restore the sludge landfill to its original state by focusing on the withdrawal, treatment, disposal, and resource utilization of landfill sludge. The research includes a comprehensive technical examination and demonstration of the sludge temporary storage area. Additionally, we aim to promote key technologies such as sludge pollution diagnosis, risk control, and resource utilization. The ultimate goal is to achieve reduction, harmlessness, stabilization, and resource utilization of the sludge stored in the temporary landfill site. The long-term landfilling of sludge under a High-Density Polyethylene (HDPE) geomembrane has led to anaerobic fermentation, producing a significant amount of toxic and harmful gases [19]. The anaerobic fermentation has resulted in changes to the properties of both the sludge and leachate, leading to higher environmental risks. Therefore, the current focus and challenges of the research involve completing the treatment and disposal of the sludge and leachate with minimal environmental impact and safely reclaiming the land resources in the storage area. This research demonstrates a complete chain of technologies, including dewatering aged landfill sludge, co-incineration in a power plant, solidified modification of sludge for use as backfill material, and the treatment process for the leachate generated during sludge dewatering. The result provides a theoretical basis and enables recommendations for the future reclamation of landfill sludge.

2. Materials and Methods

2.1. Overview of Sludge Landfill Site and Sludge Extraction Equipment

The sludge landfill site comprises 12 pits, each with a length of approximately 180 m, a width ranging from 80 to 120 m, and a depth of 8 m. To prevent the release of pollutants, half of the upper portion of the landfill cells is covered with an HDPE geomembrane. In this study, a suspended cable-based equipment system was used for the extraction of sludge from the landfill site.

The equipment consists of five main components: the sub-membrane sludge removal system, the onshore towing system, the cable winding system, the control system, and the maintenance system. The suspended cable system utilizes power to drive water pumps, generating high-pressure water flow that enters the spray pipes. The water is then sprayed out through the nozzles installed on the spray pipes, agitating the sludge at the bottom of the sedimentation pit into a turbid water-like state. This allows the sludge to flow out without opening the geomembrane, ensuring that sludge odors do not spread extensively. The sludge extraction equipment and the construction section are depicted in Figure 1.

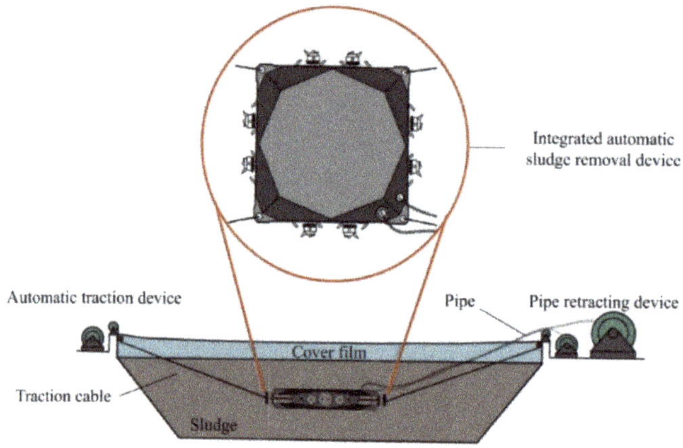

Figure 1. Suspended cable sludge removal equipment under plastic film and a construction cross-section diagram.

2.2. Materials

Due to the landfilling process, the majority of the sludge was directly deposited into the sludge pit after undergoing thickening and dewatering, resulting in a relatively high organic matter concentration and moisture content. Within the covered pit, the sludge underwent further digestion under anaerobic conditions, leading to complex changes in its physicochemical properties. Samples were collected from the aged sludge at depths of 1 m and 4 m within the covered area, and relevant indicators were tested. On-site sampling revealed that the surface layer of the test pit primarily consisted of sludge, with the sludge concentration gradually increasing from top to bottom. In some pits, the lower layers even exhibited compacted conditions. The thickness of the liquid sludge layer ranged from approximately 0.5 to 2.2 m, while the thickness of the solid sludge layer ranged from approximately 5.2 to 6.1 m. The data for sludge at different depths are presented in Table 1.

The leachate from the sludge landfill site shared certain similarities with the leachate from traditional solid waste landfills, but with higher concentrations of specific pollutants. In this study, the sludge leachate used was generated through the dewatering process of sludge that had been conditioned with chemicals and passed through a plate-and-frame filter press. Through testing and analysis of the properties of the leachate, it was found that the C/N ratio of the leachate was extremely low. The biodegradability of the leachate was poor, and the main pollutant was ammonia nitrogen. Table 2 presents the water quality of the sludge leachate and the operating conditions of the treatment equipment.

Table 1. Physicochemical properties of landfilled sludge at depths of 1 m and 4 m.

Depth	1 m	4 m
pH	7.58	7.84
Moisture content	85.14%	72.09%
Organic matter	37.70%	39.62%
Low heating value (kJ/kg)	6954	6343
C (%)	15.6	14.2
S (%)	1.47	1.62
Ca (mg/kg)	3.429×10^4	3.203×10^4
Al (mg/kg)	5.392×10^4	7.909×10^4
Fe (mg/kg)	2.771×10^4	2.717×10^4
Cl (mg/L)	1036	1478

Table 2. The water quality of the sludge leachate and the operating conditions of the treatment equipment.

Item	Treatment Standard	Influent	Effluent
pH	6–9	5.53	6.67
SS (mg/L)	400	595	98
COD_{cr} (mg/L)	n.a.	479	392
NH_3-N (mg/L)	40	1.26×10^3	15.6
TP (mg/L)	8	7.00	1.98
TN (mg/L)	n.a.	2.12×10^3	161

Notes: n.a. means not available.

The results indicated that after sludge leachate continuous treatment, the effluent water quality met the required treatment standards. The coagulation–flocculation–filtration–oxidation process employed in the experiment is feasible.

2.3. *Treatment and Disposal Methods for Landfill Sludge*

The treatment and disposal technology route for landfill sludge and leachate in this study is shown in Figure 2.

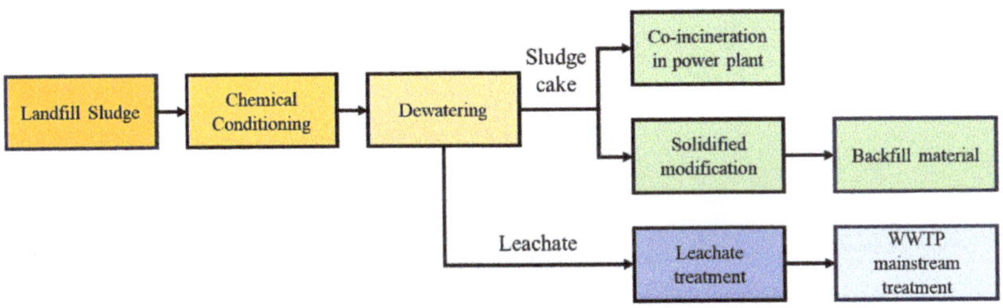

Figure 2. The treatment and disposal technology pathway for landfill sludge and leachate.

2.3.1. Chemical Conditioning and Dewatering

The main components of the chemicals used for sludge conditioning and dewatering were polyferric silicate sulfate (PFSS) and PEA. Among these, the molecular weight control of PFSS directly affects the efficacy of sludge dewatering [20]. It is crucial to select the appropriate silicon-to-iron molar ratio and quantity of hydroxy polymers. PEA is a high-molecular-weight amine-based coagulant that is in emulsion form. It is characterized by a low molecular weight, high charge density, and the ability to flocculate sludge particles. Unlike polyacrylamide, PEA is almost completely soluble in water and could not lead to clogging of filter cloths or increased viscosity of the sludge [21].

Based on the characteristics of the sludge and the performance of the deep dewatering equipment, experiments were conducted to examine the dewatering efficiency, cost-effectiveness, and safety of the dewatering agents. Sludge dewatering was carried out using a plate-and-frame filter press (04YLJ-20 Jingjin, Shandong) in the dewatering workshop, with a maximum daily sludge processing capacity of 10 t DS/day.

2.3.2. Sludge Modification

The experimental sludge used was collected from the discharge outlet of the frame filter press machine. The chemicals applied are patented agents developed independently by the Shanghai Municipal Engineering Design Institute, known as the "SHGT-16 Soil Stabilizer (NOWA-SH)". These agents belong to the category of calcium-based activator-type composite soil stabilizers. The main components of the agents are Portland cement, steel slag powder, industrial byproduct gypsum, mineral admixtures, and surfactant.

After dewatering, the water content of solid sludge was less than 60%. The sludge became solid and block-like. Before the modification process, the dehydrated sludge was crushed into powder form with a particle size not exceeding 20 mm. Based on preliminary testing of the types and dosages of chemicals, the chemicals were mixed thoroughly with the crushed sludge. Subsequently, the mixture was transferred to the sludge solidifying area, where it was shaped into piles, covered with tarpaulins, and subjected to solidification.

2.3.3. Sludge Leachate Treatment

In addition to the indicators related to carbon sources, the effluent water quality from the sludge leachate treatment process should meet the "Water Quality Standards for Discharging Wastewater into Urban Sewers" (DB31445-2009) in Shanghai [22]. Based on the primary pollutants in the leachate and the results of static tests, a combination of physical and chemical techniques was applied in the treatment. The technologies used for phosphorus removal included coagulation and sedimentation. The technologies used for ammonia nitrogen removal included flocculation, aeration, and oxidation. The specific process is detailed in Figure 3.

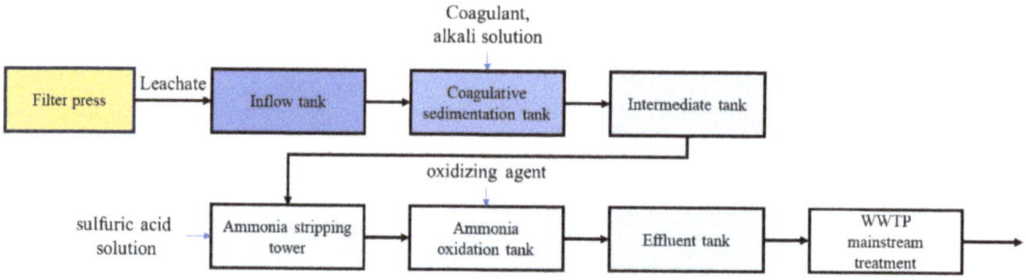

Figure 3. The experimental process flow for sludge leachate treatment.

The sludge leachate was directed from the outlet pipe of the plate-and-frame filter press into the continuous experimental influent tank. Subsequently, the leachate was pumped to the coagulation and precipitation tank. Following the application of coagulants for phosphorus removal and pH adjustment using an alkaline solution, the leachate flowed into an intermediate tank. From the intermediate tank, the leachate was pumped into the ammonia nitrogen stripping tower. After the stripping process, the treated leachate was pumped to an oxidation tank for ammonia nitrogen oxidation. Finally, the treated leachate was discharged into the effluent tank.

2.4. Analytical Method

2.4.1. pH, Organic Matter, Potassium (K), and Hygienic Indicators for Sludge

The pH, organic matter, potassium (K), and hygienic indicators in the sludge samples were determined by strictly following the Chinese standard method (CJ/T 221-2005) [23].

2.4.2. pH and COD (Chemical Oxygen Demand) for Leachate

The pH and COD in the water samples were determined by strictly following the Chinese standard methods (GB 6980-1986 [24] and GB 11914-89 [25]). The pH value was detected using an Eh-pH meter (PHS-25, Shanghai Precision and Scientific Instrument Co., Ltd., Shanghai, China) directly. The value of COD was detected using the dichromate method. Water quality detections were all accomplished on the sample collection day.

2.4.3. Heavy Metals and Heat Value of Sludge

The contents of heavy metals in the sludge were quantified by means of ICP-AES spectrometry (Agilent Corporation, Santa Clara, CA, USA). Heat value tests on sludge samples were performed according to GB/T213-2008 [26]. The sludge samples were dried for 24 h under 105 °C and then crushed to 2 mm particle size. The heat value of sludge samples (~0.6 g) was determined by employing an oxygen bomb typical calorimeter.

3. Results and Discussion

3.1. Sludge Conditioning and Dewatering

An experiment was conducted on the raw landfilled sludge with an average moisture content of 90.5% and an average organic matter content of 32.3%. The sludge was conditioned in a conditioning tank and then transported to a plate-and-frame filter press for dewatering, with the resulting sludge product being discharged into the lower sludge hopper. The properties of the dewatered sludge were analyzed and are presented in Table 3.

Table 3. Properties of dewatered sludge.

Item	Mean Value	Max. Value	Min. Value
Moisture content (%)	58.3	63.6	52.9
Organic matter (%)	32.2	35.7	28.9
Cl (mg/L)	240	354	157
Higher heating value (kcal/kg)	2005	2080	1950
Lower heating value (kcal/kg)	1800	1880	1740
Ni (mg/kg)	52.1	61.7	45.5
Cu (mg/kg)	483	521	414
Zn (mg/kg)	1074	1250	944
Cr (mg/kg)	191	200	176
Cd (mg/kg)	2.38	2.51	2.29
Pb (mg/kg)	59.6	64.8	53.7
Hg (mg/kg)	3.45	3.82	3.14
As (mg/kg)	20.0	21.8	18.6

The results indicated that the moisture content of the sludge product was controlled at around 60%. The dehydrated sludge exhibited high hardness, with most of it readily detaching automatically. The conventional chemicals used for sludge dewatering are usually PAC (polyaluminum chloride) and PFC (polymerization ferric chloride), typically containing large quantities of chlorine ions, causing severe corrosion in incineration facilities [27,28]. However, the average chloride ion concentration of the dewatered sludge was 240 mg/kg in this study. According to the Code for Investigation of Geotechnical Engineering (GB50021-2001) [29], indicating the corrosiveness of clayey soil to reinforcements in concrete structures above the groundwater level, the dewatered sludge product fell within the category of "weak corrosiveness". The organic matter content was at an average value of 32.2%. The variation range of the HHV (higher heating value) and LHV (lower heating value) showed relatively small fluctuations of 2010 kcal/kg (HHV) and 1800 kcal/kg (LHV). Comparing the heavy metal indicators in the dewatered sludge with conventional sludge disposal standards, it could be concluded that the heavy metal indicators in the test dewatered sludge cake met the standards for conventional sludge disposal. Therefore, there was no need for further treatment or disposal of heavy metals in the sludge. In summary, the use of chemicals made from PFSS and PEA for sludge dewatering and conditioning resulted in favorable equipment operation and sludge properties.

3.2. Power Plant Co-Incineration

Power plant co-incineration refers to a relatively stable and controllable sludge treatment and disposal method where sludge is co-incinerated with powdered coal in power plants. The existing sludge dewatering facilities and transfer vehicles at the WWTP could support the co-incineration of sludge in a thermal power plant.

As previous results of sludge conditioning and dewatering experiments indicated, using PFSS and PEA emulsion coagulant as conditioning agents showed a good dewatering effect. However, during incineration, the chlorine and sulfur in the raw fuels typically led to corrosion damage to the equipment, as well as air pollution [30–33]. According to the latest requirements from power plants, the chlorine and sulfur element contents in the received sludge after conditioning and dewatering should both be less than 1.2% to prevent corrosive effects on equipment. The chlorine element content in the dewatered sludge met the requirement after conditioning with these agents, but the sulfur ion content reached 1.59%. Therefore, an experiment was conducted to optimize the dewatering agent formulation for co-incineration sludge by replacing PFSS with polyaluminum silicate (PAS), as shown in Table 4.

Table 4. Chlorine and sulfur element detection results for power plant co-incineration sludge.

Reagent	Main Component	Dosage (kg/t DS)	Dry Weight Gain Ratio (%)	Moisture Content (%)	Chlorine as Received Basis (%)	Sulfur as Received Basis (%)
Original reagent	PFSS PEA	550 9	5.20	59.6	0.24	1.59
Modified reagent	PAS PEA	100–600 10–30	2.7–20	58.7	0.12	0.79

The thickness of the dewatered sludge cake was approximately 3–4 cm. The sludge cake could be easily separated and then transported to the power plant for co-incineration. A total of 149.6 tons of dehydrated sludge with approximately 60% moisture content was co-incinerated in the experiment. The results are presented in Table 5. Overall, the co-incineration process proceeded smoothly, without significant issues. Some sludge with a moisture content exceeding 60% made the feeding system slightly sticky, but it showed a relatively minor impact on the overall combustion process. To prevent problems with the feeding system during long-term operation, the sludge moisture content of the deep dewatered sludge is recommended to be below 60%.

Table 5. Power plant co-incineration results.

Power Plant	Reagent	Moisture Content (%)	Co-Incineration Amount (t)
A	PFSS + PEA PAS + PEA	58.9 57.2	13.6 48.6
B	PFSS + PEA PAS + PEA	58.6 58.2	15.4 45.1
C	PFSS + PEA PAS + PEA	63.3 62.1	12.1 15.4

In the experiments conducted at three power plants, the different reagents and varying dosages had no obvious impact on the incineration flue gas. There was no difference in smoke indicators between co-incineration and conventional coal powder incineration. Based on the analysis of the co-incineration results and the chlorine and sulfur element concentrations in the received sludge, the combination of PAS and PEA was more suitable for application in actual sludge co-incineration than the combination of PFSS and PEA.

3.3. Sludge Modification

To address the problem of insufficient processing scale in existing sludge incineration facilities, a treatment has been implemented to blend the solidified sludge with the existing embankment soil within the landfill. This treatment provides a new approach to the resource utilization of excess landfill sludge, aiming to meet land use criteria in China, including heavy metal content, organic matter, compaction, etc., to comply with the standards required for construction site backfill soil. This approach facilitates the co-treatment of sludge within the landfill, reducing the need for external transportation and additional earthworks. Feasibility testing and optimization of the modified sludge were conducted, including the types and proportions of modification agents.

3.3.1. Heavy Metal

Heavy metals in sludge products pose a potential danger that limits the use of sludge for land applications [34–36]. The heavy metal results indicated that both before and after modification, the detected concentrations for all indicators were below the requirements of standards for various types of soil, including agricultural soil, land improvement soil, garden landscaping soil, forest soil, mixed landfill soil, etc. Therefore, after modification, the risk of heavy metal pollution in the sludge when used as construction backfill soil was relatively low, making it suitable for various end-uses. Table 6 shows the heavy metal content of dewatered sludge after modification experiments.

Table 6. Heavy metal content of dewatered sludge.

Item	Dosage of Solidifying Agent		
	0	5%	7.5%
Ni (mg/kg)	55	63	33
Cu (mg/kg)	417	370	365
Zn (mg/kg)	1192	1038	1022
Cr (mg/kg)	120	104	89
Cd (mg/kg)	1.8	1.6	1.6
Pb (mg/kg)	75	67	65
Hg (mg/kg)	1.7	1.6	1.5
As (mg/kg)	5.87	5.78	5.81

3.3.2. Soluble Salt

The soluble salt content results indicated no significant difference in the soluble salt index before and after modification. According to the Code for Geotechnical Investigation of Building Foundation (GB50021-2001) [29], the corrosion levels of sulfate ions, chloride ions, and magnesium ions were determined to be weak, very weak, and weak, respectively. The comprehensive evaluation suggested weak corrosion. This implies that when used as construction backfill soil, the sludge would have a relatively minor impact on building materials. Table 7 shows the soluble salt content and the corrosion level of dewatered sludge after modification experiments.

Table 7. The soluble salt content of dewatered sludge.

Item	Batch 1	Batch 2	Corrosion Level	0% Addition	5% Addition	7.5% Addition	Corrosion Level
CO_3^{2-} (%)	0	0	n.a.	0	0	0	n.a.
HCO_3^- (%)	0.13	0.02	n.a.	0.05	0.14	0.12	n.a.
SO_4^{2-} (%)	0.24	0.51	weak	0.21	0.19	0.18	weak
Cl^- (%)	0.03	0.05	very weak	0.03	0.03	0.01	very weak
Ca^{2-} (%)	0.13	0.36	n.a.	0.37	0.39	0.35	n.a.
Mg^{2-} (%)	0.06	0.06	very weak	0.14	0.21	0.18	very weak
Na^+ (mg/kg)	359.8	327.3	n.a.	40.23	46.83	50.37	n.a.
K^+ (mg/kg)	458.1	363.7	n.a.	42.37	53.99	57.99	n.a.

Notes: n.a. means not available.

3.3.3. Organic Matter, Bearing Ratio, Compressive Strength

After a 5% solidifying agent was added, the organic matter content decreased to 27.19%, which could not meet the requirements for organic matter content in standards such as Specification for Design of Urban Road Subgrades (CJJ194-2013) [37] and Code for Construction and Acceptance of Earthwork and Blasting Engineering (GB50201-2012) [38]. Therefore, the modified sludge was not suitable for direct application in compacted fill areas. As a solution to expand the range of suitable fill materials, the modified sludge could be mixed with inorganic materials, such as lime-treated soil, to reduce the organic matter content.

The bearing ratio is a typical indicator used to evaluate the strength of subgrade soil and pavement materials [39]. The unconfined compressive strength test measures the ultimate strength of a specimen under axial pressure without lateral confinement. The results of bearing ratio tests and unconfined compressive strength tests under different proportions of stabilizing agents are shown in Figure 4. Without a solidifying agent, the bearing ratio of the sludge product was 31%. The bearing ratio of the sludge increased to 53% after 5% solidifying agent was added and further to 57% with a 7.5% proportion. Sludge without a solidifying agent had a very low unconfined compressive strength. As the proportion of stabilizing agents increased, the 7-day unconfined compressive strength of the sludge specimens showed a significant increasing trend. This result indicates that the modification treatment significantly enhanced the strength of the sludge.

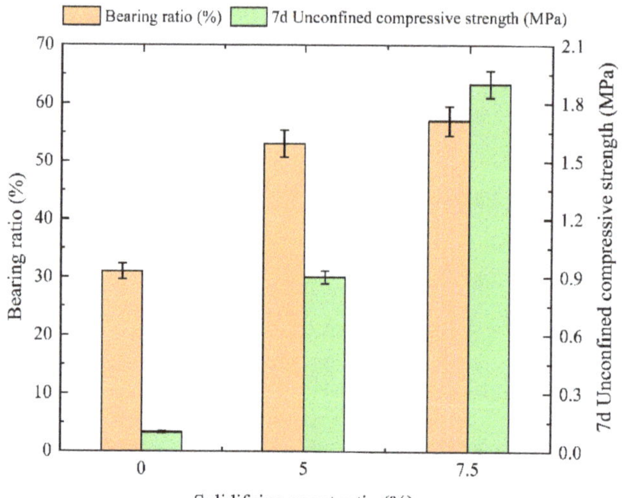

Figure 4. Dewatered sludge bearing ratio and unconfined compressive strength results.

3.3.4. Apparent Compaction Effect of Sludge

The visual appearance of the compacted sludge after rolling is depicted in Figure 5. When no solidifying agent was added, the sludge exhibited a loose texture with significant elasticity during the compaction process, making it challenging to compact. Additionally, the sludge tended to adhere to the compactor roller, resulting in a rough and cracked surface after compaction. However, after adding 5% and 7.5% solidifying agent, the compressive strength of the sludge significantly improved. This improvement alleviated the issue of adhesion to the roller during compaction, leading to denser and smoother compacted sludge with a more even surface. The apparent quality after compaction improved with a higher dosage of the chemical agent.

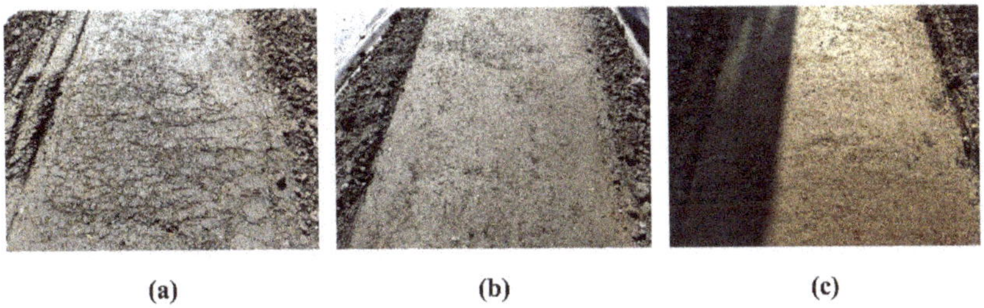

Figure 5. Visual appearance after compaction of dewatered sludge: (**a**) solidifying agent addition ratio of 0%; (**b**) solidifying agent addition ratio of 5%; (**c**) solidifying agent addition ratio of 7.5%.

3.3.5. Compaction Test Results

The compaction degree, also known as the compaction density, refers to the percentage represented by the ratio of the dry density of soil or other road construction materials after compaction to the standard maximum dry density [40]. Proper compaction is essential to ensure the strength, stiffness, stability, and smoothness of roadbed and pavement layers, thus extending the service life of the roadbed and pavement. The results for the compaction degree are illustrated in Figure 6.

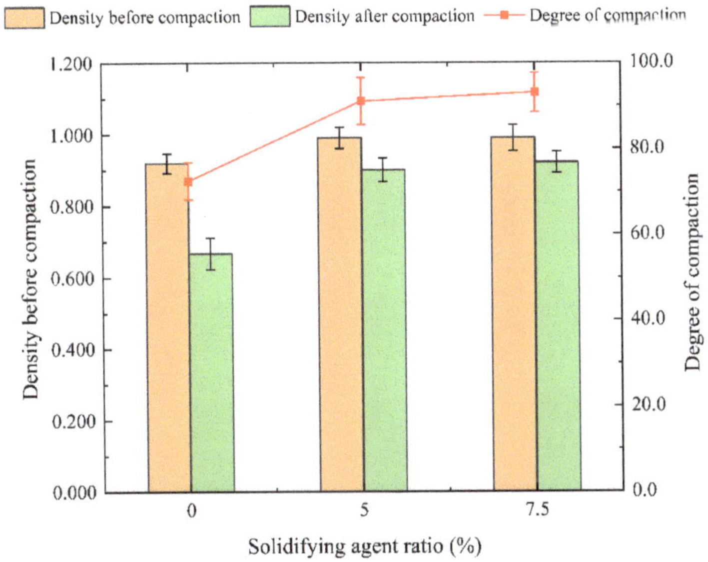

Figure 6. Sludge compaction test results.

When no solidifying agent was added, the compaction degree of the sludge was 72.5%. After adding 5% and 7.5% solidifying agent, the compaction degree of the sludge increased by more than 90%, meeting the compaction requirements for backfill soil above pipelines according to the Code for Construction and Acceptance of Water and Sewerage Pipeline Works (GB 50268-2008) [41].

In summary, the detected concentrations of heavy metals and soluble salts in the sludge before and after modification both met the requirements for construction backfill soil. After adding 5% and 7.5% solidifying agent, the organic matter content in the sludge remained relatively high, but the bearing ratio and 7-day unconfined compressive strength were significantly improved. The modified sludge is generally suitable for use as backfill soil above pipelines.

3.4. Leachate Treatment

The coagulation and precipitation unit, as a pretreatment processor before ammonia nitrogen stripping, primarily adjusted the pH value and reduced the total phosphorus and suspended solids in the sludge leachate. The total phosphorus concentration of the sludge leachate influent was relatively low, and after dosing with the phosphorus removal agent, it generally met the treatment target requirements.

The stripping unit was mainly used to remove ammonia nitrogen. By adjusting the pH value and adding sulfuric acid solution, ammonia nitrogen was removed by blowing air at room temperature. More than 60% of the ammonia nitrogen in the sludge leachate was removed through stripping. The variations of pH value and the concentration of ammonia nitrogen during stripping and oxidation processes are depicted in Figure 7.

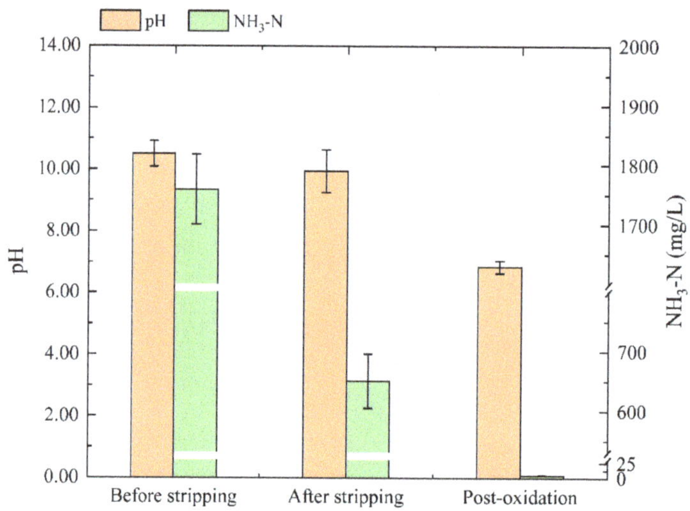

Figure 7. The ammonia nitrogen stripping and oxidation effect on the sludge press leachate.

The oxidation unit was applied to treat the remaining ammonia nitrogen. Sodium hypochlorite was added to oxidize and remove ammonia nitrogen, ensuring that the effluent's ammonia nitrogen remained consistently within treatment standards. The results indicated that the oxidation unit effectively removed the remaining ammonia nitrogen from the stripping tower's effluent, and the effluent's ammonia nitrogen consistently met treatment requirements. The actual chlorine dosage was higher than the theoretical dosage, primarily due to the presence of organic nitrogen and reducible substances in the sludge filter liquor. Additionally, the continuous unit showed some removal of COD in the effluent, suggesting that the oxidation unit cooperatively removed some of the COD.

Additionally, due to the acidic nature of the solid sodium hypochlorite used in the experiments, different amounts of sodium hydroxide were added into the oxidation unit to ensure that the effluent pH value met treatment requirements. In practical applications, a ready-made 10% sodium hypochlorite solution was used, which might have varying levels of free chlorine and is highly alkaline. When oxidizing with the ready-made 10% sodium hypochlorite solution, the pH value might remain unchanged or increase. Therefore, the pH value of the effluent after oxidation might exceed a value of 9. To meet treatment requirements, the pH value of the sludge leachate after stripping and oxidation should be kept within the desired range by using an acidic solution. Finally, the treated leachate was recycled back to the mainstream treatment of the WWTP. The pH of the effluent was controlled between 7 and 9, as it could serve as an alkalinity supplement for wastewater treatment.

4. Conclusions and Prospects

Due to the historical "emphasize wastewater and underestimate sludge" approach in the construction of wastewater treatment plants in China, the development of sludge treatment and disposal has been slow. Sludge landfilling thus used to be the priority method for sludge management. This research on the treatment of landfill sludge, conducted at a WWTP, suggests the feasibility of the overall technical route of sludge extraction, conditioning and dewatering, co-incineration at power plants, and solidification for backfilling. Both the combination of PFSS and PEA and the combination of PAS and PEA as coagulant aids were able to reduce the sludge moisture content to below 60%. The use of conditioning agents such as PAS and PEA in the dewatering and co-incineration process did not reveal any significant problems regarding the equipment. The contents of various heavy metals in the modified sludge met the relevant standards for various types of construction land. However, practical implications are rarely seen in China because the organic matter content of the final modification sludge exceeds the standard of 8%. The soluble salt contents of sludge before and after solidification and modification were not much different; the corrosion grade was low; and the corrosion of concrete, steel, and other building materials was weak. The results of the modification experiment illustrated that the modified sludge could be used as a backfill material in construction areas without requirements for organic matter. This process provides a new approach to sludge resource utilization.

All technologies for landfill sludge and the associated leachate treatment were feasible for meeting the wastewater discharge standards. These research findings provide valuable engineering experience and solutions for the reprocessing and resource utilization of existing landfill sludge. Nevertheless, these processes are associated with high energy consumption and costs, and they result in the wastage of nitrogen and phosphorus resources in the wastewater. It is recommended that in future research, emphasis should be placed on analyzing the possibility of nitrogen and phosphorus recovery and utilization from percolate. Simultaneously, from the perspective of energy conservation, an investigation into carbon neutralization technology for high-concentration ammonia-containing wastewater is suggested.

Author Contributions: Writing—Original Draft Preparation, Y.Y.; Writing—Review and Editing, Y.Y., J.D., X.Z., J.L. and H.C.; Data Curation, G.Z., J.D., Y.F., H.C., Y.L. and J.N.; Methodology, L.D. All authors have read and agreed to the published version of the manuscript.

Funding: This study was sponsored by Shanghai Sailing Program (21YF1443900) and Shanghai Science and Technology Innovation Project (21DZ1209800). This study was supported by Shanghai Municipal Engineering Design Institute (Group) Co., Ltd. (grant number K2023K015).

Data Availability Statement: Data are contained within the article.

Conflicts of Interest: Author Yifeng Yang, Author Jingshuai Luan, Author Xin Zhang, Author Jiong Du, Author Lei Dong, Author Yong Fan, Author He Cui, and Author Yubo Li were employed by Shanghai Municipal Engineering Design Institute (Group) Co., Ltd.. Author Jing Nie was employed by Shanghai Chengtou Water Engineering Project Management Co., Ltd. Author Gang Zhao was employed by Shanghai Urban Construction Design & Research Institute Groups Co., Ltd. All authors declare that the research was conducted in the absence of any commercial or financial relationships that could be construed as a potential conflict of interest.

Abbreviations

WWTP, wastewater treatment plant; HDPE, High-Density Polyethylene; PFSS, polyferric silicate sulfate; PEA, polyetheramine; COD, Chemical Oxygen Demand; PAC, polyaluminum chloride; PFC, polymerization ferric chloride; HHV, higher heating value; LHV, lower heating value; PAS, polyaluminum silicate.

References

1. Lee, L.H.; Wu, T.Y.; Shak, K.P.Y.; Lim, S.L.; Ng, K.Y.; Nguyen, M.N.; Teoh, W.H. Sustainable approach to biotransform industrial sludge into organic fertilizer via vermicomposting: A mini-review. *J. Chem. Technol. Biotechnol.* **2018**, *93*, 925–935. [CrossRef]
2. Xian, C.; Gong, C.; Lu, F.; Wu, H.; Ouyang, Z. The evaluation of greenhouse gas emissions from sewage treatment with urbanization: Understanding the opportunities and challenges for climate change mitigation in China's low-carbon pilot city, Shenzhen. *Sci. Total Environ.* **2023**, *855*, 158629. [CrossRef] [PubMed]
3. Zhang, Q.H.; Yang, W.N.; Ngo, H.H.; Guo, W.S.; Jin, P.K.; Dzakpasu, M.; Yang, S.J.; Wang, Q.; Wang, X.C.; Ao, D. Current status of urban wastewater treatment plants in China. *Environ. Int.* **2016**, *92–93*, 11–22. [CrossRef] [PubMed]
4. Zhou, G.; Gu, Y.; Yuan, H.; Gong, Y.; Wu, Y. Selecting sustainable technologies for disposal of municipal sewage sludge using a multi-criterion decision-making method: A case study from China. *Resour. Conserv. Recycl.* **2020**, *161*, 104881. [CrossRef]
5. An, K.; Zhuang, D.; Lin, W.; Argilaga, A.; Chen, Y.; Zhan, L. Field Treatment of Storage Sludge and Stability Analysis of Overlying Municipal Waste Landfilling. *Appl. Sci.* **2021**, *11*, 12102. [CrossRef]
6. Ololade, O.O.; Mavimbela, S.; Oke, S.A.; Makhadi, R. Impact of Leachate from Northern Landfill Site in Bloemfontein on Water and Soil Quality: Implications for Water and Food Security. *Sustainability* **2019**, *11*, 4238. [CrossRef]
7. Ogawa, A.; Ono, S.; Onoda, H. Environmental and economic evaluation of mechanical biological treatment system for municipal waste considering the political framework in ichihara city. *Appl. Sci.* **2021**, *11*, 10296. [CrossRef]
8. Xiao, H.; Li, K.; Zhang, D.; Tang, Z.; Niu, X.; Yi, L.; Lin, Z.; Fu, M. Environmental, energy, and economic impact assessment of sludge management alternatives based on incineration. *J. Environ. Manag.* **2022**, *321*, 115848. [CrossRef]
9. Liu, H.; Qiao, H.; Liu, S.; Wei, G.; Zhao, H.; Li, K.; Weng, F. Energy, environment and economy assessment of sewage sludge incineration technologies in China. *Energy* **2023**, *264*, 126294. [CrossRef]
10. Gao, P.; Xu, W.; Sontag, P.; Li, X.; Xue, G.; Liu, T.; Sun, W. Correlating microbial community compositions with environmental factors in activated sludge from four full-scale municipal wastewater treatment plants in Shanghai, China. *Appl. Microbiol. Biotechnol.* **2016**, *100*, 4663–4673. [CrossRef]
11. Zhao, G.; Tang, J.; Zhou, C.; Wang, C.; Mei, X.; Wei, Y.; Xu, J. A Megacity-Scale Analysis of Sludge Management and Carbon Footprint in China. *Pol. J. Environ. Stud.* **2022**, *31*, 2451–2460. [CrossRef]
12. Ma, S.; Zhou, C.; Pan, J.; Yang, G.; Sun, C.; Liu, Y.; Chen, X.; Zhao, Z. Leachate from municipal solid waste landfills in a global perspective: Characteristics, influential factors and environmental risks. *J. Clean. Prod.* **2022**, *333*, 130234. [CrossRef]
13. Zhang, F.; Peng, Y.; Wang, Z.; Jiang, H. High-efficient nitrogen removal from mature landfill leachate and waste activated sludge (WAS) reduction via partial nitrification and integrated fermentation-denitritation process (PNIFD). *Water Res.* **2019**, *160*, 394–404. [CrossRef] [PubMed]
14. De Carluccio, M.; Fiorentino, A.; Rizzo, L. Multi-barrier treatment of mature landfill leachate: Effect of Fenton oxidation and air stripping on activated sludge process and cost analysis. *J. Environ. Chem. Eng.* **2020**, *8*, 104444. [CrossRef]
15. Dos Santos, H.A.P.; de Castilhos Júnior, A.B.; Nadaleti, W.C.; Lourenço, V.A. Ammonia recovery from air stripping process applied to landfill leachate treatment. *Environ. Sci. Pollut. Res.* **2020**, *27*, 45108–45120. [CrossRef] [PubMed]
16. Bueno, R.d.F.; Faria, J.K.; Uliana, D.P.; Liduino, V.S. Simultaneous removal of organic matter and nitrogen compounds from landfill leachate by aerobic granular sludge. *Environ. Technol.* **2021**, *42*, 3756–3770. [CrossRef] [PubMed]
17. Yuan, Y.; Liu, J.; Gao, B.; Sillanpää, M.; Al-Farraj, S. The effect of activated sludge treatment and catalytic ozonation on high concentration of ammonia nitrogen removal from landfill leachate. *Bioresour. Technol.* **2022**, *361*, 127668. [CrossRef] [PubMed]
18. Miao, L.; Yang, G.; Tao, T.; Peng, Y. Recent advances in nitrogen removal from landfill leachate using biological treatments—A review. *J. Environ. Manag.* **2019**, *235*, 178–185. [CrossRef] [PubMed]
19. Gao, M.; Li, S.; Zou, H.; Wen, F.; Cai, A.; Zhu, R.; Tian, W.; Shi, D.; Chai, H.; Gu, L. Aged landfill leachate enhances anaerobic digestion of waste activated sludge. *J. Environ. Manag.* **2021**, *293*, 112853. [CrossRef]
20. Yoo, M.J.; Kim, H.W.; Yoo, B.M.; Park, H.B. Highly soluble polyetheramine-functionalized graphene oxide and reduced graphene oxide both in aqueous and non-aqueous solvents. *Carbon* **2014**, *75*, 149–160. [CrossRef]
21. Feng, Q.; Guo, K.; Gao, Y.; Liu, B.; Yue, Q.; Shi, W.; Feng, C.; Zhou, J.; Wang, G.; Gao, B. Effect of coagulation treatment on sludge dewatering performance: Application of polysilicate and their mechanism. *Sep. Purif. Technol.* **2022**, *301*, 121954. [CrossRef]
22. *DB31/T 445-2009*; Discharge Standard for Municipal Sewerage System. Shanghai Municipal Bureau of Quality Supervision: Shanghai, China, 2009.
23. *CJ/T 221-2005*; Determination Method for Municipal Sludge in Wastewater Treatment Plant. Ministry of Construction of the People's Republic of China: Beijing, China, 2005.
24. *GB 6920-1986*; Water Quality; Determination of pH Value; Glass Electrode Method. Ministry of Ecology and Environment of the People's Republic of China: Beijing, China, 1986.
25. *GB 11914-1989*; Water Quality-Determination of the Chemical Oxygen Demand-Dichromate Method. Ministry of Ecology and Environment of the People's Republic of China: Beijing, China, 1989.
26. *GB/T 213-2008*; Determination of Calorific Value of Coal. General Administration of Quality Supervision, Inspection and Quarantine of the People's Republic of China: Beijing, China, 2008.
27. Cao, B.; Zhang, T.; Zhang, W.; Wang, D. Enhanced technology based for sewage sludge deep dewatering: A critical review. *Water Res.* **2021**, *189*, 116650. [CrossRef] [PubMed]

28. Zhu, Y.; Li, H.; Yang, P.; Li, D.; Wang, Z.; Qi, Y.; Zhang, J. Aluminum Speciation in Polymerized Aluminum Chloride: Roles and Chloride Ion Migration in Sludge Dewatering. *J. Environ. Chem. Eng.* **2023**, *12*, 111749. [CrossRef]
29. *GB 50021-2001*; Code for Investigation of Geotechnical Engineering. Ministry of Construction of the People's Republic of China: Beijing, China, 2002.
30. Ma, Y.; Peng, Y.; Wang, X. Improving nutrient removal of the AAO process by an influent bypass flow by denitrifying phosphorus removal. *Desalination* **2009**, *246*, 534–544. [CrossRef]
31. *DB31/1291-2021*; Emission Standard of Air Pollutants for Coal and Sludge Co-Fired Power Plant. Shanghai Municipal Bureau of Quality Supervision: Shanghai, China, 2021.
32. Liang, Y.; Xu, D.; Feng, P.; Hao, B.; Guo, Y.; Wang, S. Municipal sewage sludge incineration and its air pollution control. *J. Clean. Prod.* **2021**, *295*, 126456. [CrossRef]
33. Wang, T.; Ma, H.; Ren, L.; Chen, Z.; Chen, S.; Liu, J.; Mei, M.; Li, J.; Xue, Y. Insights into in-situ sulfur retention by co-combustion of dyeing sludge and wood sawdust. *J. Clean. Prod.* **2021**, *323*, 129114. [CrossRef]
34. Geng, H.; Xu, Y.; Zheng, L.; Gong, H.; Dai, L.; Dai, X. An overview of removing heavy metals from sewage sludge: Achievements and perspectives. *Environ. Pollut.* **2020**, *266*, 115375. [CrossRef] [PubMed]
35. Naz, A.; Chowdhury, A.; Chandra, R.; Mishra, B.K. Potential human health hazard due to bioavailable heavy metal exposure via consumption of plants with ethnobotanical usage at the largest chromite mine of India. *Environ. Geochem. Health* **2020**, *42*, 4213–4231. [CrossRef]
36. Latosińska, J.; Kowalik, R.; Gawdzik, J. Risk assessment of soil contamination with heavy metals from municipal sewage sludge. *Appl. Sci.* **2021**, *11*, 548. [CrossRef]
37. *CJJ 194-2013*; Specification for Design of Urban Road Subgrades. People's Republic of China Ministry of Housing and Urban-Rural Development: Beijing, China, 2013.
38. *GB 50201-2012*; Code for Construction and Acceptance of Earthwork and Blasting Engineering. General Administration of Quality Supervision, Inspection and Quarantine of the People's Republic of China: Beijing, China, 2012.
39. Ahmad, M.; Al-Zubi, M.A.; Kubińska-Jabcoń, E.; Majdi, A., Al-Mansob, R.A.; Sabri, M.M.S.; Ali, E.; Naji, J.A.; Elnaggar, A.Y.; Zamin, B. Predicting California bearing ratio of HARHA-treated expansive soils using Gaussian process regression. *Sci. Rep.* **2023**, *13*, 13593. [CrossRef]
40. Shah, S.A.R.; Mahmood, Z.; Nisar, A.; Aamir, M.; Farid, A.; Waseem, M. Compaction performance analysis of alum sludge waste modified soil. *Constr. Build. Mater.* **2020**, *230*, 116953. [CrossRef]
41. *GB 50268-2008*; Code for Construction and Acceptance of Water and Sewerage Pipeline Works. People's Republic of China Ministry of Housing and Urban-Rural Development: Beijing, China, 2008.

water

MDPI

Article

Delving into the Impacts of Different Easily Degradable Carbon Sources on the Degradation Characteristics of 2,4,6-Trichlorophenol and Microbial Community Properties

Jianguang Wang [1,2,3,*], Haifeng Fang [1,3], Shiyi Li [1,3] and Hailan Yu [1,3,*]

1 PowerChina Huadong Engineering Corporation Limited, Hangzhou 311122, China
2 National Engineering Laboratory for Advanced Municipal Wastewater Treatment and Reuse Technology, Beijing University of Technology, Beijing 100124, China
3 Huadong Eco-Environmental Engineering Research Institute of Zhejiang Province, Hangzhou 311122, China
* Correspondence: wjg909090@163.com (J.W.); yu_hl@hdec.com (H.Y.)

Abstract: In chlorophenol wastewater treatment, adding easily degradable carbon sources, such as methanol, ethanol, sodium acetate, and sodium propionate, significantly improves the chlorophenol removal efficiency. This study systematically compares these conventional carbon sources in different sequencing batch reactors to understand their specific effects on both 2,4,6-trichlorophenol (2,4,6-TCP) degradation efficiency and microbial abundance. In a 35-day experiment, as a carbon source, ethanol exhibited a lower 2,4,6-TCP degradation concentration (77.56 mg/L) than those of methanol, sodium acetate, and sodium propionate, which achieved higher degradation concentrations: 123.89 mg/L, 170.96 mg/L, and 151.79 mg/L, respectively. As a carbon source, sodium acetate enhanced extracellular polymeric substance production (200.80 mg/g·VSS) by microorganisms, providing protection against the toxicity of chlorophenol and resulting in a higher 2,4,6-TCP removal concentration. Metagenomics identified crucial metabolic genes, including *PcpA*, *chqB*, *Mal-r*, *pcaI*, *pcaF*, and *fadA*. The abundance of genera containing the *chqB* gene correlated positively with the metabolic capacity for 2,4,6-TCP. Moreover, small molecular carbon sources such as methanol, sodium acetate, and sodium propionate promoted the enrichment of genera with functional genes.

Keywords: 2,4,6-trichlorophenol; easily degradable carbon sources; functional gene; microbial community

1. Introduction

2,4,6-trichlorophenol (2,4,6-TCP) is a crucial chemical raw material that is widely utilized in various industrial sectors, such as synthesis, papermaking, printing and dyeing, and plastic production [1]. However, industrial wastewater containing 2,4,6-TCP is discharged in large quantities due to inadequate treatment, posing a new threat to aquatic ecosystems. The hazard of 2,4,6-TCP arises from its high toxicity and bioaccumulation characteristics, making it an environmentally high-risk compound [2]. It is particularly carcinogenic to humans and animals, leading it to be classified as a priority pollutant in many countries [3,4].

In comparison to physical and chemical methods, biological methods exhibit advantages in the treatment of chlorophenol wastewater, including strong applicability, high processing capacity, and minimal secondary pollution. However, biological methods, particularly the activated sludge method, face two major challenges in the degradation of toxic organic compounds: firstly, the slow growth and metabolism of microorganisms due to the effects of toxicity, and secondly, the lack of microbial growth and metabolism-requiring carbon sources in wastewater with toxic compounds. Due to the constraints of toxicity factors, the inflow concentration of chlorophenol wastewater is not likely to be excessively high. This results in chlorophenols and their intermediates not providing sufficient carbon sources for microbial growth, leading to continuous loss of activated sludge biomass and a decline in biomass, which makes it challenging for the reactor to operate [5]. The bioco-metabolism method can effectively address this issue. Many wastewater streams containing chlorophenols, including monochlorophenols, dichlorophenols, and trichlorophenols, have indeed implemented biological co-metabolism degradation approaches [6–12]. This method not only provides necessary carbon sources and energy for microbial growth but also reduces the toxic inhibition of chlorophenols on activated sludge bacteria [13–15].

Currently, literature reports predominantly focus on studying the impact of the addition of a single carbon source on the microbial degradation of chlorophenolic pollutants and the microbial community. For example, studies have investigated the effects of sodium acetate or glucose as a sole carbon source on the degradation of phenol, 4-chlorophenol, and 2,4-dichlorophenol [11,12,16–20]. However, there were few attempts to compare the influences of different organic molecules on the degradation of chlorophenols, especially those of easily degradable carbon sources, such as methanol, ethanol, and sodium acetate. Furthermore, in previous studies, there has been a lack of research from the perspective of the conditioning of activated sludge and the operation of reactors on the mechanism of the impact of small molecular carbon sources on the cultivation of bacteria for degrading 2,4,6-TCP. Therefore, further research is needed to explore the effects of carbon sources with different molecular weights on the enrichment of functional bacteria and the stability of reactor operation during the 2,4,6-TCP degradation process.

Different wastewater qualities could significantly alter microbial communities and abundance [21]. The phyla *Proteobacteria, Actinobacteria*, and *Firmicutes* are considered the main phyla responsible for degrading chlorophenols [22]. However, it is currently unclear whether the type of carbon source can promote the growth of such chlorophenol-degrading bacteria in the process of 2,4,6-TCP degradation.

Against this background, the main content of this study includes the following: (1) studying the impacts of carbon sources with different molecular weights on the microbial degradation of 2,4,6-TCP; (2) exploring the changes in microbial diversity and the influence on functional microbial communities after adding different carbon sources during the conditioning process; (3) evaluating the potential correlation between the characteristics of activated sludge and the type of carbon source. This study conducted long-term conditioning experiments using conventional carbon sources with different molecular weights, such as methanol, ethanol, sodium acetate, and sodium propionate. High-throughput and metagenomic techniques were employed to analyze the potential relationship between the microbial community in activated sludge and the type of carbon source. The findings of this study can offer valuable data support for the selection of carbon sources during the treatment process of phenolic wastewater in practice.

2. Materials and Methods

2.1. Reactor and Operation

The sequencing batch reactor (SBR), which served as a biochemical reaction apparatus, comprised a total of five SBRs in this study. Among these, four SBRs were supplemented with distinct carbon sources (methanol, ethanol, sodium acetate, and sodium propionate) (Sinopharm Chemical Reagent Co. Ltd., Shanghai, China), while one SBR operated without the addition of any carbon sources (only 2,4,6-TCP(Sinopharm Chemical Reagent Co., Ltd., Shanghai, China). The effective volume for each SBR was consistently maintained at 3 L. Operating under constant temperature conditions of 28 ± 0.5 °C, the SBRs underwent two cycles per day. This cycle encompassed several phases: a 5-min period for feeding synthetic wastewater, followed by a 600-min aerobic reaction phase with dissolved oxygen maintained at 5 ± 0.5 mg/L. Subsequently, a 60-min settling phase was followed by a 5-min discharge of supernatant, with a volumetric exchange ratio of 50%. Finally, a 50-min idling phase concluded the cycle. The solid residence time of 30 days was upheld by discharging 50 mL of mixed activated sludge from each SBR in every cycle.

2.2. Seed Sludge and Water

The activated sludge used for the experimental inoculation was sourced from the secondary sedimentation tank of the Gaobeidian Wastewater Treatment Plant in Beijing.

The experimental setup involved the use of artificially prepared influent, comprising 2,4,6-TCP, carbon sources, and trace nutrients. Methanol (Met), ethanol (Eth), sodium acetate (Sa), and sodium propionate (Sp) were employed as carbon sources, with an influent concentration of 300 mgCOD/L. The influent concentration of 2,4,6-TCP was incrementally elevated from low concentrations, with the dosing concentration slightly exceeding the degradable concentration of the activated sludge to maintain a certain level of selective pressure. The composition of trace nutrients primarily adhered to the components detailed in the work by Wang, J. et al. [7].

2.3. Batch Experiment

The activated sludge used in the batch experiments was obtained from the stable phase of a long-term experiment in the SBR. Batch experiments were conducted under constant temperature at 28 °C, with dissolved oxygen at 4–5 mgO_2/L and a magnetic stirrer set at a speed of 200 rpm.

The specific steps of the batch experiments involved studying the degradation characteristics of 2,4,6-TCP by activated sludge cultivated with different carbon sources. Parameters such as the 2,4,6-TCP removal efficiency, dechlorination capability, and mineralization ability were investigated. To eliminate interference from chloride ions in the nutrient elements, $CaCl_2 \cdot 2H_2O$ was removed from the water and replaced with ultrapure water. The addition of each of the four carbon sources was set at 300 mgCOD/L, and the influent concentration of 2,4,6-TCP ranged from 44 to 47 mg/L.

Samples were collected at 60-min intervals, with each sample consisting of 10 mL of mixed sludge. After low-speed centrifugation at 4000 rpm, the samples were filtered through a 0.22 μm polyethersulfone membrane. The treated samples were then analyzed using liquid chromatography, ion chromatography, and a TOC analyzer to determine the concentrations of 2,4,6-TCP, chloride ions, and TOC, respectively.

2.4. Analytical Methods

2.4.1. The Analysis of the Microbial Community

This investigation involved assessing variations in EPS, PN, and PS content under different carbon source conditions, as described in Reference [10].

During the long-term cultivation period in the SBR, mixed activated sludge samples were collected for an in-depth analysis of the microbial community, as described in Reference [23]. The raw sequence data generated through high-throughput sequencing were duly submitted to the NCBI under the sequence read accession number PRJNA707254.

2.4.2. Water Quality Testing

The water quality indicators encompassed 2,4,6-TCP, total organic carbon (TOC), and chloride ions, with their quantification being performed through distinct methodologies. High-performance liquid chromatography (HPLC, Waters 1525, Milford, MA, USA) was employed for the analysis of 2,4,6-TCP, while TOC was measured using a TOC analyzer (Elementar vario TOC, Frankfurt, Germany). The detection of chloride ions was conducted through ion chromatography (Metrohm 883 Basic IC plus, Herisau, Switzerland), as detailed in Reference [23].

The conventional water quality parameters, including COD, mixed-liquor suspended solids (MLSSs), SV_{30} (settling velocity in 30 min), and the sludge volume index (SVI), were assessed using the standard methods outlined in Reference [24].

In this study, water quality sampling was conducted using triplicate samples for each sampling point.

3. Results and Discussion

3.1. Long-Term Acclimatization Characteristics of Activated Sludge

The carbon source could alter the microbial community, thereby influencing the capacity for the degradation of target pollutants [21]. Figure 1 illustrates the long-term degradation characteristics of activated sludge in different carbon source conditions when degrading 2,4,6-TCP. It describes the concentrations of influent, effluent, and degradable 2,4,6-TCP. The SBR had been inoculated with activated sludge lacking any chlorophenol degradation capabilities before operation. This sludge had initially been used for nitrogen and phosphorus removal in municipal wastewater treatment, exhibiting rich population diversity and microbial communities conducive to the selection and acclimatization of trichlorophenol-degrading bacteria [7].

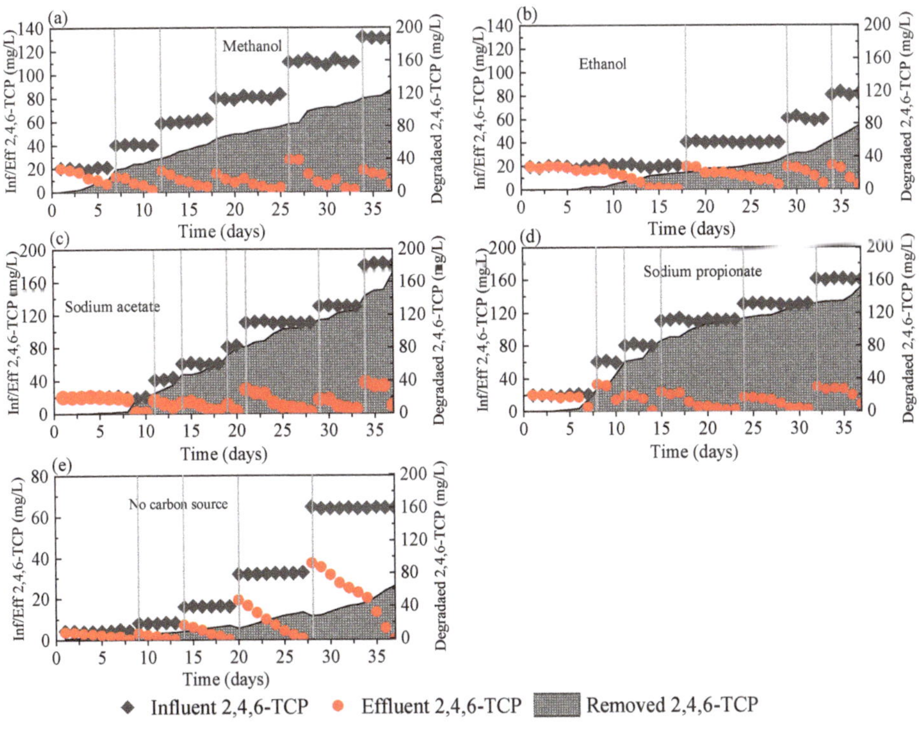

Figure 1. The domesticated performance of 2,4,6-TCP with the addition of different carbon sources ((**a**) Methanol; (**b**) Ethanol; (**c**) Sodium acetate; (**d**) Sodium propionate; (**e**) No carbon source).

Considering the biological toxicity of 2,4,6-TCP, a gradient-increasing dosing approach was adopted. When the 2,4,6-TCP concentration was 10 mg/L or 20 mg/L, except for the SBR utilizing ethanol as a carbon source, which had a longer adaptation period, the other SBRs achieved the degradation of low-concentration chlorophenols in a relatively short time. The 2,4,6-TCP was gradually increased until each SBR reached the maximum degradation concentration. During the stable operational phase, the maximum degradation concentrations of 2,4,6-TCP were as follows: 123.89 mg/L (methanol), 77.56 mg/L (ethanol), 170.96 mg/L (sodium acetate), 151.79 mg/L (sodium propionate), and 58.72 mg/L (no carbon source). With the exception of ethanol, small organic molecules as carbon sources all achieved relatively high 2,4,6-TCP degradation concentrations, especially in the cases of sodium acetate and sodium propionate as carbon sources. The SBR that did not receive additional carbon sources removed 58.72 mg/L 2,4,6-TCP in the short term. However, the degradable 2,4,6-TCP gradually decreased with the SBR's operation. This decline could potentially be attributed to the reduction in the activated sludge concentration, leading to a decrease in the concentration of 2,4,6-TCP degradation. In conclusion, the use of sodium acetate as a carbon source is likely to yield higher concentrations of 2,4,6-TCP degradation compared to other carbon sources.

Figure 2 illustrates the changes in the MLSSs and settling characteristics within the SBRs. It was observed that the SBR without additional carbon sources experienced a rapid reduction in initial MLSSs from 3000 mg/L to 1000 mg/L. In contrast, the SBRs with added carbon sources maintained a higher microbial biomass level and exhibited a gradual upward trend.

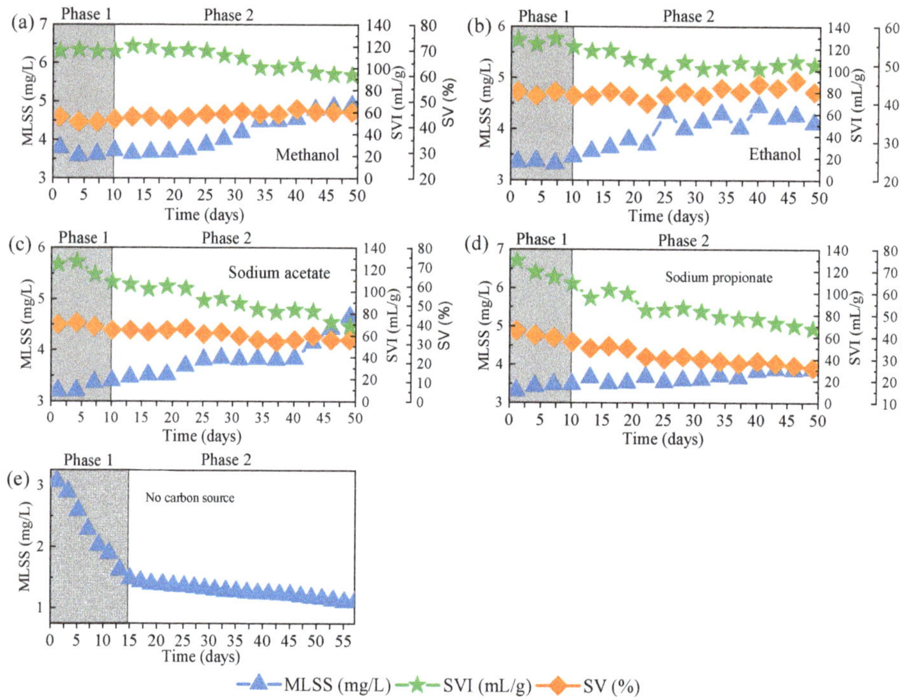

Figure 2. MLSSs and settling performance of each SBR in long-term operation ((**a**) Methanol; (**b**) Ethanol; (**c**) Sodium acetate; (**d**) Sodium propionate; (**e**) No carbon source).

The settling characteristics of activated sludge directly influenced the operational performance of the SBRs during the settling phase. As depicted in Figure 2, the addition of small molecular carbon sources contributes to maintaining favorable sludge settling. However, the use of starch as a carbon source results in inferior settling characteristics for an SBR, with an SVI close to 200 mL/g [7]. The 300 mgCOD/L carbon source leads to a gradual increase in sludge concentration in the SBR, but it has not yet reached a complete steady-state operation. Therefore, further optimization and adjustment of the carbon source dosage are needed to achieve optimal performance. The MLSS and SVI indicators can provide feedback on the operational status of an SBR. Based on the results obtained, it is observed that the use of sodium acetate and sodium propionate as carbon sources results in lower SVI values, which is beneficial for the sedimentation of activated sludge and the discharge of effluent from the SBR.

Additionally, the effluent COD did not exhibit significant fluctuations during the long-term operational process, as illustrated in Figure 3. The influent COD was primarily contributed by the added carbon sources, and the average effluent COD for each SBR was as follows: 37.8 mg/L (methanol), 36.2 mg/L (ethanol), 38.2 mg/L (sodium acetate),

40.7 mg/L (sodium propionate), and 10.5 mg/L (no carbon source). These values were consistently maintained at relatively low levels, indicating that different carbon sources had no significant impacts on the effluent COD from the SBRs.

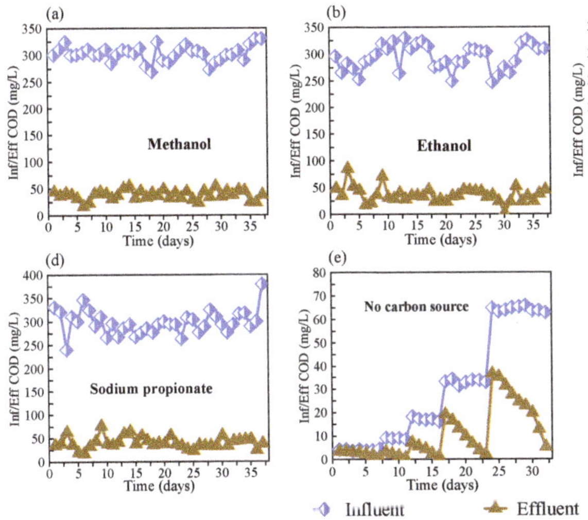

Figure 3. The average influent and effluent CODs of the SBRs in long-term operation ((**a**) Methanol; (**b**) Ethanol; (**c**) Sodium acetate; (**d**) Sodium propionate; (**e**) No carbon source).

3.2. The Mineralization and Dechlorination of 2,4,6-TCP

In Figure 4, the degradation, dechlorination, and TOC removal of 2,4,6-TCP are depicted over a typical cycle. At the end of the typical cycle, no 2,4,6-TCP was detected, indicating that the sludge acclimated with various carbon sources could effectively remove 2,4,6-TCP. The theoretical dechlorination concentration was calculated based on the chlorine content in the 2,4,6-TCP molecule. The detected chloride ion in the effluent was found to be almost identical to the theoretical chlorine concentration, suggesting complete dechlorination. A comparison revealed that the activated sludge acclimated with different carbon sources could achieve complete dechlorination of 2,4,6-TCP.

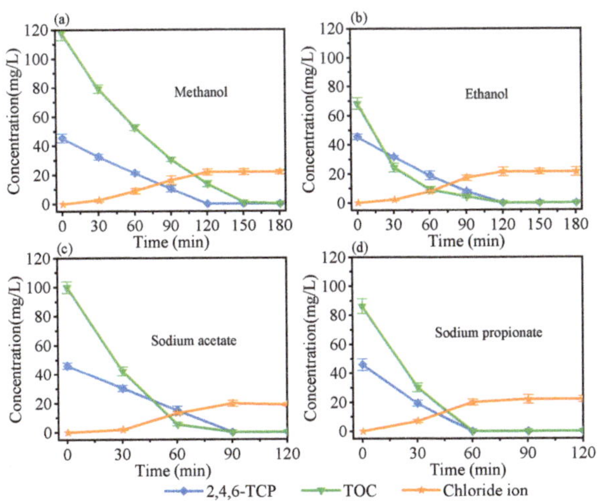

Figure 4. Batch tests of 2,4,6-TCP mineralization with different carbon sources ((**a**) Methanol; (**b**) Ethanol; (**c**) Sodium acetate; (**d**) Sodium propionate).

Furthermore, the removal efficiency of TOC in the effluent from the SBRs exceeded 95%. The inability to achieve a 100% removal rate might have been associated with suspended microorganisms in the effluent. The TOC removal rate and chloride ion data indicated that activated sludge acclimated with different carbon sources could effectively achieve the harmless degradation of 2,4,6-TCP.

3.3. The EPS Content of the Activated Sludge

In the biological treatment of toxic wastewater, EPS played a role in protecting microbial cells from external toxic substances while also enhancing the removal efficiency of activated sludge for toxic compounds [10]. The influent water quality was a key factor influencing the content and composition of EPS [25].

In Figure 5, it is evident that the activated sludge, after acclimatization (excluding the sludge without a carbon source), exhibited an increase in EPS. This suggested that activated sludge, by generating a higher amount of EPS, aimed to mitigate the toxic effects of 2,4,6-TCP on microbial cells. The activated sludge without the addition of a carbon source had the lowest total EPS, measuring only 59.69 mg/g·VSS. This was attributed to the lack of carbon sources in the system, leading to a reduction in EPS production, or to microbes utilizing EPS as a carbon source in the absence of an external carbon source. Wang, J. et al. [7] utilized starch as the carbon source for 2,4,6-TCP degradation, resulting in the production of a higher amount of EPS by activated sludge, reaching 285.81 mg/g·VSS.

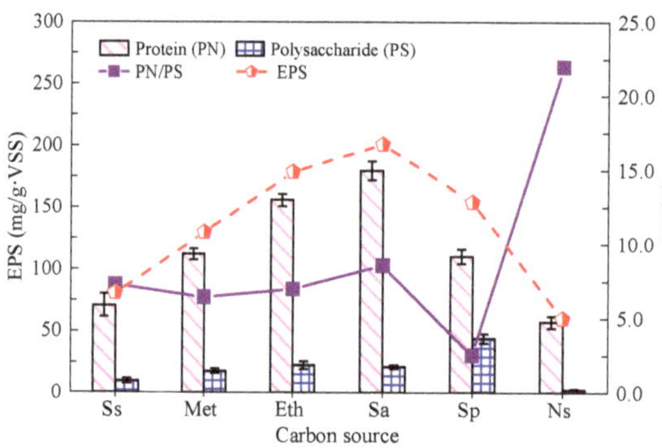

Figure 5. EPS concentration of 2,4,6-TCP-degrading sludge using different carbon sources (Ss: seed sludge; Met: methanol; Eth: ethanol; Sa: sodium acetate; Sp: sodium propionate; Ns: no substrate).

The main components of EPS are proteins and polysaccharides, with proteins playing a crucial role in the extracellular hydrolysis process of microorganisms. For activated sludge with low-molecular-weight organic compounds as carbon sources, the protein in EPS was lower than that in cases where high-molecular-weight organic compounds served as carbon sources. Among them, the protein in the sodium acetate group was the highest. Considering that the sodium acetate group achieved the highest removal of 2,4,6-TCP as a carbon source and that sodium acetate could be directly utilized by activated sludge without undergoing hydrolysis, the proteins may have directly contributed to the 2,4,6-TCP degradation.

The content of polysaccharides in EPS is related to hydrophilicity, where a smaller PN/PS value indicates stronger hydrophilicity [26]. Higher hydrophilicity allowed for sufficient contact between microbial cells and 2,4,6-TCP, facilitating the degradation process. Activated sludge with better settling characteristics often accompanied a lower PN/PS. Under the no-addition condition, the PN/PS value of EPS reached 22, consistently with the poor settling performance. Simultaneously, the polysaccharide level in EPS was at a lower level (2.6 mg/g·VSS), leading to reduced cell aggregation capabilities. This was a significant factor contributing to the substantial loss of sludge in the SBR reactor without the addition of a carbon source during the later stages of cultivation.

3.4. Bacterial Abundance and Functional Gene Analysis

3.4.1. Influences of Different Carbon Sources on Bacterial Abundance

As depicted in Figure 6, the microbial community at the phylum level with different carbon sources is illustrated. At the phylum level, a total of 14 phyla were detected, and the proportions of these phyla varied significantly with the different carbon sources. According to literature reports, phyla such as *Proteobacteria*, *Actinobacteria*, *Firmicutes*, and *Saccharibacteria* have been found to have higher proportions in phenol- and 4-chlorophenol-degrading bacteria [18,22,27–31]. This study exclusively employed 2,4,6-TCP as the target pollutant and similarly observed higher proportions of the four aforementioned phyla: Under the no-addition condition, these four phyla collectively accounted for 93.36% of all detected phyla. Under different carbon source conditions, the abundances of these four phyla were 95.92% (methanol), 90.94% (ethanol), 71.89% (sodium acetate), and 81.25% (sodium propionate), respectively, which were significantly higher than those in the inoculated activated sludge. This indicated that at the phylum level, the chlorophenol-degrading microbial community was similar.

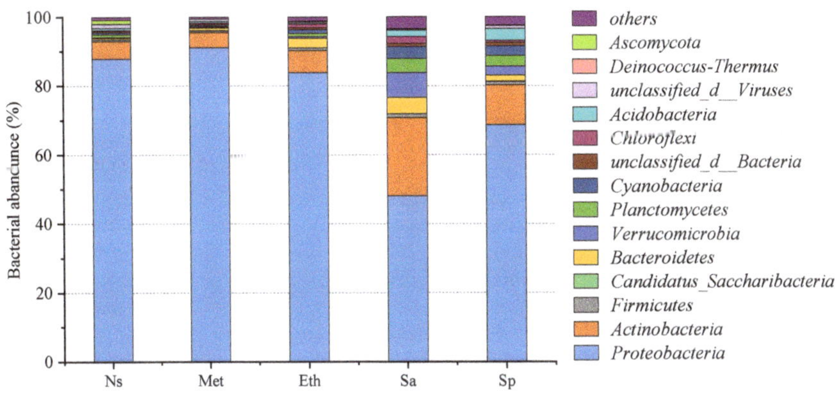

Figure 6. Bacterial community at the phylum level with different carbon sources (Ns: no substrate; Met: methanol; Eth: ethanol; Sa: sodium acetate; Sp: sodium propionate).

As shown in Figure 7, at the genus level, the dominant bacterial genera under different carbon source conditions were significantly different. The dominant genera and their abundances were 19.16% *Sphingomonas* (no carbon source), 20.40% *Ralstonia* (methanol), 18.68% *Sphingomonas* (ethanol), 16.53% *Mycobacterium* (sodium acetate), and 16.62% *Variovorax* (sodium propionate). The genus *Sphingomonas* is known for its ability to degrade 2,6-dichlorophenol, 2,4,6-TCP, 2,3,4,6-tetrachlorophenol, and pentachlorophenol [32,33]. With no carbon source or with ethanol as a carbon source, the enrichment of *Sphingomonas* as a dominant genus was promoted. *Ralstonia* is a common dominant genus in the metabolism of chlorophenolic compounds [34–36], and in this study, methanol increased its abundance to 20.4%. The dominant genus with the addition of sodium propionate (*Variovorax*) has not been reported to have relevant chlorophenol-degrading capabilities. *Mycobacterium*, the genus with the second-highest abundance after *Variovorax*, played a crucial role in the degradation of monochlorophenols [37,38], and sodium acetate promoted its dominance as a genus. Different carbon sources significantly altered the microbial community, and although some genera are commonly associated with chlorophenol metabolism, their high abundance can only suggest their potential for 2,4,6-TCP metabolism. To further verify the capabilities for 2,4,6-TCP metabolism of the mentioned genera, we conducted further analyses from a genetic perspective.

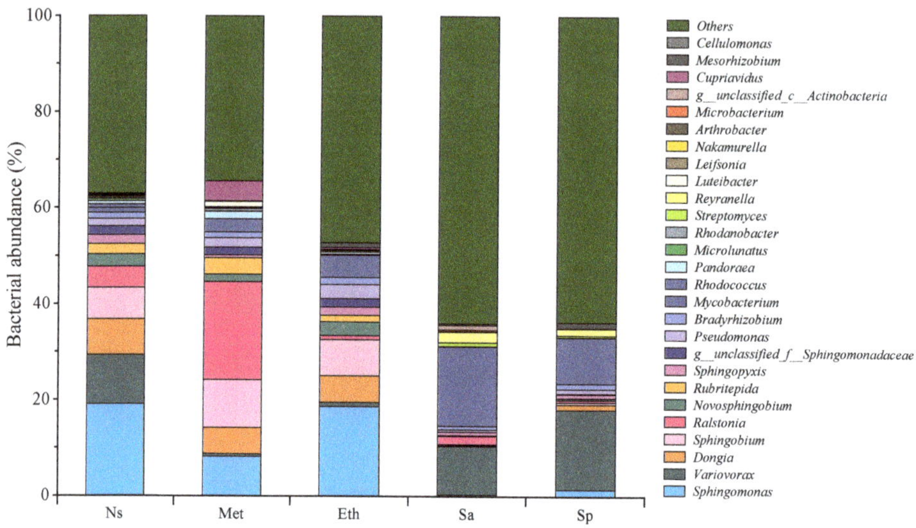

Figure 7. Bacterial community at the genus level with different carbon sources.

3.4.2. The Impacts of Different Carbon Sources on the Abundance of Functional Genes

As shown in Figure 8, the abundance of functional genes related to 2,4,6-TCP metabolism under different carbon source conditions is illustrated. The abundance of functional genes at the front end of the 2,4,6-TCP metabolic pathway was relatively low, while the abundance of functional genes closer to the back end of the metabolic pathway was higher. The abundance of *fadA* was consistently above 100,000 hits, indicating that at the front end of the metabolic pathway, where 2,4,6-TCP and its toxic intermediates are present, fewer microorganisms possess metabolic capabilities, resulting in significantly lower gene abundance. In contrast, at the back end of the metabolic pathway, where the toxicity of the intermediates is lower, they can serve as carbon sources for more microorganisms, leading to a higher abundance of functional genes.

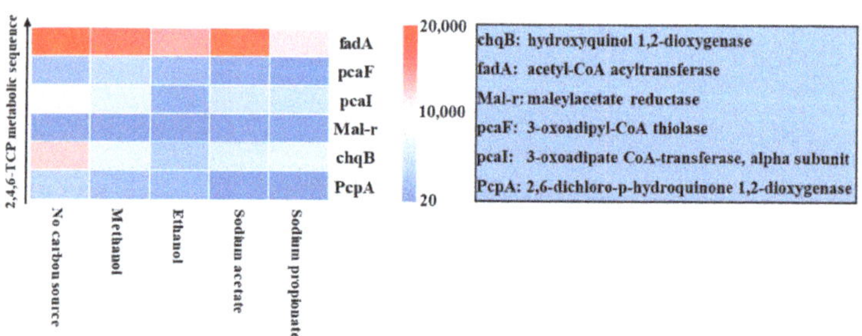

Figure 8. Heat map of gene abundance for 2,4,6-TCP degradation with different carbon sources.

As shown in Figure 9, the total abundance of functional genes under different carbon source conditions is depicted. Under the no-carbon-source condition, the gene abundance reached 42,858 hits, which was higher than that in the cases with added carbon sources. However, due to the low biomass under the condition without adding carbon sources, it was challenging to maintain a satisfactory 2,4,6-TCP degradation performance. Although adding carbon sources reduced the abundance of functional genes related to chlorophenol degradation, it increased microbial biomass. This indicates that both microbial abundance and the functional genes' abundance jointly determined the effectiveness of microbial degradation of 2,4,6-TCP.

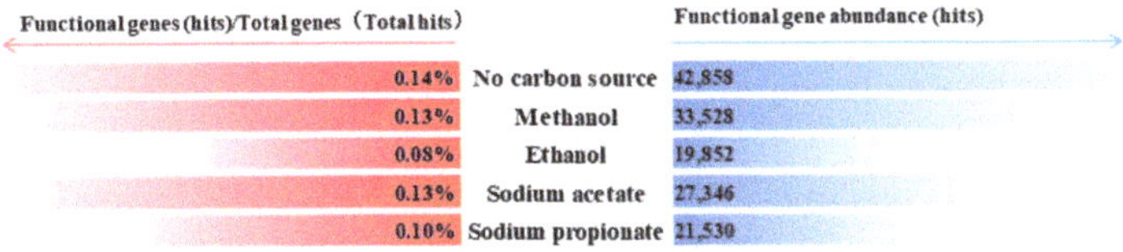

Figure 9. Comparison of the total gene abundance in 2,4,6-TCP degradation under different carbon sources.

3.4.3. Distribution Characteristics of Functional Genes in Different Microbial Communities

The abundance of functional genes did not exhibit a significant correlation with the effectiveness of 2,4,6-TCP degradation. Consequently, an analysis was conducted on the abundance of microbial communities containing specific genes, as illustrated in Figure 10. Several key genes in the metabolic pathway of 2,4,6-TCP, including *PcpA*, *chqB*, *Mal-r*, *pcaI*, *pcaF*, and *fadA*, were considered. Additionally, it was noted that the toxicity of products at the front end of the metabolic pathway was higher, gradually decreasing or becoming non-toxic as the reaction progressed. Combining the degradation concentrations of 2,4,6-TCP under different carbon source conditions, it was observed that the abundance of microbial communities containing *chqB* exhibited a significant positive correlation with the degradation rate of 2,4,6-TCP (correlation coefficient: 0.61, $p < 0.01$). The proportions of microbial communities containing other specific genes showed correlation coefficients with the degradation rate of 2,4,6-TCP of less than 0. Therefore, the abundance of microbial communities containing the *chqB* gene was positively correlated with the degradation rate of 2,4,6-TCP. Methanol, sodium acetate, and sodium propionate as carbon sources facilitated the enrichment of these microbial communities, enabling the removal of higher concentrations of 2,4,6-TCP.

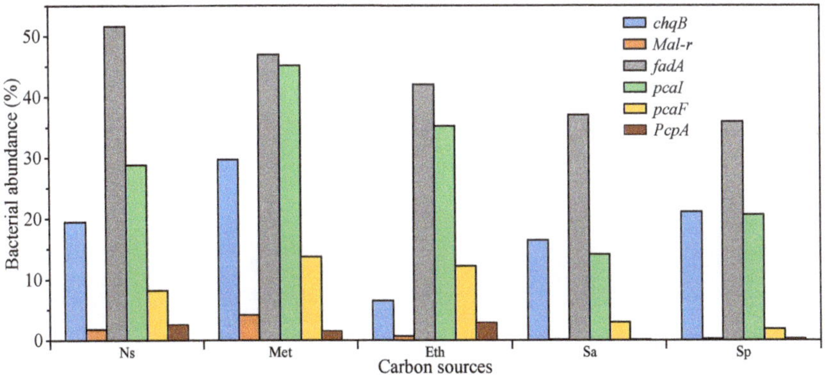

Figure 10. Abundance of bacteria containing specific functional genes.

4. Conclusions

Under different carbon source conditions, varying degrees of 2,4,6-TCP degradation were achieved by altering the microbial community. In comparison to hard-to-degrade carbon sources, easily degradable co-metabolic carbon sources demonstrated higher concentrations of 2,4,6-TCP removal. Specifically, activated sludge supplemented with methanol, sodium acetate, and sodium propionate as carbon sources achieved degradation concentrations of 123.89 mg/L, 170.96 mg/L, and 151.79 mg/L, respectively, surpassing those of other carbon sources. From the perspective of 2,4,6-TCP removal efficiency, sodium acetate appears to be the most suitable as a carbon source in the treatment of actual phenolic wastewater. Not only does it yield higher concentrations of 2,4,6-TCP removal, but it also enhances the overall performance of the SBR's operation. When compared to scenarios without the addition of carbon sources, all four carbon sources were found to significantly increase the functional gene abundance related to 2,4,6-TCP degradation, including *PcpA*, *chqB*, *Mal-r*, *pcaI*, *pcaF*, and *fadA*. The abundance of genera containing the chqB gene demonstrates a strong correlation with the metabolic capacity of 2,4,6-TCP. Small molecular carbon sources such as methanol, sodium acetate, and sodium propionate can facilitate the enrichment of genera harboring functional genes. However, this study solely focused on the effects of adding different carbon sources on 2,4,6-TCP removal efficiency and microbial community abundance. The underlying mechanisms of different carbon sources' profound impacts require further exploration to provide guidance for the effective treatment of actual phenolic wastewater.

Author Contributions: Conceptualization, J.W.; data curation, J.W.; formal analysis, J.W., H.F. and S.L.; writing—original draft, J.W.; writing—review and editing, J.W. and H.Y. All authors have read and agreed to the published version of the manuscript.

Funding: This research was supported by the scientific program of PowerChina Huadong Engineering Corporation Limited (KY2022-HS-02-20).

Data Availability Statement: Data are contained within the article.

Conflicts of Interest: Author Jianguang Wang was employed by the company PowerChina Huadong Engineering Corporation Limited. The remaining authors declare that the research was conducted in the absence of any commercial or financial relationships that could be construed as potential conflicts of interest.

References

1. Khan, M.Z.; Mondal, P.K.; Sabir, S. Bioremediation of 2-chlorophenol containing wastewater by aerobic granules-kinetics and toxicity. *J. Hazard. Mater.* **2011**, *190*, 222–228. [CrossRef]
2. Sze, M.F.F.; Mckay, G. An adsorption diffusion model for removal of para-chlorophenol by activated carbon derived from bituminous coal. *Environ. Pollut.* **2010**, *158*, 1669–1674. [CrossRef]
3. Barik, A.J.; Gogate, P.R. Hybrid treatment strategies for 2,4,6-trichlorophenol degradation based on combination of hydrodynamic cavitation and AOPs. *Ultrason. Sonochemistry* **2018**, *40*, 383–394. [CrossRef] [PubMed]
4. Xu, R.; Cui, J.; Tang, R.; Li, F.; Zhang, B. Removal of 2,4,6-trichlorophenol by laccase immobilized on nano-copper incorporated electrospun fibrous membrane-high efficiency, stability and reusability. *Chem. Eng. J.* **2017**, *326*, 647–655. [CrossRef]
5. Wang, C.C.; Lee, C.M.; Kuan, C.H. Removal of 2,4-dichlorophenol by suspended and immobilized Bacillus insolitus. *Chemosphere* **2000**, *41*, 447–452. [CrossRef]
6. Assadi, A.; Alimoradzadeh, R.; Movahedyan, H.; Amin, M.M. Intensified 4-chlorophenol biodegradation in an aerobic sequencing batch reactor: Microbial and kinetic properties evaluation. *Environ. Technol. Innov.* **2021**, *21*, 101243. [CrossRef]
7. Wang, J.; Sun, Z. Effects of different carbon sources on 2,4,6-trichlorophenol degradation in the activated sludge process. *Bioprocess Biosyst. Eng.* **2020**, *43*, 2143–2152. [CrossRef]
8. Machado, L.M.M.; Lutke, S.F.; Perondi, D.; Godinho, M.; Oliveira, M.L.S.; Collazzo, G.C.; Dotto, G.L. Treatment of effluents containing 2-chlorophenol by adsorption onto chemically and physically activated biochars. *J. Environ. Chem. Eng.* **2020**, *8*, 104473. [CrossRef]
9. Miao, M.; Zhang, Y.; Shu, L.; Zhang, J.; Kong, Q.; Li, N. Development and characterization of the 2,4,6-trichlorophenol (2,4,6-TCP) aerobic degrading granules in sequencing batch airlift reactor. *Int. Biodeterior. Biodegrad.* **2014**, *95*, 61–66. [CrossRef]
10. Tian, Y.; Zhang, J.; Wu, D.; Li, Z.; Cui, Y. Distribution variation of a metabolic uncoupler, 2,6-dichlorophenol (2,6-DCP) in long-term sludge culture and their effects on sludge reduction and biological inhibition. *Water Res.* **2013**, *47*, 279–288. [CrossRef]
11. Ziagova, M.; Kyriakou, G.; Liakopoulou-Kyriakides, M. Co-metabolism of 2,4-dichlorophenol and 4-Cl-m-cresol in the presence of glucose as an easily assimilated carbon source by Staphylococcus xylosus. *J. Hazard. Mater.* **2009**, *163*, 383–390. [CrossRef]
12. Wang, S.; Liu, X.; Zhang, H.; Gong, W.; Sun, X.; Gao, B. Aerobic granulation for 2,4-dichlorophenol biodegradation in a sequencing batch reactor. *Chemosphere* **2007**, *69*, 769–775. [CrossRef] [PubMed]
13. Reardon, K.F.; Mosteller, D.C.; Rogers, J.B.; Duteau, N.M.; Kim, K. Biodegradation kinetics of aromatic hydrocarbon mixtures by pure and mixed bacterial cultures. *Environ. Health Perspect.* **2002**, *110*, 1005–1011. [CrossRef]
14. Luo, W.; Zhu, X.; Chen, W.; Duan, Z.; Wang, L.; Zhou, Y. Mechanisms and strategies of microbial cometabolism in the degradation of organic compounds-chlorinated ethylenes as the model. *Water Sci. Technol.* **2014**, *69*, 1971–1983. [CrossRef] [PubMed]
15. Chaudhuri, B.K.; Wiesmann, U. Enhanced anaerobic degradation of benzeneby enrichment of mixed microbial cultureand optimization of the culture medium. *Appl. Microbiol. Biotechnol.* **1995**, *43*, 178–187. [CrossRef]

16. Poggi-Varaldo, H.M.; Barcenas-Torres, J.D.; Moreno-Medina, C.U.; Garcia-Mena, J.; Garibay-Orijel, C.; Rios-Leal, E.; Rinderknecht-Seijas, N. Influence of discontinuing feeding degradable cosubstrate on the performance of a fluidized bed bioreactor treating a mixture of trichlorophenol and phenol. *J. Environ. Manag.* **2012**, *113*, 527–537. [CrossRef] [PubMed]
17. Carucci, A.; Milia, S.; De Gioannis, G.; Piredda, M. Acetate-fed aerobic granular sludge for the degradation of 4-chlorophenol. *J. Hazard. Mater.* **2009**, *166*, 483–490. [CrossRef]
18. Zhao, J.; Li, Y.; Chen, X.; Li, Y. Effects of carbon sources on sludge performance and microbial community for 4-chlorophenol wastewater treatment in sequencing batch reactors. *Bioresour. Technol.* **2018**, *255*, 22–28. [CrossRef]
19. Ma, J.; Quan, X.; Yang, Z.; Li, A. Biodegradation of a mixture of 2,4-dichlorophenoxyacetic acid and multiple chlorophenols by aerobic granules cultivated through plasmid pJP4 mediated bioaugmentation. *Chem. Eng. J.* **2012**, *181*, 144–151. [CrossRef]
20. Carucci, A.; Milia, S.; Cappai, G.; Muntoni, A. A direct comparison amongst different technologies (aerobic granular sludge, SBR and MBR) for the treatment of wastewater contaminated by 4-chlorophenol. *J. Hazard. Mater.* **2010**, *177*, 1119–1125. [CrossRef]
21. Zhang, T.; Shao, M.; Ye, L. 454 Pyrosequencing reveals bacterial diversity of activated sludge from 14 sewage treatment plants. *ISME J.* **2012**, *6*, 1137–1147. [CrossRef] [PubMed]
22. Gomez-Acata, S.; Vital-Jacome, M.; Perez-Sandoval, M.V.; Navarro-Noya, Y.E.; Thalasso, F.; Luna-Guido, M.; Conde-Barajas, E.; Dendooven, L. Microbial community structure in aerobic and fluffy granules formed in a sequencing batch reactor supplied with 4-chlorophenol at different settling times. *J. Hazard. Mater.* **2018**, *342*, 606–616. [CrossRef] [PubMed]
23. Wang, J.; Sun, Z. Successful application of municipal domestic wastewater as a co-substrate in 2,4,6-trichlorophenol degradation. *Chemosphere* **2021**, *280*, 130707. [CrossRef]
24. Apha. *Standard Methods for the Examination of Water and Wastewater*, 24th ed.; United Book Press: Washington, DC, USA, 1998.
25. Li, X.Y.; Yang, S.F. Influence of loosely bound extracellular polymeric substances (EPS) on the flocculation, sedimentation and dewaterability of activated sludge. *Water Res.* **2007**, *41*, 1022–1030. [CrossRef]
26. Xu, C.; Zhang, S.; Chuang, C.; Miller, E.J.; Schwehr, K.A.; Santschi, P.H. Chemical composition and relative hydrophobicity of microbial exopolymeric substances (EPS) isolated by anion exchange chromatography and their actinide-binding affinities. *Mar. Chem.* **2011**, *126*, 27–36. [CrossRef]
27. Vetrovsky, T.; Steffen, K.T.; Baldrian, P. Potential of cometabolic transformation of polysaccharides and lignin in lignocellulose by soil Actinobacteria. *PLoS ONE* **2014**, *9*, e89108. [CrossRef]
28. Kindaichi, T.; Yamaoka, S.; Uehara, R.; Ozaki, N.; Ohashi, A.; Albertsen, M.; Nielsen, P.H.; Nielsen, J.L. Phylogenetic diversity and ecophysiology of Candidate phylum Saccharibacteria in activated sludge. *FEMS Microbiol. Ecol.* **2016**, *92*, fiw078. [CrossRef]
29. Liang, J.; Fang, X.; Lin, Y.; Wang, D. A new screened microbial consortium OEM2 for lignocellulosic biomass deconstruction and chlorophenols detoxification. *J. Hazard. Mater.* **2018**, *347*, 341–348. [CrossRef] [PubMed]
30. Baek, S.; Kim, K.; Yin, C.; Jeon, C.O.; Im, W.; Kim, K.; Lee, S. Isolation and characterization of bacteria capable of degrading phenol and reducing nitrate under low-oxygen conditions. *Curr. Microbiol.* **2003**, *47*, 462–466. [CrossRef]
31. Ju, F.; Zhang, T. Novel microbial populations in ambient and mesophilic biogas-producing and phenol-degrading consortia unraveled by high-throughput sequencing. *Microb. Ecol.* **2014**, *68*, 235–246. [CrossRef]
32. Mannisto, M.K.; Tiirola, M.A.; Puhakka, J.A. Degradation of 2,3,4,6-tetrachlorophenol at low temperature and low dioxygen concentrations by phylogenetically different groundwater and bioreactor bacteria. *Biodegradation* **2001**, *12*, 291–301. [CrossRef] [PubMed]
33. Rutgers, M.; Breure, A.M.; van Andel, J.G.; Duetz, W.A. Growth yield coefficients of *Sphingomonas* sp. strain P5 on various chlorophenols in chemostat culture. *Appl. Microbiol. Biotechnol.* **1997**, *48*, 656–661. [CrossRef]
34. Leonard, D.; Lindley, N.D. Growth of Ralstonia eutropha on inhibitory concentrations of phenol: Diminished growth can be attributed to hydrophobic perturbation of phenol hydroxylase activity. *Enzym. Microb. Technol.* **1999**, *25*, 271–277. [CrossRef]
35. Baggi, G.; Cavalca, L.; Francia, P.; Zangrossi, M. Chlorophenol removal from soil suspensions: Effects of a specialised microbial inoculum and a degradable analogue. *Biodegradation* **2004**, *15*, 153–160. [CrossRef] [PubMed]
36. Matus, V.; Sanchez, M.A.; Martinez, M.; Gonzalez, B. Efficient degradation of 2,4,6-trichlorophenol requires a set of catabolic genes related to tcp genes from Ralstonia eutropha JMP134(pJP4). *Appl. Environ. Microbiol.* **2003**, *69*, 7108–7115. [CrossRef] [PubMed]
37. Burback, B.L.; Perry, J.J. Biodegradation and biotransformation of groundwater pollutant mixtures by *Mycobacterium vaccae*. *Appl. Environ. Microbiol.* **1993**, *59*, 1025–1029. [CrossRef]
38. Burback, B.L.; Perry, J.J.; Rudd, L.E. Effect of environmental-pollutants and their metabolites on a soil mycobacterium. *Appl. Microbiol. Biotechnol.* **1994**, *41*, 134–136. [CrossRef]

water

MDPI

Article

Occurrence, Fate, and Mass Balance Analysis of Organophosphate Flame Retardants in a Municipal Wastewater Treatment Plant in Hunan Province, China

Yang Liu [1,2], Yang Song [1,2], Haipu Li [1,2,*] and Zhaoguang Yang [1,2]

[1] Center for Environment and Water Resources, College of Chemistry and Chemical Engineering, Central South University, Changsha 410083, China; liuyangso00@163.com (Y.L.); trustwh2010@163.com (Y.S.); zgyang@csu.edu.cn (Z.Y.)

[2] Key Laboratory of Hunan Province for Water Environment and Agriculture Product Safety, Changsha 410083, China

* Correspondence: lihaipu@csu.edu.cn; Tel.: +86-073188876961

Abstract: The occurrence, distribution, removal, and mass loadings of common organophosphate flame retardants (OPFRs) in an advanced municipal wastewater treatment plant (WWTP) were comprehensively investigated. The OPFRs were mainly partitioning in the dissolved phase, and the total concentrations ranged from 1364 to 1701 ng/L in influent, 678~1064 in effluent, and 177~470 ng/g dw in residual sludge. Tributoxyethyl phosphate and tris(2-chloroethyl) phosphate were the abundant compounds in both the dissolved phase and adsorbed phase. The removal frequencies and mechanisms of the OPFRs were highly associated with the properties of compounds. According to the mass balance analysis, 14.9%, 13.0%, and 11.2% of the total OPFR loads were removed in the traditional treatment, tertiary treatment, and to the sludge, respectively. The mass loadings and environmental emissions of the OPFRs were 0.67~291 μg/d/person and 0.57~107 μg/d/person, respectively. The effluent discharged from the WWTP posed ecological risks to the receiving river, which requires being paid more attention.

Keywords: organophosphate flame retardants; municipal wastewater treatment plant; mass balance analysis; mass loadings; environmental emissions

1. Introduction

In recent years, the production and consumption of organophosphate flame retardants (OPFRs) have grown significantly due to the restricted application of brominated flame retardants. OPFRs have been widely used in plastics, building materials, textiles, electronic products, lubricate oil, and other industrial products [1]. The global consumption of OPFRs increased to 1 million tons in 2018 [2], and the growth rate in China could achieve 15% annually [3]. OPFRs are used by physically adding them to the product without chemical bonding, which allows for their easy release into the environment [4]. As a result, they are widely present in a range of environmental media and even in living organisms. Numerous studies have been reported on the occurrence of OPFRs in water [4–7], air [8–10], dust [10–12], sediment [2,4,13], soil [14,15], and biota samples [16,17]. Given the high detection frequency and potential toxicity to organisms, OPFRs might pose a potential threat to ecology and humans, which need to be paid attention to.

A wastewater treatment plant (WWTP) is the final treatment site for pollutants in wastewater. Traditional pollutants like COD, BOD, and total suspended solid (TSS) collect here and are eventually removed through a sequence of treatments [18]. Nevertheless, several studies have indicated that the removal efficiencies of OPFRs by a WWTP are limited [19–21]. As a result, the residual OPFRs may be released into the environment along with effluent or residual sludge, making a WWTP the main source of OPFRs into the environment rather than the elimination site.

Currently, several studies have been carried out to study the concentration level and removal efficiency of OPFRs in a WWTP [18,22–24]. Yin et al. [22] investigated the concentration and distribution of seven OPFRs in water samples from a WWTP, the total removal rate was found to be 57.2%, and the average concentrations of influent and effluent were 978.2 ± 166.5 ng/L and 418.3 ± 12.0 ng/L, respectively. Kim et al. [20] researched the removal efficiencies of OPFRs in a WWTP from New York State, the removal efficiencies ranged from negative values to about 60%, showing incomplete removal and a significant difference in OPFRs. However, the behavior and emissions of OPFRs in the various treatment stages in a WWTP have not been thoroughly investigated and reported [25–27]. Liang and Liu [25] performed the mass flow and mass balance analysis in an advanced municipal WWTP to unveil the potential removal mechanisms. Additionally, the behavior of pollutants in the WWTP would have been affected by a variety of factors, including the population, climate, and WWTP treatment conditions. Wang et al. [28] investigated the occurrence of OPFRs in 25 municipal WWTPs across China and found that the removal frequencies of OPFRs using the same treatment process might vary significantly in different districts. Therefore, more efforts should be made to study the fate of OPFRs in a WWTP.

In this study, we investigate the occurrence, behavior, and removal of 12 common OPFRs in a municipal WWTP in Changsha, Hunan Province, which has a typical Anaerobic/Anoxic/Oxic bioreactor and an advanced treatment stage. Both the dissolved phase and adsorbed phase (suspended particulate matter and sludge) were involved in the analysis to comprehensively assess the fate of OPFRs in the WWTP. The mass balance analysis was introduced to study the removal mechanisms. The mass loadings and environmental emissions were also calculated to evaluate the consumption and pollution emissions of OPFRs in this area for the first time.

2. Materials and Methods

2.1. Chemicals and Standards

Twelve common OPFRs were set as the target compounds in this study, including tri-isobutyl phosphate (TIBP), tri-nbutyl phosphate (TNBP), tributoxyethyl phosphate (TBOEP), tris(2-ethylhexyl) phosphate (TEHP), triphenyl phosphate (TPHP), tricresyl phosphate (TMPP), cresyl diphenyl phosphate (CDP), 2-ethylhexyl diphenyl phosphate (EHDPP), tris(2-chloroethyl) phosphate (TCEP), tris(2-chloroethyl) phosphate (TCIPP), tris(1,3-dichloro-2-propyl) phosphate (TDCIPP), and triphenylphosphine oxide (TPPO). Among them, TNBP and EHDPP were purchased from Aladdin (Shanghai, China), the other ten target OPFRs were purchased from Macklin (Shanghai, China). Deuterated TNBP-d27 and TPHP-d15 were used as the surrogate standards and bought from Toronto Research Chemicals Inc. (Toronto, ON, Canada). Detailed information on the compounds is listed in Table S1.

2.2. Study Plant and Sample Collection

The municipal WWTP was located in Changsha, Hunan Province, China. The service area of the plant was 62.98 km^2 with about 9,815,000 residents. The treatment process scheme of the WWTP included four main stages: (1) primary treatment (screen and grit chamber); (2) secondary treatment (Anaerobic/Anoxic/Oxic treatment and secondary clarifier); (3) tertiary treatment (high-efficient sedimentation tank, deep-bed filter, and UV disinfection); (4) sludge dewatering system (Figure 1). Among the stages, stage 1 and stage 2 were the traditional treatment process. During the sampling period, the average daily capacity of the plant was about 430,000 m^3/d, and the sludge production was about 250 t/d (wet weight, contained 80% moisture).

The sampling campaigns were conducted in September 2020. The wastewater samples, including influent, primary treatment effluent, secondary treatment effluent, and tertiary treatment effluent (also the final effluent), were collected in a 2.5 L amber glass bottle. The sludge samples were collected after the sludge dewatering system. The sampling points are shown in Figure 1. All of the samples were kept in a cooler and immediately transported to the lab for further analysis.

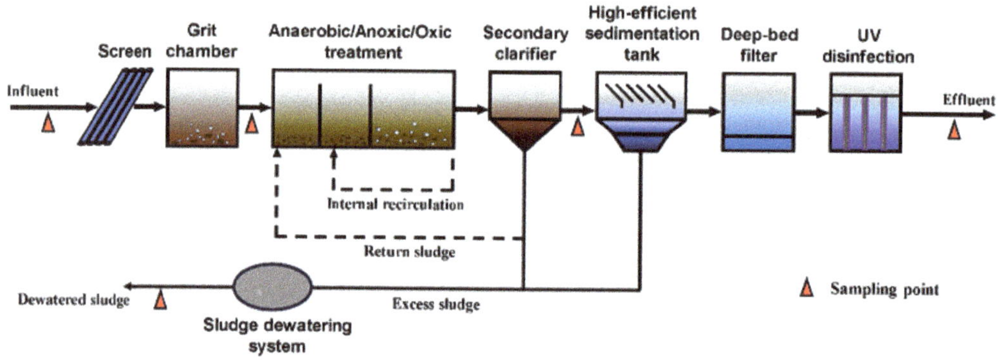

Figure 1. Schematic diagram of the studied wastewater treatment plant.

2.3. Sample Preparation

The wastewater samples were filtered using glass fiber filters (GF/F, Whatman, Kent, UK), which were pre-treated in a muffle furnace at 450 °C for 4 h. The solid interceptions were collected as suspended particulate matter (SPM) samples and also used to further calculate the TSS. The preparation of filtered water samples was conducted according to our previous study [5] with some modifications. Briefly, the water samples with surrogate standards (TNBP-d27 and TPHP-d15) were passed through the HLB cartridges (6 mL, 200 mg, ANPEL, Shanghai, China) and the target compounds were extracted using acetonitrile from the loaded HLB cartridges. The acetonitrile eluent was collected and concentrated to 1 mL for instrument analysis. The freeze-dried solid samples (SPM and sludge) were spiked with surrogate standards (TNBP-d27 and TPHP-d15), and then ultrasonic-assisted extracted for 15 min using acetonitrile (10 mL) as the ex-traction solution. The extractant was obtained by centrifugation, and the extraction process was repeated three times. A total of 30 mL of the collected extractant was concentrated and redissolved in 100 mL of ultra-pure water. The subsequent operation is the same as the extraction process of water samples.

The determination of 12 target OPFRs was performed on a liquid chromatography system (HPLC, Agilent 1260, Santa Clara, CA, USA) coupled with a triple quadrupole mass spectrometer (MS/MS, Agilent 6460, Santa Clara, CA, USA). The separation of target OPFRs was performed on the Poroshell 120EC-C18 column (50 mm × 4.6 mm i.d., 2.7 μm, Santa Clara, CA, USA). The column temperature was 30 °C, and the injection volume of samples was 5 μL. Gradient elution was performed using a binary mobile phase consisting of 0.1% (*v*/*v*) formic acid (A) and acetonitrile (B). The elution gradients are listed in Table S2. Using the multiple reaction monitoring (MRM) in positive ionization mode to quantify the target OPFRs in the samples, the optimized MS parameters were set as follows: the source temperature was 330 °C; the source gas flow was 8 mL/min; the nebulizer gas pressure was 40 psi. The optimized mass spectrum parameters of target OPFRs are listed in Table S3.

2.4. QA/QC

The equipment that might be in direct contact with the samples was thoroughly washed with methanol and ultra-pure water before use to avoid introducing contamination. The internal standard method was used to quantify the target OPFRs, and the recoveries of TNBP-d27 and TPHP-d15 were 91.7 ± 10.1% and 94.6 ± 4.7% for the water samples, and 98.1 ± 5.9% and 95.5 ± 9.7% for the solid samples, respectively. The limits of method quantification (LOQ) for the target OPFRs were defined as 10 times the signal-to-noise ratio, and the LOQ values of the water samples and solid samples were 0.005~0.05 μg/L and

0.06~3.89 μg/kg dw, respectively (Table S4). The recoveries and matrix effects of the water samples and solid samples are listed in Table S5. For instrument analysis, a solvent blank and a standard sample of specific concentration were detected every 10 samples to monitor the operating status of the instrument.

2.5. Data Analysis

The mass balance analysis for the OPFRs could be calculated as follows:

$$M_{influent/effluent} = C_{dissolved} \times Q \times 10^{-6} + C_{adsorbed} \times Q \times C_{TSS} \times 10^{-9} \quad (1)$$

$$M_{sludge} = C_{sludge} \times P_s \times 10^{-6} \quad (2)$$

$$M_{influent} = M_{effluent} + M_{sludge} + M_{loss} \quad (3)$$

$$M_{loss\text{-}TT} = M_{influent} - M_{se,effluent} - M_{sludge} \quad (4)$$

$$M_{loss\text{-}AT} = M_{se,effluent} - M_{effluent} \quad (5)$$

where $C_{dissolved}$ (ng/L), $C_{adsorbed}$ (ng/g, dw), and C_{sludge} (ng/g, dw) are the concentrations of OPFRs in the aqueous phase, SPM, and residual sludge, respectively; Q (m^3/d) is the daily water follow of the plant; P_s (kg/d, dw) is the average daily sludge output of the plant; $M_{influent}$, $M_{se,effluent}$, $M_{effluent}$, and M_{sludge} (g/d) represented the mass loads of OPFRs in influent, secondary treatment effluent, tertiary treatment effluent, and residual sludge, respectively; among them, the influent, secondary treatment effluent, and tertiary treatment effluent load contain both OPFRs dissolved in water and adsorbed on suspended particles; M_{loss} (g/d) is the mass load loss of OPFRs during the wastewater treatment process, which can be considered as the loss caused by biodegradation and/or adsorption, including the $M_{loss\text{-}TT}$ (the loss occurred in the traditional treatment process) and the loss $M_{loss\text{-}AT}$ (the loss occurred in the advanced treatment process stage).

The total removal efficiency of OPFRs (R_M) could be calculated as follows:

$$R_M = \frac{M_{influent} - \left(M_{effluent} + M_{sludge}\right)}{M_{influent}} \times 100\% \quad (6)$$

Furthermore, the per capita consumption of OPFRs can be estimated by the pollution mass loadings of the WWTP influent, and the environmental emissions of OPFRs discharged from the WWTP can infer the total amount of pollution discharged in the region.

$$M_{load} = \frac{M_{inffluent} \times 10^9}{N_s} \quad (7)$$

$$E = \frac{\left(M_{effluent} + M_{sludge}\right) \times 10^9}{N_s} \quad (8)$$

where M_{load} (μg/d/person) is the per capita pollution mass loadings of influent water, E (μg/d/person) is the per capita environmental emissions, and N_s (person) is the total population served by the plant, which is 981,500 people in this study.

2.6. Ecological Risk Assessment

The risk quotient (RQ) method was used to assess the risk of residual OPFR discharge in wastewater to the aquatic environment.

$$RQ = \frac{MEC}{PNEC} \quad (9)$$

where MEC is the concentration of OPFRs (ng/L) in the effluent water of the WWTP, and PNEC is the predicted concentration of no effect (ng/g). To estimate the possible ecological threat caused by the total OPFRs, the risk quotient RQ_{mix} is calculated, which is the sum of the RQ for each OPFRs [29].

3. Results and Discussion

3.1. Occurrence of OPFRs in Wastewater Treatment

OPFRs in water and adsorbed on SPM were detected in water samples collected from the WWTP. The results showed that all the 12 target pollutants were detected at least once (Figure 2, Tables S8 and S9).

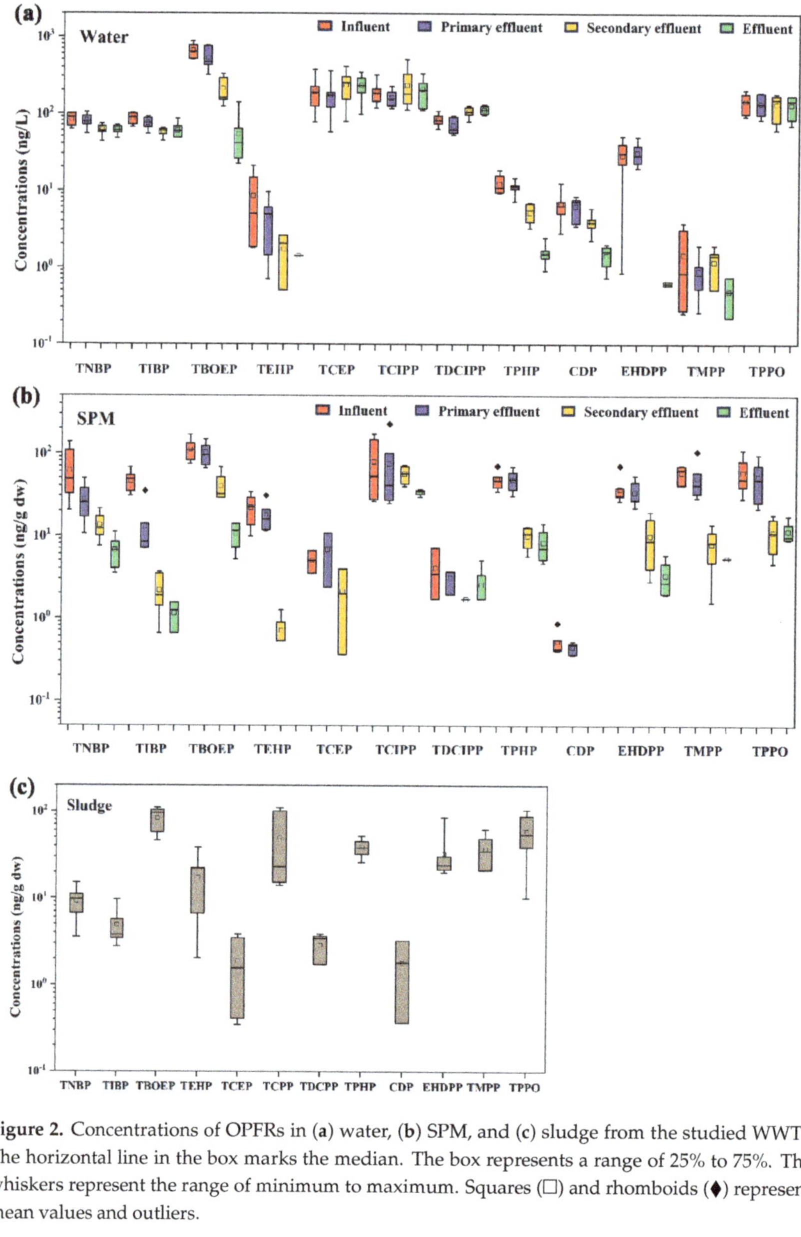

Figure 2. Concentrations of OPFRs in (**a**) water, (**b**) SPM, and (**c**) sludge from the studied WWTP. The horizontal line in the box marks the median. The box represents a range of 25% to 75%. The whiskers represent the range of minimum to maximum. Squares (□) and rhomboids (♦) represent mean values and outliers.

In the water of the influent sample, TBOEP (499~866 ng/L, mean 661 ± 126 ng/L) was the most abundant compound, accounting for about 44% of OPFRs in the dissolved phase, followed by TCEP (76.8~376 ng/L. mean 190 ± 90 ng/L) and TCIPP (118~320 ng/L, mean 191 ± 60 ng/L). Most of the compounds had high detection frequencies (DF > 50%), indicating the incomplete removal of OPFRs in the WWTP. TCEP (97.8~348 ng/L, 232 ± 76.8 ng/L) and TCIPP (110~336 ng/L, mean 207 ± 72.6 ng/L) were the most abundant compounds in the water of the effluent sample, accounting for 27% and 23% of the total OPFR concentration, respectively. Several studies from Spain [30], Germany [31], the United States [20], Greece [26], and a WWTP in Beijing [25] all indicated that TBOEP, TCEP, and TCIPP were the most abundant individual OPFRs, which was consistent with the results of this study. TBOEP has a variety of applications in home improvement materials, such as floor polish, added to paint or glue [7]; TCIPP and TCEP are widely used as flame retardants for polyurethane foams and other materials [1]. They had been widely detected in indoor dust, which was confirmed to be an important source of pollutants in domestic sewage [7]. Therefore, certain TBOEP, TCEP, and TCIPP were easily able to enter the urban sewage network through indoor dust or residents' flushing water. The total concentration of OPFRs (∑OPFRs) in the influent and effluent ranged from 1364 to 1701 ng/L and from 678 to 1064 ng/L, respectively. Compared with other countries and regions, both the individual OPFRs and ∑OPFRs in sewage in this study are at a relatively low level (Table S10).

The OPFRs of the SPM in the influent and effluent are listed in Table S9. TBOEP (71.8~168 ng/g, mean 108 ± 32.4 ng/g) and TCIPP (25.9~171 ng/g, mean 79.1 ± 56.2 ng/g) were the most important compounds in the SPM of the influent. However, TCEP with a high content in the aquatic phase has a lower content, which might be related to the physicochemical properties of the OPFRs with a lower n-octanol/water partition coefficient (log K_{OW} = 1.44) and higher solubility (W_S = 7000 mg/L), making the substance more likely to appear in the aquatic phase. In addition, TNBP, TPPO, and TMPP also had relatively high detected concentrations in the SPM of the influent, and the mean concentrations were 61.9 ± 40.3, 59.3 ± 25.7, and 58.6 ± 11.8 ng/g dw, respectively. ∑OPFRs in the SPM of the influent was 405~717 ng/g dw, while that in the effluent was 5.07~76.9 ng/g dw. The concentrations of all compounds in the SPM of the effluent decreased significantly, and the detection frequency of TMPP was only 14%, while TEHP, TCEP, and CDP were not detected. Because the effluent from the WWTP has been processed by deep treatment processes, the suspended particles were almost removed (removal frequency > 99.5%), so the OPFR concentrations on the SPM in the effluent also decreased. At present, the relevant studies on the OPFR concentration of SPM are limited, the result in this study was lower than that in WWTPs in Thessaloniki, Greece [7], and the residue level was the same as that in a WWTP in Beijing [25].

Most of the target OPFRs had high detection frequencies in the residual sludge, except CDP, which had a detection frequency of 29%. TBOEP (46.0~111 ng/g dw, mean 83.0 ± 23.4 ng/g) was again the most important compound, followed by TPPO (10.2~104 ng/g dw, mean 60.0 ± 30.9 ng/g dw) and TCIPP (14.0~110 ng/g dw, mean 49.7 ± 39.4 ng/g dw). ∑OPFRs in the residual sludge ranged from 177 to 470 ng/g dw, which was the same as that of a WWTP in Beijing [25] and other sewage treatment plants in Henan Province [32], but much lower than that reported in Spain [23], the United States [20], and Greece [26].

3.2. Distributions and Removal Efficiencies of OPFRs

Understanding the distribution patterns of OPFRs between the dissolved phase (water) and adsorbed phase (solid) in wastewater treatment systems helps investigate the path and mechanism of pollutant removal. The distribution of pollutants in the two phases may be related to various factors, such as the load of pollutants in the influents, the partitioning of pollutants in each phase, and the properties of organic matter itself, such as persistence [33]. The OPFRs of the adsorbed phase were converted into ng/L, to facilitate direct comparison with the OPFRs of the dissolved phase. It was found that in this study, individual OPFRs except TPHP were mainly located in the dissolved phase, and the adsorbed phase only accounted for 9.77~29.6%. The fraction of OPFRs in the adsorbed phase was further decreased along with the treatment process. According to the results, the OPFRs were mainly dissolved in the aquatic phase, and only a small extent of OPFRs were removed by adsorbing onto the SPM in the secondary treatment stage. For TEHP, TPHP, and TMPP, which were more hydrophobic, the fractions of the adsorbed phase in the influent were high, while they were eliminated as the solid phases in the secondary effluent were removed. Therefore, the adsorption of SPM and sludge might be an important way for the removal of these OPFRs. However, the fractions of OPFRs in the adsorbed phases in the effluent for two WWTPs in Greece were still above 20% [26], and the difference might be caused by the specificity of the source and composition of the sewage and the sludge.

The removal efficiencies of OPFRs in each stage of the WWTP are shown in Figure 3. The total removal efficiency of OPFRs was 39.1% ± 9.58%, and the removal efficiencies of each OPFR were significantly different. Among them, the removal efficiencies of Aryl-OPFRs (TPHP, CDP, EHDPP, and TMPP) were all above 85%, while those of Halo-OPFRs (TCEP, TCIPP, and TDCIPP) were all negative. Alkyl-OPFRs (TIBP, TNBP, TBOEP, and TEHP) differed from each other greatly. The removal efficiency of TEHP, which had long branched chains in its molecular structure, was high, while the removal efficiencies of TNBP and TIBP were about 30%. The negative removal efficiencies of Halo-OPFRs in WWTPs have also been reported in other areas [20,26,34,35]. In this study, the fractions of Halo-OPFRs in the adsorbed phase were low, implying limited removal efficiencies by adsorption to solid. As reported, Halo-OPFRs were recalcitrant to biodegradation [25], photodegradation [6], and hydrolyzation [36]; therefore, the negative removal efficiencies of Halo-OPFRs might be associated with their resistance to transformation and formation from precursor compounds [20,25]. Additionally, Halo-OPFRs are widely used as the flame retardant and plasticizer in the plastic materials of WWTP; the Halo-OPFRs might be released during the treatment process, resulting in a higher effluent concentration [25,37,38]. However, as the pollutant concentrations of influent may vary greatly within a day, the negative removal efficiency might also be attributed to the imperfect sampling schemes [26].

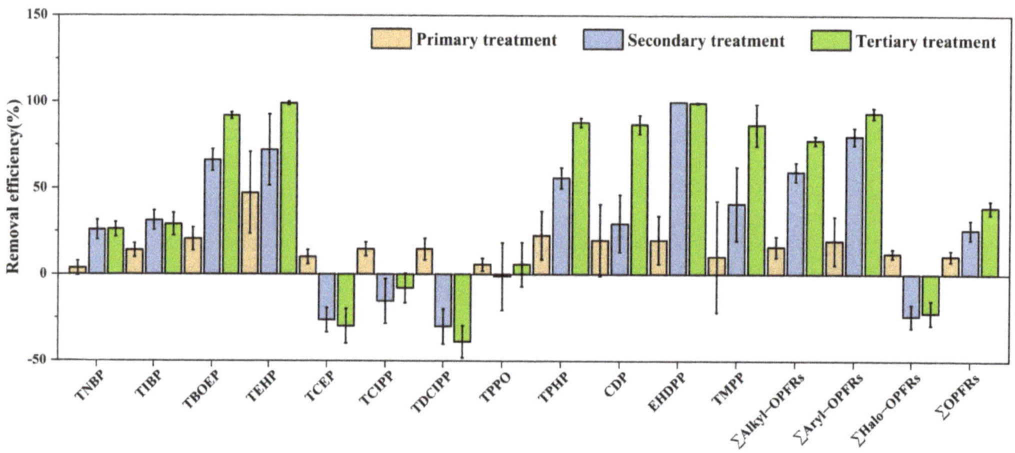

Figure 3. Removal efficiencies of OPFRs in different stages of WWTP.

Comparing the removal efficiencies of different stages of the wastewater treatment process, the removal of most OPFRs (especially Aryl-OPFRs) mainly occurred in the secondary biological treatment stage through adsorption or biodegradation. In the tertiary treatment stage, the removal frequencies of most OPFRs were further increased. As Alkyl-OPFRs are considered to be photostable without absorption bands at 200 to 400 nm [39], the increase in the removal frequency of TEHP at this process stage might be caused by adsorption and interception at the high-efficient sedimentation tank and deep-bed filter.

3.3. *Mass Balance Analysis*

Mass balance analysis is an effective way to investigate the removal mechanism of OPFRs in WWTPs and can reflect the true trend of OPFRs in WWTPs. The influent and effluent mass loads of OPFRs in the WWTP were calculated (Figure 4). The influent load ($M_{influent}$) was used as the system input, while the system output included effluent ($M_{effluent}$), dehydrated sludge (M_{sludge}), traditional treatment process (primary and secondary treatment) losses ($M_{loss\text{-}TT}$), and tertiary treatment losses ($M_{loss\text{-}AT}$).

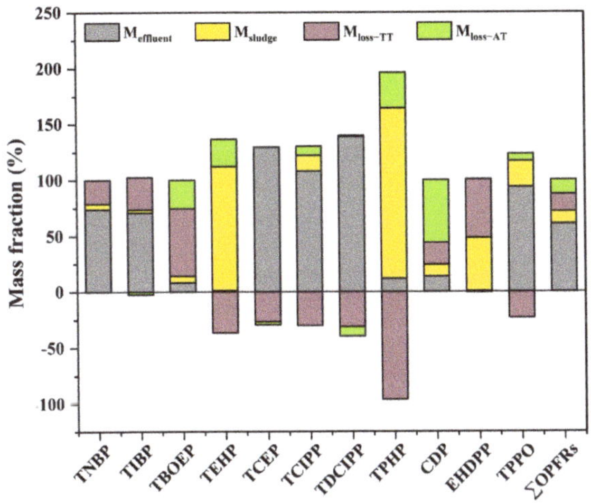

Figure 4. Mass balance analysis of OPFRs between effluent, sludge, and loss during the studied WWTP.

The mass fraction of ∑OPFRs in the final effluent of the WWTP accounted for 60.9 ± 8.96% of the $M_{influent}$, and only 11.2 ± 3.68% of the total load was transferred into the sludge. Mass loads lost in the traditional treatment process and tertiary treatment process were 14.9 ± 13.4% and 13.0 ± 11.2%, respectively. Most OPFRs, especially Halo-OPFRs, were not effectively removed in the wastewater treatment process and were discharged into the environmental water body. The removal processes of TNBP, TIBP, TBOEP, and EHDPP mainly occurred in traditional processes, indicating that biodegradation/biotransformation played an important role in this process. Most TEHP and TPHP and a portion of EHDPP were transferred to the sludge, indicating that they are mainly removed by adsorption. Except for CDP, other OPFRs had limited removal effectiveness in the tertiary treatment stage. In addition, TMPP was detected in large quantities in sludge and limited in influent water, which may be due to the instantaneous sampling method, which could not detect real-time changes in concentration and hydraulic retention time during treatment [26].

3.4. *Mass Loadings and Environmental Emissions*

The per capita daily OPFR pollution mass loadings and environmental emissions were calculated based on the total concentrations of OPFRs in the dissolved phase of sewage, the adsorbed phase on suspended particulate matter, and the sludge.

As shown in Figure 5, the daily pollution mass loadings of each OPFR in the WWTP involved in this study ranged from 0.67 to 291 μg/d/person. TBOEP (290 ± 67.7 μg/d/person), TCEP (85.9 ± 41.1 μg/d/person), TCIPP (83.9 ± 27.5 μg/d/person), and TPPO (64.7 ± 19.7 μg/d/person) were the main pollutants. The higher mass loadings of these pollutants might be related to their higher yields [20]. The per capita environmental emissions ranged from 0.57 to 107 μg/d/person, with the highest emission of TCEP (107 ± 45.1 μg/d/person). It was followed by TCIPP (101 ± 32.7 μg/d/person), TPPO

(70.7 ± 19.0 μg/d/person), and TDCIPP (50.6 ± 11.4 μg/d/person). Although TBOEP was in a high concentration level in the influent, its environmental emissions were reduced to 40.3 ± 15.5 μg/d/person due to the effective removal in the WWTP.

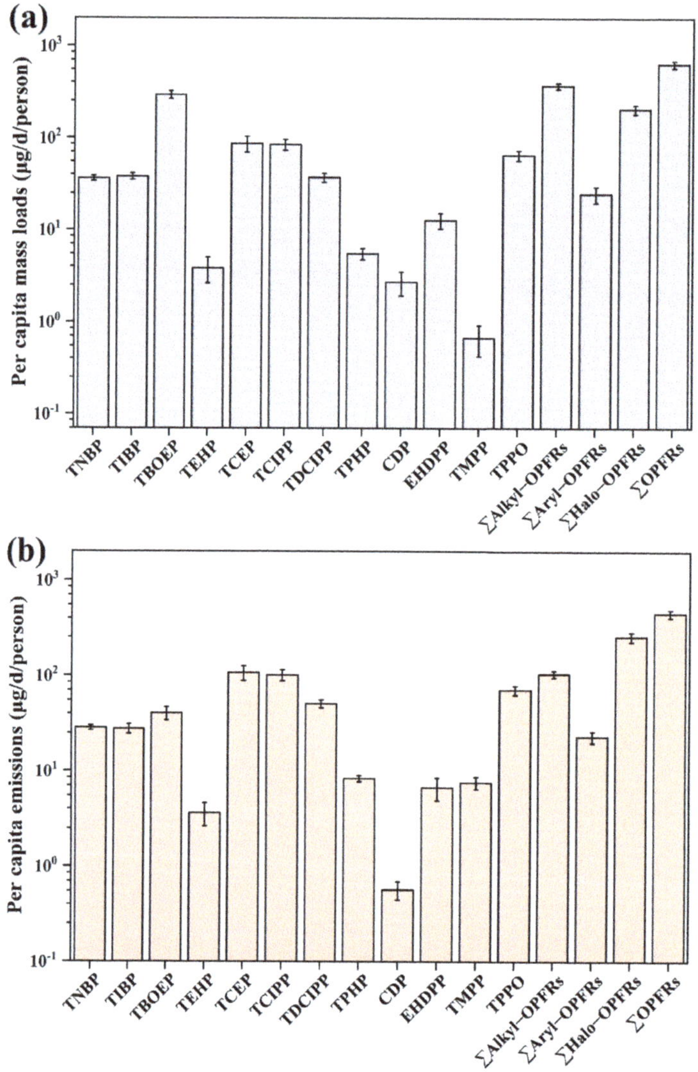

Figure 5. (**a**,**b**) Mass loadings and environmental emissions of the OPFRs in the studied WWTP.

Few literatures have paid attention to the pollution mass loadings and environmental emissions of OPFRs in WWTPs. According to reports, the pollution mass loadings of OPFRs in this study were lower than those in other areas. A study on two sewage treatment plants in Greece showed that the pollution mass loadings of individual OPFRs in this area ranged from 20 μg/d/person (tripropyl phosphate, TPP) to 540 μg/d/person (TBOEP) [26]. The mass loadings of sewage plants in Australia and the United States could reach 850~2860 μg/d/person and 20~28,700 μg/d/person, respectively [20,40].

Compared with other regions, the average daily environmental emissions of OPFRs per capita in this study were also at a low level. The emissions of total OPFRs were

2100 μg/d/person, which takes into account only the content in the dissolved phase [40]. Kim estimated the environmental emissions of a sewage plant in the United States [20]. The average daily emissions of TCIPP in the WWTP were the highest at 5120 μg/d/person, followed by TBOEP (3720 μg/d/person) and TDCIPP (2890 μg/d/person), which were much higher than the results of this study.

3.5. Ecological Risk Assessment

Figure 6 shows the potential ecological risks of effluent from the studied WWTP. Four levels of ecological risk could be identified based on the RQ values: $RQ \leq 0.1$, no risk; $0.1 < RQ \leq 1$, medium risk; $RQ > 1$, high risk [41].

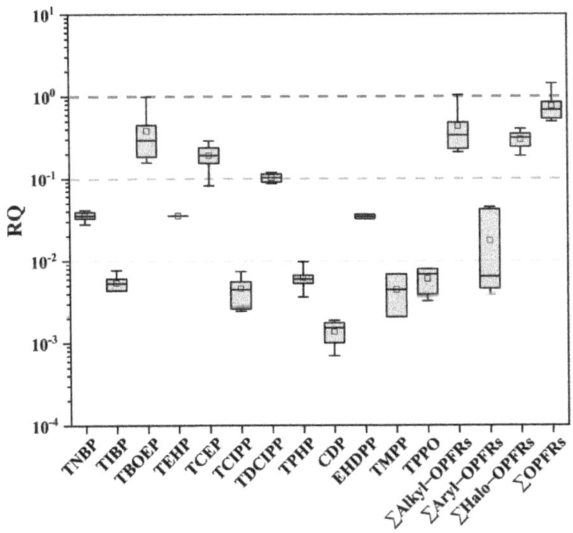

Figure 6. Estimated RQ values of individual and total OPFRs from the effluent. Squares (□) represent mean values. The dash lines in red, yellow, and green are located at values of 1.0, 0.1, and 0.01 for RQ, respectively.

The majority of individual OPFRs posed no to low ecological risk. TBOEP, TCEP, and TDCIPP required special attention due to their medium ecological risks. The mixed ecological risk (RQ_{mix}) of 12 OPFRs was close to the boundary of $RQ = 1$, indicating that there might be ecological threats. As a result, it is necessary to pay attention to the ecological security of the receiving river's water environment, especially during the dry season when the dilution effect of the river is further diminished.

4. Conclusions

Twelve common OPFRs were universally detected in both the dissolved phase and adsorbed phase in the studied WWTP. The mean concentration ranges were 1.47~661 ng/L (dissolved phase) in the influent, 0.14~232 ng/L (dissolved phase) in the effluent, and nd~83.0 ng/g dw adsorbed onto the sludge, which were all at relatively low levels compared to other reports. TBOEP and TCIPP were the most abundant individual OPFRs. The distribution and partitioning of individual OPFRs were significantly different, and was associated with their physicochemical properties. The removal efficiency of the total OPFRs was 39.1%, and Halo-OPFRs present a negative removal efficiency. The removal of OPFRs in the wastewater treatment could be attributed to biodegradation/biotransformation, adsorption onto the sludge, and physical adsorption in the tertiary treatment stage. Mass loadings and environmental emissions were 0.67~291 μg/d/person and 0.57~107 μg/d/person, respectively. The effluent of the studied WWTP might cause an ecological risk to the receiving river.

Supplementary Materials: The following supporting information can be downloaded at: https://www.mdpi.com/article/10.3390/w16111462/s1, Table S1: physicochemical information of the target OPFRs; Table S2: LC conditions for the target OPFRs; Table S3: the retention times and optimized MS/MS transitions of target OPFRs; Table S4: linearity, limits of quantitation (LOQs), and validated analytical method of target OPFRs; Table S5: matrix effects and recoveries (%, n = 5) of target OPFRs.; Table S6: the water quality parameters in the influent and effluent water; Table S7: predicted no-effective concentration (PNEC) based on effective concentration 50 or lethal concentration 50 (EC50 or LC50); Table S8: occurrence of target OPFRs in the dissolved phase of influent and effluent; Table S9: occurrence of target OPFRs in the adsorbed phase of influent, effluent, and sludge; Table S10: the occurrence of OPFRs in influent (ng/L), effluent (ng/L), and sludge (ng/g dw) from WWTP around the world. References [42–48] are cited in the Supplementary Materials.

Author Contributions: Conceptualization, Y.L. and H.L.; methodology, Y.L. and Y.S.; investigation, Y.L. and Y.S.; writing—original draft preparation, Y.L.; writing—review and editing, Y.L. and H.L.; visualization, Y.L.; project administration, Z.Y.; funding acquisition, Z.Y. All authors have read and agreed to the published version of the manuscript.

Funding: This research was funded by the Special Fund for Agro-scientific Research in the Public Interest of China, No. 201503108 and the Hydraulic Science & Technology Project of Hunan Province (2017-230-13).

Data Availability Statement: Data are contained within the article and Supplementary Materials.

Conflicts of Interest: The authors declare no conflicts of interest.

References

1. van der Veen, I.; de Boer, J. Phosphorus flame retardants: Properties, production, environmental occurrence, toxicity and analysis. *Chemosphere* **2012**, *88*, 1119–1153. [CrossRef]
2. Fu, J.; Fu, K.; Hu, B.; Zhou, W.; Fu, Y.; Gu, L.; Zhang, Q.; Zhang, A.; Fu, J.; Jiang, G. Source identification of organophosphate esters through the profiles in proglacial and ocean sediments from Ny-Ålesund, the Arctic. *Environ. Sci. Technol.* **2023**, *57*, 1919–1929. [CrossRef] [PubMed]
3. Zhu, K.; Sarvajayakesavalu, S.; Han, Y.; Zhang, H.; Gao, J.; Li, X.; Ma, M. Occurrence, distribution and risk assessment of organophosphate esters (OPEs) in water sources from Northeast to Southeast China. *Environ. Pollut.* **2022**, *307*, 119461. [CrossRef] [PubMed]
4. Li, W.; Yuan, Y.; Wang, S.; Liu, X. Occurrence, spatiotemporal variation, and ecological risks of organophosphate esters in the water and sediment of the middle and lower streams of the Yellow River and its important tributaries. *J. Hazard. Mater.* **2023**, *443*, 130153. [CrossRef] [PubMed]
5. Liu, Y.; Chen, L.; Li, H.; Song, Y.; Yang, Z.; Cui, Y. Occurrence of organophosphorus flame retardants in Xiangjiang River: Spatiotemporal variations, potential affecting factors, and source apportionment. *Chemosphere* **2024**, *355*, 141822. [CrossRef] [PubMed]
6. Li, S.; Wan, Y.; Wang, Y.; He, Z.; Xu, S.; Xia, W. Occurrence, spatial variation, seasonal difference, and ecological risk assessment of organophosphate esters in the Yangtze River, China: From the upper to lower reaches. *Sci. Total Environ.* **2022**, *851*, 158021. [CrossRef] [PubMed]
7. Cristale, J.; Oliveira Santos, I.; Umbuzeiro, G.d.A.; Fagnani, E. Occurrence and risk assessment of organophosphate esters in urban rivers from Piracicaba watershed (Brazil). *Environ. Sci. Pollut. Res.* **2021**, *28*, 59244–59255. [CrossRef] [PubMed]
8. Lao, J.-Y.; Lin, H.; Qin, X.; Ruan, Y.; Leung, K.M.; Zeng, E.Y.; Lam, P.K. Insights into the atmospheric persistence, transformation, and health implications of organophosphate esters in urban ambient air. *Environ. Sci. Technol.* **2022**, *56*, 12003–12013. [CrossRef] [PubMed]
9. Suhring, R.; Diamond, M.L.; Scheringer, M.; Wong, F.; Pucko, M.; Stern, G.; Burt, A.; Hung, H.; Fellin, P.; Li, H. Organophosphate esters in Canadian Arctic air: Occurrence, levels and trends. *Environ. Sci. Technol.* **2016**, *50*, 7409–7415. [CrossRef] [PubMed]
10. Tao, F.; Sellström, U.; De Wit, C.A. Organohalogenated flame retardants and organophosphate esters in office air and dust from Sweden. *Environ. Sci. Technol.* **2019**, *53*, 2124–2133. [CrossRef]
11. Yadav, I.C.; Devi, N.L.; Zhong, G.; Li, J.; Zhang, G.; Covaci, A. Occurrence and fate of organophosphate ester flame retardants and plasticizers in indoor air and dust of Nepal: Implication for human exposure. *Environ. Pollut.* **2017**, *229*, 668–678. [CrossRef] [PubMed]
12. Li, W.; Shi, Y.; Gao, L.; Wu, C.; Liu, J.; Cai, Y. Occurrence, distribution and risk of organophosphate esters in urban road dust in Beijing, China. *Environ. Pollut.* **2018**, *241*, 566–575. [CrossRef] [PubMed]

13. Liao, C.; Kim, U.-J.; Kannan, K. Occurrence and distribution of organophosphate esters in sediment from northern Chinese coastal waters. *Sci. Total Environ.* **2020**, *704*, 135328. [CrossRef] [PubMed]
14. Cui, K.; Wen, J.; Zeng, F.; Li, S.; Zhou, X.; Zeng, Z. Occurrence and distribution of organophosphate esters in urban soils of the subtropical city, Guangzhou, China. *Chemosphere* **2017**, *175*, 514–520. [CrossRef] [PubMed]
15. Wang, Y.; Yao, Y.; Li, W.; Zhu, H.; Wang, L.; Sun, H.; Kannan, K. A nationwide survey of 19 organophosphate esters in soils from China: Spatial distribution and hazard assessment. *Sci. Total Environ.* **2019**, *671*, 528–535. [CrossRef] [PubMed]
16. Han, L.; Sapozhnikova, Y.; Nuñez, A. Analysis and occurrence of organophosphate esters in meats and fish consumed in the United States. *J. Agric. Food Chem.* **2019**, *67*, 12652–12662. [CrossRef] [PubMed]
17. Pantelaki, I.; Voutsa, D. Occurrence, analysis and risk assessment of organophosphate esters (OPEs) in biota: A review. *Mar. Pollut. Bull.* **2020**, *160*, 111547. [CrossRef]
18. Zeng, X.; Liu, Z.; He, L.; Cao, S.; Song, H.; Yu, Z.; Sheng, G.; Fu, J. The occurrence and removal of organophosphate ester flame retardants/plasticizers in a municipal wastewater treatment plant in the Pearl River Delta, China. *J. Environ. Sci. Health Part A-Toxic/Hazard. Subst. Environ. Eng.* **2015**, *50*, 1291–1297. [CrossRef]
19. Lian, M.; Lin, C.; Li, Y.; Hao, X.; Wang, A.; He, M.; Liu, X.; Ouyang, W. Distribution, partitioning, and health risk assessment of organophosphate esters in a major tributary of middle Yangtze River using Monte Carlo simulation. *Water Res.* **2022**, *219*, 118559. [CrossRef]
20. Kim, U.-J.; Oh, J.K.; Kannan, K. Occurrence, removal, and environmental emission of organophosphate flame retardants/plasticizers in a wastewater treatment plant in New York State. *Environ. Sci. Technol.* **2017**, *51*, 7872–7880. [CrossRef]
21. Iqbal, M.; Syed, J.H.; Katsoyiannis, A.; Malik, R.N.; Farooqi, A.; Butt, A.; Li, J.; Zhang, G.; Cincinelli, A.; Jones, K.C. Legacy and emerging flame retardants (FRs) in the freshwater ecosystem: A review. *Environ. Res.* **2017**, *152*, 26–42. [CrossRef] [PubMed]
22. Yin, H.; Luo, Y.; Song, J.; Li, S.; Lin, S.; Xiong, Y.; Fang, S.; Tang, J. Pollution characteristics and emissions of typical organophosphate esters of a wastewater treatment plant. *Environ. Sci. Pollut. Res.* **2022**, *29*, 25892–25901. [CrossRef] [PubMed]
23. Cristale, J.; Ramos, D.D.; Dantas, R.F.; Junior, A.M.; Lacorte, S.; Sans, C.; Esplugas, S. Can activated sludge treatments and advanced oxidation processes remove organophosphorus flame retardants? *Environ. Res.* **2016**, *144*, 11–18. [CrossRef] [PubMed]
24. Pang, L.; Yang, P.; Zhao, J.; Zhang, H. Comparison of wastewater treatment processes on the removal efficiency of organophosphate esters. *Water Sci. Technol.* **2016**, *74*, 1602–1609. [CrossRef]
25. Liang, K.; Liu, J. Understanding the distribution, degradation and fate of organophosphate esters in an advanced municipal sewage treatment plant based on mass flow and mass balance analysis. *Sci. Total Environ.* **2016**, *544*, 262–270. [CrossRef] [PubMed]
26. Pantelaki, I.; Voutsa, D. Occurrence and removal of organophosphate esters in municipal wastewater treatment plants in Thessaloniki, Greece. *Environ. Res.* **2022**, *214*, 113908. [CrossRef] [PubMed]
27. Zhang, D.; Li, S.; Zhu, F.; Li, C.; Xu, Y.; Qing, D.; Wang, J. The influence of an upgrade on the reduction of organophosphate flame retardants in a wastewater treatment plant. *Chemosphere* **2020**, *256*, 126895. [CrossRef] [PubMed]
28. Wang, S.; Qian, J.; Zhang, B.; Chen, L.; Wei, S.; Pan, B. Unveiling the Occurrence and Potential Ecological Risks of Organophosphate Esters in Municipal Wastewater Treatment Plants across China. *Environ. Sci. Technol.* **2023**, *57*, 1907–1918. [CrossRef] [PubMed]
29. Lian, M.; Wang, J.; Wang, B.; Xin, M.; Lin, C.; Gu, X.; He, M.; Liu, X.; Ouyang, W. Spatiotemporal variations and the ecological risks of organophosphate esters in Laizhou Bay waters between 2019 and 2021: Implying the impacts of the COVID-19 pandemic. *Water Res.* **2023**, *233*, 119783. [CrossRef]
30. Rodríguez, I.; Calvo, F.; Quintana, J.; Rubi, E.; Rodil, R.; Cela, R. Suitability of solid-phase microextraction for the determination of organophosphate flame retardants and plasticizers in water samples. *J. Chromatogr. A* **2006**, *1108*, 158–165. [CrossRef]
31. Rodil, R.; Quintana, J.B.; Reemtsma, T. Liquid chromatography–tandem mass spectrometry determination of nonionic organophosphorus flame retardants and plasticizers in wastewater samples. *Anal. Chem.* **2005**, *77*, 3083–3089. [CrossRef] [PubMed]
32. Pang, L.; Yuan, Y.; He, H.; Liang, K.; Zhang, H.; Zhao, J. Occurrence, distribution, and potential affecting factors of organophosphate flame retardants in sewage sludge of wastewater treatment plants in Henan Province, Central China. *Chemosphere* **2016**, *152*, 245–251. [CrossRef]
33. Marklund, A.; Andersson, B.; Haglund, P. Organophosphorus flame retardants and plasticizers in Swedish sewage treatment plants. *Environ. Sci. Technol.* **2005**, *39*, 7423–7429. [CrossRef] [PubMed]
34. Xu, L.; Hu, Q.; Liu, J.; Liu, S.; Liu, C.; Deng, Q.; Zeng, X.; Yu, Z. Occurrence of organophosphate esters and their diesters degradation products in industrial wastewater treatment plants in China: Implication for the usage and potential degradation during production processing. *Environ. Pollut.* **2019**, *250*, 559–566. [CrossRef]
35. Sun, J.; Liu, Q.; Zhang, R.; Xing, L. Organophosphate esters in rural wastewater along the Yangtze River Basin: Occurrence, removal efficiency and environmental implications. *J. Environ. Manag.* **2023**, *345*, 118830. [CrossRef]
36. Su, G.; Letcher, R.J.; Yu, H. Organophosphate flame retardants and plasticizers in aqueous solution: pH-dependent hydrolysis, kinetics, and pathways. *Environ. Sci. Technol.* **2016**, *50*, 8103–8111. [CrossRef]
37. Rodil, R.; Quintana, J.B.; López-Mahía, P.; Muniategui-Lorenzo, S.; Prada-Rodríguez, D. Multi-residue analytical method for the determination of emerging pollutants in water by solid-phase extraction and liquid chromatography–tandem mass spectrometry. *J. Chromatogr. A* **2009**, *1216*, 2958–2969. [CrossRef] [PubMed]
38. Hahladakis, J.N.; Velis, C.A.; Weber, R.; Iacovidou, E.; Purnell, P. An overview of chemical additives present in plastics: Migration, release, fate and environmental impact during their use, disposal and recycling. *J. Hazard. Mater.* **2018**, *344*, 179–199. [CrossRef]

39. Cristale, J.; Dantas, R.F.; De Luca, A.; Sans, C.; Esplugas, S.; Lacorte, S. Role of oxygen and DOM in sunlight induced photodegradation of organophosphorous flame retardants in river water. *J. Hazard. Mater.* **2017**, *323*, 242–249. [CrossRef]
40. O'Brien, J.W.; Thai, P.K.; Brandsma, S.H.; Leonards, P.E.; Ort, C.; Mueller, J.F. Wastewater analysis of Census day samples to investigate per capita input of organophosphorus flame retardants and plasticizers into wastewater. *Chemosphere* **2015**, *138*, 328–334. [CrossRef]
41. Xing, R.; Zhang, P.; Zheng, N.; Ji, H.; Shi, R.; Ge, L.; Ma, H. Organophosphate esters in the seawater of the Bohai Sea: Environmental occurrence, sources and ecological risks. *Mar. Pollut. Bull.* **2023**, *191*, 114883. [CrossRef] [PubMed]
42. Verbruggen, E.; Rila, J.; Traas, T.; Posthuma-Doodeman, C.; Posthumus, R. *Environmental Risk Limits for Several Phosphate Esters, with Possible Application as Flame Retardant*; RIVM Rapport 601501024; National Institute for Public Health and the Environment: Bilthoven, The Netherlands, 2006.
43. NORMAN. NORMAN Ecotoxicology Database—Lowest PNECs. 2022. Available online: https://www.norman-network.com/nds/ecotox/lowestPnecsIndex.php (accessed on 1 May 2024).
44. Lian, M.; Lin, C.; Wu, T.; Xin, M.; Gu, X.; Lu, S.; Cao, Y.; Wang, B.; Ouyang, W.; Liu, X. Occurrence, spatiotemporal distribution, and ecological risks of organophosphate esters in the water of the Yellow River to the Laizhou Bay, Bohai Sea. *Sci. Total Environ.* **2021**, *787*, 147528. [CrossRef] [PubMed]
45. Liu, Y.; Song, N.; Guo, R.; Xu, H.; Zhang, Q.; Han, Z.; Feng, M.; Li, D.; Zhang, S.; Chen, J. Occurrence and partitioning behavior of organophosphate esters in surface water and sediment of a shallow Chinese freshwater lake (Taihu Lake): Implication for eco-toxicity risk. *Chemosphere* **2018**, *202*, 255–263. [CrossRef] [PubMed]
46. European Commission. *European Union Risk Assessment Report: Tris (2-chloroethyl) Phosphate, TCEP*; European Commission: Luxembourg, 2009.
47. Shi, Y.; Gao, L.; Li, W.; Wang, Y.; Liu, J.; Cai, Y. Occurrence, distribution and seasonal variation of organophosphate flame retardants and plasticizers in urban surface water in Beijing, China. *Environ. Pollut.* **2016**, *209*, 1–10. [CrossRef]
48. Green, N.; Schlabach, M.; Bakke, T.; Brevik, E.; Dye, C.; Herzke, D.; Huber, S.; Plosz, B.; Remberger, M.; Schøyen, M. *Screening of Selected Metals and New Organic Contaminants 2007. Phosphorus Flame Retardents, Polyfluorinated Organic Compounds, Nitro-PAHs, Silver, Platinum and Sucralose in Air, Wastewater Treatment Falcilities, and Freshwater and Marine Recipients*; Norsk Institutt for Vannforskning: Oslo, Norway, 2008.

water

MDPI

Article

Research on Intelligent Chemical Dosing System for Phosphorus Removal in Wastewater Treatment Plants

Xi Lu [1,2], Song Huang [1], Haichen Liu [1,*], Fengwei Yang [1], Ting Zhang [1] and Xinyu Wan [3]

1 Shanghai Investigation, Design and Research Institute Co., Ltd., No. 65 Linxin Road, Changning District, Shanghai 200050, China; lu_xi1@ctg.com.cn (X.L.); huang_song1@ctg.com.cn (S.H.); yang_fengwei@ctg.com.cn (F.Y.); zhang_ting1@ctg.com.cn (T.Z.)

2 Three Gorges Smart Water Technology Co., Ltd., No. 65 Linxin Road, Changning District, Shanghai 200050, China

3 YANGTZE Eco-Environment Engineering Research Center, China Three Gorges Corporation, No. 234 Yanjiang Avenue, Jiang'an District, Wuhan 430010, China; wan_xinyu@ctg.com.cn

* Correspondence: liu_haichen@ctg.com.cn

Abstract: Whether the phosphorus removal chemical in wastewater treatment plants (WWTPs) can be accurately dosed not only affects the compliance of the effluent total phosphorus but also has a huge impact on sludge production and energy consumption during the wastewater treatment process. For the effluent from the secondary sedimentation tank of a wastewater treatment plant in southern China, based on experimental screening of the optimal pH value, chemical types and concentrations of chemicals, coagulation time, etc., a dynamic dosage prediction feedforward model for chemical phosphorus removal agents in the effluent from the secondary sedimentation tank of the WWTPs was developed to predict the most economical dosage of the chemicals. Meanwhile, combined with the adaptive fuzzy neural network P feedback control algorithm, dynamic real-time control of chemical dosing was achieved. Through micro-control design, a software model for signal collection and feedback in a specific phosphorus removal scenario was formed, and an automatic control system for chemical dosing was ultimately developed for a WWTP in a city in southern China. After stable operation for two months, the system achieved a 100% compliance rate for effluent total phosphorus (TP) concentration and a 67% improvement in effluent stability, helping the wastewater treatment plant achieve stable and precise control of the phosphorus removal process in the secondary sedimentation tank effluent, which is conducive to further promoting its implementation of low-carbon pathways.

Keywords: wastewater treatment plant; phosphorus removal; prediction model; intelligent chemical dosing

1. Introduction

For a long time, phosphorus has been one of the focal points in wastewater treatment plants (WWTPs). However, phosphorus removal in wastewater is a complex process, involving multiple operational units such as biological tanks and secondary sedimentation tanks [1]. This complexity arises from a multitude of influencing variables, making it difficult to achieve desired phosphorus removal outcomes [2]. Due to often insufficient biological phosphorus removal efficiency, recent years have seen widespread scholarly attention towards chemically-based methods for controlling effluent total phosphorus [3–6]. These methods primarily involve the addition of metal salts to the aerobic zone to induce particle precipitation, achieving phosphorus removal by discharging excess sludge containing particulate phosphorus [7–9]. However, the effectiveness of this method is influenced by factors such as pH, temperature, and redox conditions [10,11], as the metal salts added to the wastewater participate in both precipitation and chemical coagulation reactions [12]. Consequently, current chemical phosphorus removal in WWTPs often relies heavily on the empirical experience of operators, resulting in excessive dosing of metal coagulants [13]. Nevertheless, studies indicate that with increasing doses of metal salts for chemical phosphorus removal, the residual phosphorus concentration in the wastewater gradually decreases, but this relationship is not linear [14,15]. Excessive dosage of agents increases sludge production, leading to increased carbon emissions during sludge treatment and disposal processes [14,16]. The control of phosphorus removal chemical dosage directly affects whether effluent water quality meets discharge standards and corresponding energy saving and carbon emission reduction, making it one of the urgent research directions in wastewater treatment plants.

With the rapid development of data acquisition techniques and intelligent control technologies in wastewater treatment processes [13], research on intelligent methods for controlling effluent total phosphorus (TP) has been widely conducted [17–19]. However, many current intelligent control strategies for effluent TP still face issues such as considering limited variables that affect phosphorus removal efficiency and poor phosphorus removal performance [20,21]. Therefore, how to design an effective controller, in consideration of both the mechanism of the chemical phosphorus removal process and the comprehensive influencing factors during the process, remains a challenging issue [22]. Adaptive control and predictive control are based on the construction of accurate mathematical models for controlled systems, thus the methodology depends heavily on the quality of the simulated system and can only achieve good performance when the model variation is small or the model operates under stable conditions [23,24]. Fuzzy control, independent of precise mathematical models, exhibits higher robustness [25]. Proportional integral derivative (PID) controllers are the most commonly used controllers in the industry [26], being simple, widely applicable, and providing performance close to optimal [27]. However, choosing suitable PID gains for nonlinear systems is still challenging, and traditional PID controllers act poorly with significant time delays [28–30]. Therefore, an adaptive fuzzy neural network PID controller is proposed in this study.

This paper focuses on the mathematical model of chemical dosing and designs a feedforward and feedback regulation system based on the adaptive PID control theory. An automatic control system for phosphorus removal chemical dosing was developed for a WWTP in a southern city in China. The goal of the system was to predict effluent quality based on real-time online monitoring data, adjust operational parameters promptly, and ultimately achieve fully automatic control of stable effluent TP, promoting the development of urban wastewater treatment plants towards energy-saving and carbon emission reduction. The novelty of the chemical phosphorus removal model combining feedforward and feedback control strategies lies in its integrated use of both control strategies to enhance the system's control accuracy and adaptability. Firstly, the model used in this paper can improve simulation accuracy, the feedforward control can predict and compensate for upcoming changes, while the feedback control can correct errors that have already occurred. When used in combination, they can more precisely control the dosage of chemical reagents. Secondly, the model has strong adaptability. By monitoring data in real-time, the system can promptly respond to changes in water quality, automatically adjust operational parameters, and enhance the system's adaptability and robustness. Moreover, this controller combines the learning capability of neural networks with the reasoning capability of fuzzy logic to handle uncertainty and nonlinearity in the wastewater treatment process.

2. Materials and Methods

2.1. Overview of the Case WWTP Process

A WWTP in southern China is designed with a capacity of 70,000 m^3/d and serves an area of 45.36 km^2 and a population of 0.25 million people. The main process adopts a modified Anaerobic-Anoxic-Oxic (AAO) process (as shown in Figure 1). The tertiary treatment includes a high-efficiency sedimentation tank and a cloth-media filter. Polyaluminum chloride (PAC) (Baore Chemical Co., Ltd., Nanjing, China), magnetic powder, and polyacrylamide (PAM) are dosed, with dosing points located at the high-efficiency sedimentation tank. The effluent quality meets the Class A standard of the "Discharge standard of pollutants for municipal wastewater treatment plant" (GB18918-2002) [31]. According to the operating data of the WWTPs in the past three years (Table 1), the actual biological phosphorus removal efficiency was 50–55%, and the TP concentration in the effluent of the secondary sedimentation tank fluctuated between 1.2–1.8 mg/L. To achieve the final goal of the Class A discharge standard (TP $\leq$ 0.5 mg/L), the current semi-manual chemical dosing system suffers from unstable pre-biological treatment and requires more advanced control strategies.

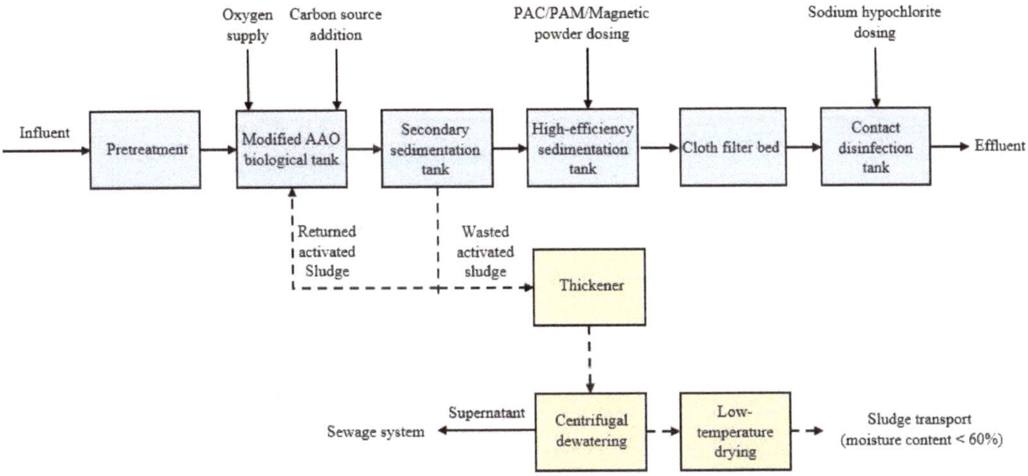

Figure 1. Process flow diagram of the case WWTP.

Table 1. Wastewater quality indicators.

Water Quality Parameters		COD (mg/L)	BOD_5 (mg/L)	SS (mg/L)	NH_4-N (mg/L)	TN (mg/L)	TP (mg/L)
Influent	Design value	240	120	200	35	30	3.5
	Actual value	93~197	56~107	34~93	13~25	7~21	2.6~3.3
Effluent	Discharge standard	40	10	10	35	5(8)	0.5
	Actual value	5~11	1~1.14	2.7~4.2	5~10	0.13~0.42	1.2~1.8

Currently, only the TP online monitoring equipment (Endress+Hauser China, Shanghai, China) is installed at the influent and effluent points of the plant, lacking process phosphorus monitoring. This inability to grasp the phosphorus fluctuation in the effluent of the secondary sedimentation tank in good time leads to the inability to accurately adjust and control the dosing system. It is preliminarily believed that there is excessive dosing of PAC.

2.2. Pilot-Scale Experimental Setup

The pilot-scale high-efficiency sedimentation reactor has four systems, i.e., the coagulation and precipitation system, sludge recirculation system, chemical dosing and control system, and online monitoring and control system (Figure 2). The coagulation and precipitation system is primarily designed based on the existing high-efficiency sedimentation tank (scaled down by 1:1000), with an influent flowrate of 35 m^3/d. Its internal structure comprises a primary coagulation zone, secondary coagulation zone, flocculation zone, and sedimentation zone. The sludge recirculation system transports a portion of sludge from the bottom of the sludge zone to the coagulation zone using a peristaltic pump

(Chongqing Jieheng Peristaltic Pump Co., Ltd., Chongqing, China), while the remaining sludge is discharged externally by another peristaltic pump. The chemical dosing and control system consists of two chemical-dissolving buckets, two gear flow meters (Shanghai Cixi Instrument Co. Ltd., Shanghai, China), two diaphragm metering pumps (NEWDOSE, Beijing, China), and other accessories, e.g., dampers, and back pressure regulators. All the electronic components (devices, instruments, and accessories) are connected to the online monitoring and control system. The online monitoring and control system includes a local power distribution and control cabinet, a remote server and a web/mobile interactive interface. It is able to collect and upload (1) local/remote control status, (2) all the device and instrument working status and alarm signals, (3) influent flowrate and valve opening, (4) influent and effluent phosphate (PO_4^{3-}), pH and temperature, (5) chemical dosing flowrate, (6) returned and wasted chemical sludge flowrates, (7) stirring speeds of five mixers. Furthermore, it could also remotely set the stirring speeds, flowrates and valve opening, as well as switch on/off the devices and clean faults. Two phosphate analyzers (Shandong Greencare Precision Instrument Co., Ltd., Shandong, China) employ the spectrophotometric determination of phosphate by the molybdenum blue method specified in GB11893-89 [32] and HJ670-2013 [33]. The phosphate is automatically sampled and detected every 40 min.

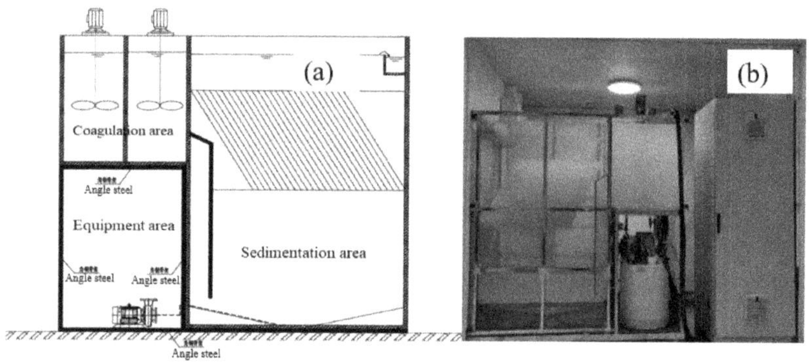

Figure 2. High-efficiency sedimentation tank, (**a**) cross-sectional view, (**b**) photo of the pilot set.

2.3. Pilot-Scale Experimental Plan

A series of accompanying pilot-scale experiments were performed by using the actual effluent from the secondary clarifier of the case WWTP. The pilot influent TP ranged from 0.62 to 1.88 mg/L in 2022 and 2023. The concentrated PAC liquid (2.5%) was made by adding 4.17 kg of PAC solid powder (30%) into the 50 L bucker with a stirring speed of 70 r/min. During the experimental period, only PAC was used as the phosphorus removal agent, without the addition of magnetite powder and PAM. The experiments are divided into four stages: (1) trial operation stage (I), (2) constant dosing stage (II), (3) feedforward dosing stage (III), and (4) adaptive feedforward-feedback dosing stage (IV).

3. Optimization of Chemical Selection and Initial Dosing Amount

3.1. Laboratory Test for Chemical Selection

In order to test the phosphorus removal performance for four commonly used agents (PAC, $FeCl_3$, polyaluminium ferric chloride (PAFC), and polysilicate aluminum ferric (PSAF)), solutions with different mass concentrations (20 mg/L, 40 mg/L, 60 mg/L, 80 mg/L, 120 mg/L, 160 mg/L, and 200 mg/L) were prepared, respectively. The results indicated that: (1) at low concentrations ($\leq$60 mg/L), the phosphorus removal rate is proportional to the dosage concentration; (2) at the same concentration, the phosphorus removal effectiveness is in the order of $FeCl_3$, PSAF, PAC, and PAFC. However, due to increased effluent turbidity caused by $FeCl_3$ and the high price of PSAF, PAC was finally chosen as the phosphorus removal chemical for this study, which is consistent with the phosphorus removal chemical used in the case WWTP. More details about these experiments can be found in [34].

3.2. Determination of the Optimal Dosage for Pilot-Scale Chemical

During the constant dosing stage (II), the effective PAC dosage was gradually increased (4, 6, 8, 10, 12 mg Al_2O_3/L), and the influent PO_4^{3-} concentration (actual effluent from the secondary sedimentation tank) fluctuated between 0.8–1.2 mg/L (Figure 3). As the dosing concentration increased, the effluent PO_4^{3-} concentration gradually decreased, and the phosphate removal amount increased. However, due to the limited height of the pilot reactor, the absence of magnetite powder and PAM, and the lack of a post-filtration device, the increase in suspended solids caused by sludge flotation would affect the effluent PO_4^{3-} concentration, resulting in slightly lower dosing efficiency of the pilot reactor compared to the actual tank. To achieve the Class A standard for effluent TP, the dosage concentration of the pilot reactor needs to reach 8–10 mg Al_2O_3/L. With the stepwise increase in the dosing concentrations, the effluent PO_4^{3-} concentrations varied from 0.6 to 0.2 mg P/L. During the whole experimental period, the influent pH was maintained between 6.24~7.24, and the effluent pH was maintained between 6.21~7.27 without pH adjustment.

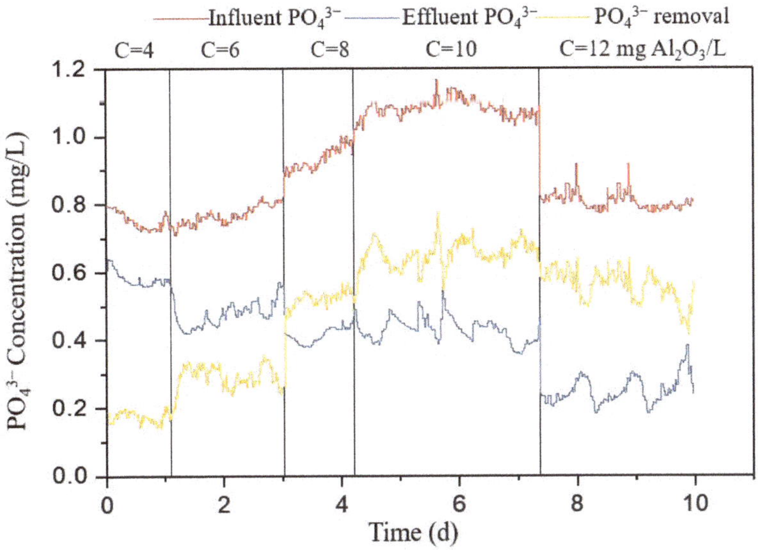

Figure 3. Performance of the pilot-scale setup at different dosing concentrations.

4. Feedforward–Feedback Compound Control Model for Phosphorus Removal Agent Dosage

4.1. Feedforward Dosage Model

When the phosphorus removal agent is PAC ($Al_n(OH)_mCl_{3n-m}$, with effective substance calculated as Al_2O_3), the reaction between PAC and PO_4^{3-} is described as follows [35]:

$$Al_2(OH)_4^{2+} + H_nPO_4^{(3-n)-} \rightarrow Al_2(OH)_3PO_4 \downarrow + (n-1)H^+ \quad (1)$$

The dosage of PAC is mainly influenced by wastewater components, the relative concentration of metal salts and phosphate ions, and the type of phosphate ions, pH, and other ligands such as sulfates, carbonates, fluorides, and organic matter. When the Al/P molar ratio is slightly higher than the stoichiometric coefficient, the dosage is linearly related to the effluent PO_4^{3-} concentration. However, when the Al/P molar ratio is far higher than the stoichiometric coefficient, excessive aluminum could form aluminum hydroxide precipitate at the same time. If pH is not corrected in advance, increasing the dosage of metal salt coagulants will further lower the pH of the sewage, forming soluble complexes such as $AlH_2PO_4^{2+}$, and thus leading to a rapid increase in PO_4^{3-} concentration after an initial decrease.

In the previous studies, the commonly used empirical formulas to describe the relationship between dosage and PO_4^{3-} concentration are mostly investigated under relatively high effluent PO_4^{3-} concentrations, rather than under low effluent PO_4^{3-} concentrations. The empirical formulas that solely consider chemical precipitation will significantly underestimate the total chemical dosage, especially when the effluent PO_4^{3-} concentration is relatively low. However, although both the adsorption mechanism and chemical precipitation mechanism are considered, the above-mentioned mechanisms could not be differentiated from other processes such as ion exchange, surface complexation of phosphates and metal hydroxide colloids. Furthermore, if PAC is overdosed, the mechanism of the reaction would change and further lead to a decrease in the model accuracy.

During this study, the pH range of the influent and effluent was relatively stable and within the optimal pH range for aluminum coagulant-based phosphorus removal. Therefore, the influence of pH could be ignored and the relationship between phosphate removal and dosage concentration is established as shown in Figure 4.

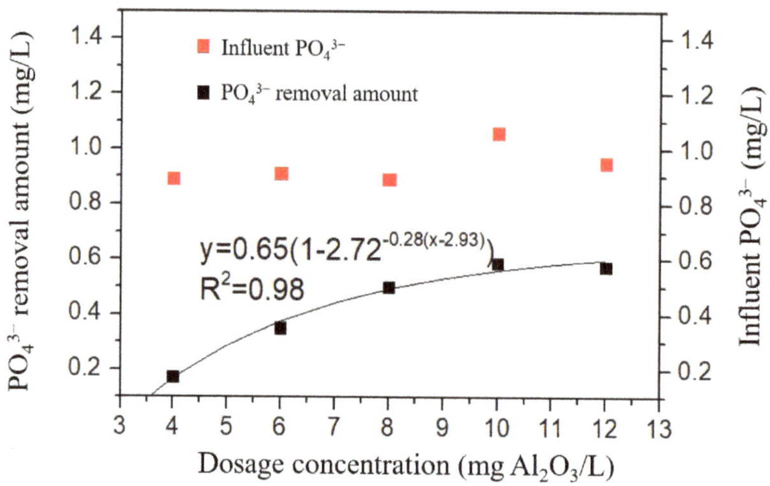

Figure 4. Effects of PAC dosage concentration on phosphorus removal performance.

The original dosage model (Equation (2)) adjusts the dosage based on the influent flowrate at a certain dosage concentration. It enables timely adjustments of the dosage amount according to the changes in the influent flowrate, making it a relatively simple and direct feedforward control method. However, if the influent PO_4^{3-} concentration varies in a wider range, a fixed value for the dosage rate could not react sufficiently and needs to be adjusted based on experience and expertise. Further modifications are needed to decide the dosage concentration C to work under more comprehensive conditions.

$$q_c = \frac{QC}{\rho w_c} \quad (2)$$

where:

q_c represents the instantaneous flowrate of the coagulant, measured in mL/h;
Q represents the influent flowrate, measured in L/h;
C represents the dosage concentration of the coagulant in water, measured in g/m^3;
ρ represents the density of the coagulant, which is 1000 kg/m^3;
w_c represents the effective content of the coagulant, which is 2.5%.

Based on the relationship between the dosage concentration C and the phosphate removal Figure 4, the following equation is established:

$$C = 2.93 - \frac{1}{0.27} \times \ln\left(1 - \frac{\Delta TP}{0.65}\right) \tag{3}$$

Finally, the feedforward equation is established as follows:

$$q_c = \frac{Q}{\rho w_c} \cdot \left(2.93 - \frac{1}{0.27} \times \ln\left(1 - \frac{P_i - P_{eset}}{0.65}\right)\right) \tag{4}$$

where:

P_i represents the inflow $PO_4{}^{3-}$ concentration, measured in g/m^3;

P_{eset} represents the setpoint value of the effluent $PO_4{}^{3-}$ concentration, measured in g/m^3.

4.2. Adaptive Fuzzy Neural Network P Feedback Controller

In order to achieve precise control of effluent $PO_4{}^{3-}$ under complex environmental conditions and ensure stable and safe compliance with effluent TP standards, a new adaptive fuzzy neural network P feedback control system is developed (Figure 5). The proposed controller comprises a neural network and fuzzy feedback control. The neural network uses an adaptive algorithm to tune the dosing rules in the fuzzy interface.

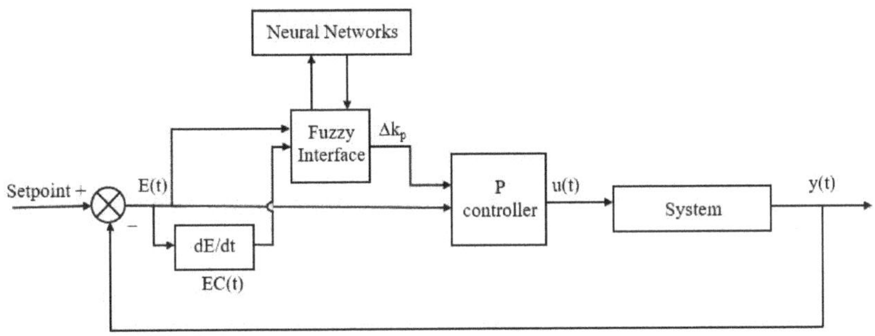

Figure 5. Adaptive fuzzy neural network P feedback control system structure for chemical phosphorus removal.

The fuzzy interface utilized a Mamdani-type fuzzy controller as the core controller. In the Mamdani-fuzzy controller, the trigonometric functions are used as membership functions, and error (e) and error rate (ec) are controller inputs. Fuzzy reasoning is employed to infer the correction amount for the P controller parameter ΔK_P (proportional gain).

The neural network was employed to tune the dosing rules of the phosphorus removal agent (shape of membership functions), i.e., the center points of the membership functions, width vectors, and connection weights of the output layer. This system combines the learning capability of neural networks with the reasoning capability of fuzzy logic, enabling better handling of uncertainty and nonlinearity. Through this system, controller parameters can be dynamically adjusted based on real-time and historical data to adapt to continuously changing environmental conditions, achieving precise control of effluent TP.

5. Application of Intelligent Chemical Dosing Control System in Case WWTP

5.1. System Design

The system architecture is an advanced wastewater treatment solution that integrates real-time monitoring, data analysis, autonomous learning, and intelligent control, focusing on efficiently removing phosphorus from wastewater (Figure 6). By deploying various monitoring devices, the system collects key parameters in real-time, such as the influent flowrates, influent and effluent PO_4^{3-} for feedforward and feedback control, and utilizes the cloud server for data processing and model analysis. The intelligent control system adjusts the dosage of chemicals every minute through dosing pumps with frequency converter based on the results of data analysis, optimizing both biological phosphorus removal and chemical phosphorus removal processes. The whole system covers the entire process from AAO biological tanks to disinfection, ensuring the efficiency and stability of wastewater treatment. Additionally, it possesses autonomous learning capabilities to adapt to different operating conditions and changes in water quality, thereby contributing to environmental protection.

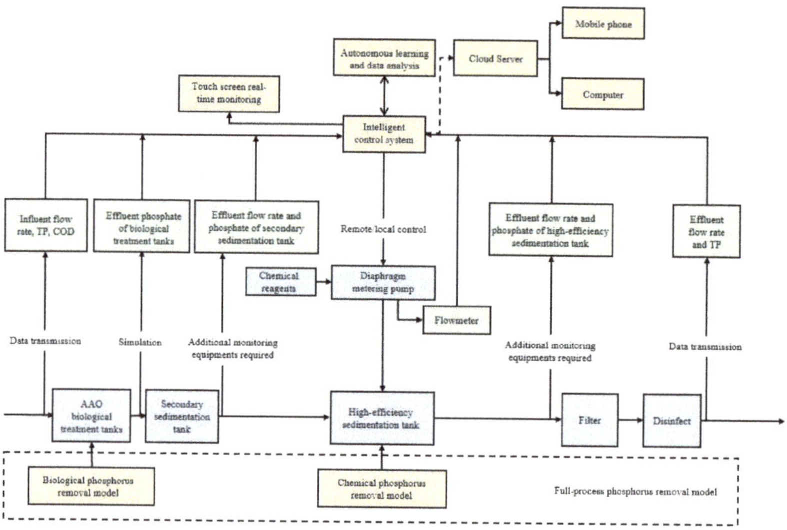

Figure 6. Chemical phosphorus removal intelligent control design structure.

5.2. Implementation of Application Interfaces

The system, developed using C#, encompasses a comprehensive suite of features that cater to the needs of modern WWTPs. It includes both web and mobile interfaces that provide a range of functionalities such as displaying key monitoring indicators, alerting users to equipment malfunctions, enabling remote control, and offering data analysis capabilities. The following is a breakdown of the system's components and their roles:

Step 1 Initialization of configuration files

Set up the necessary configuration settings that the system requires to operate. This includes parameters for device communication, user access, and system preferences.

Step 2. Initialization of database

Prepare the database for storing and retrieving data. This is crucial for maintaining records of operational metrics, system logs, and historical data for analysis.

Step 3. Initialization of WebSocket (WS) and Message Queuing Telemetry Transport (MQTT) task processors

These protocols are used for real-time, bi-directional communication between the server and clients. WS is often used for web applications, while MQTT is a lightweight messaging protocol ideal for IoT devices.

Step 4. Starting MQTT server

The MQTT server is launched to handle the publish/subscribe messaging pattern, allowing the system to efficiently distribute messages to different parts of the infrastructure.

Step 5. Starting WS server

The WS server is initiated to provide a full-duplex communication channel over a single long-lived connection, which is particularly useful for real-time data transmission.

Step 6. Starting HTTP server

The HTTP server is started to manage web requests and responses, allowing users to interact with the system via web browsers.

Step 7. Alarm data change notifications

The system is designed to alert users when there are significant changes in alarm data, such as critical equipment failures or breaches in operational parameters.

Step 8. Real-time monitoring of key indicators

Users can view real-time data for various operational indicators, providing immediate insights into the plant's performance.

Step 9. Real-time value upload for indicators

The system supports the continuous upload of real-time values for the monitored indicators, ensuring that the latest data are always available for analysis.

Step 10. Remote control

Allows users to remotely control equipment and processes within the plant, enabling adjustments to be made from a distance.

Step 11. Control reply

After a remote control command is issued, the system provides feedback to confirm the execution of the command and to report any status changes.

5.3. Implementation of an Upper Computer Program

The system, implemented in Python 3.7, includes a variety of intelligent control and data management functions, specifically:

Step 1. Local control

Allows the system to directly control devices within the local network, reducing latency and improving response speed.

Step 2. Remote data upload

The switch and analog data obtained from the device can be uploaded remotely to a central database for centralized management and analysis.

Step 3. Remote control

Enables control of the device over the internet or a dedicated network, without geographical limitations.

Step 4. Automatic chemical dosing algorithm

The system automatically adjusts the amount of chemicals added based on real-time data, optimizing the treatment process for improved efficiency and accuracy.

Key components and workflow of the system are as follows:

Step 1. Modbus RTU connection: Establishes a connection with local devices via the Modbus RTU protocol for real-time monitoring and control.

Step 2. Data acquisition and device control: After obtaining switch and analog data from the device, the system can perform corresponding control operations.

Step 3. Database storage: The acquired device data are stored in a database for historical records, trend analysis, and fault diagnosis.

Step 4. Scheduled data upload: The system automatically uploads data every full hour to ensure continuity and completeness of the data.

Step 5. Remote monitoring program

- Initializes MQTT client: Sets up the MQTT protocol client for communication with remote devices or servers.
- Sets Connection information: Configures connection parameters for the MQTT client, such as server address, port, and client ID.
- Subscribes on connection: Automatically subscribes to relevant topics upon successful connection to receive control messages.
- Parses information and controls devices: Parses receive information and execute corresponding device control commands based on the parsed results.

Step 6. Automatic chemical dosing calculation

The system runs the automatic chemical dosing algorithm on a separate thread, calculating and adjusting the amount of chemicals added based on real-time monitoring data, achieving automatic control.

5.4. Implementation of Dosing Algorithm Program

In the feedforward control stage, the algorithm utilizes real-time data monitoring to predict and adjust the dosage in advance to anticipate changes in water quality. The feedforward algorithms could be switched based on whether the following data could be acquired and trusted, including the influent flowrate, influent and effluent TP or PO_4^{3-} concentrations. Additionally, the system can calculate the treatment capacity of the reagents in real time and dynamically adjust the dosage according to actual conditions to achieve optimal phosphorus removal performance.

In the feedback control stage, the algorithm sets multiple control objectives and corresponding proportional gain variations (ΔKp) based on fuzzy logic control, which are used to implement graded feedback control according to different treatment stages.

In this system (Figure 7), besides precise operations in the feedforward and feedback control stages, neural network technology is introduced to optimize fuzzy logic control rules, further enhancing phosphorus removal efficiency. During the training process, the neural network continuously adjusts the weights and biases in the network through forward and backward propagation algorithms to minimize the error between the actual output and the desired output. Through this learning process, the neural network can automatically adjust key parameters such as the proportional gain variation (ΔKp) and membership functions in the fuzzy controller to adapt to changing water quality conditions and treatment requirements.

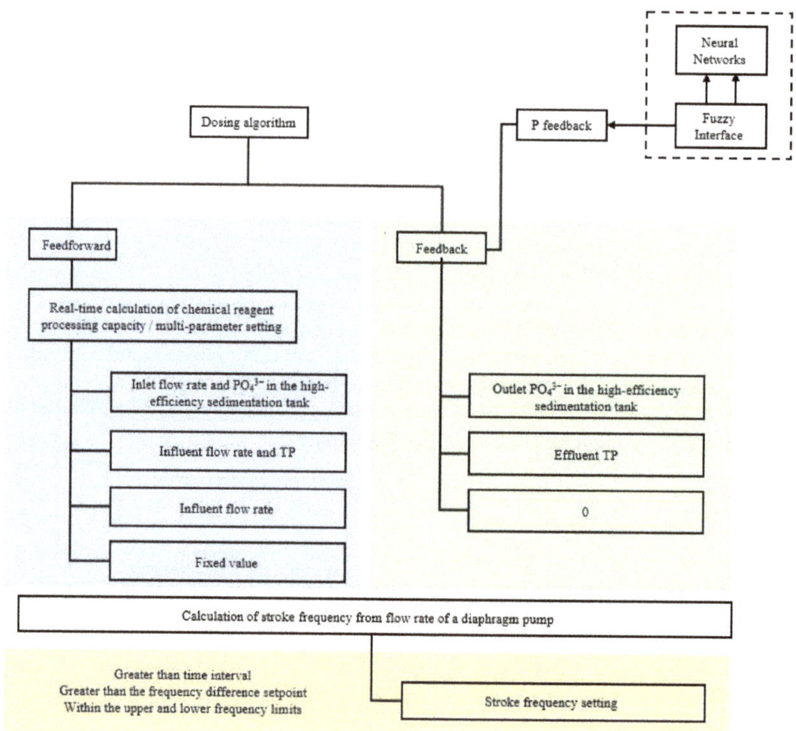

Figure 7. Phosphorus removal chemical dosing algorithm design.

6. Results of Intelligent Phosphorus Removal Operation with Automatic Dosing

Comparison before and after the implementation of intelligent control algorithms indicates that despite a gradual increase in influent PO_4^{3-} concentration from 0.8 mg/L to approximately 1.2 mg/L, the stability of effluent has improved (Figure 8). Previously, the effluent PO_4^{3-} concentration fluctuated between 0.3–0.6 mg/L, mainly due to semi-manual operations, which lacked sufficient response to real-time changes in influent conditions. After the implementation of intelligent control algorithms, the fluctuation range was narrowed to between 0.4–0.5 mg/L. The dosage can be dynamically adjusted based on real-time data, resulting in more precise and efficient phosphorus removal, with a stability improvement of 67%.

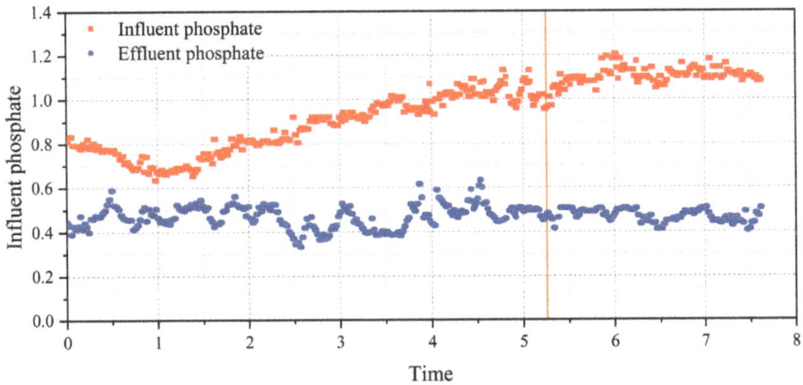

Figure 8. Comparison between semi-manual and intelligent automatic dosing.

7. Conclusions

(1) At low concentrations (≤60 mg/L), the phosphorus removal efficiency of the four phosphorus removal chemicals is in the following order: $FeCl_3$, PSAF, PAC, and PAFC.

(2) The mathematical chemical dosing model for phosphorus removal in the high-efficiency sedimentation tank is as follows: the feedforward dosage is a function of the influent flowrate and the effluent TP from the secondary sedimentation tank. Additionally, the effluent TP is continuously monitored and used as feedback to adjust the dosage of the chemicals in real time to ensure stable compliance.

(3) To ensure compliance with effluent standards, traditional dosing methods of phosphorus removal chemicals are relatively fixed and conservative. With the implementation of an automatic control system, dosing can be adjusted more accurately and flexibly in real-time according to changes in influent water quality and quantity. It is estimated that this can improve effluent stability by 67%.

(4) Automatic control of phosphorus removal chemicals is easily achievable through modifications in actual production operations. Moreover, due to its favorable economic effects, it is worth promoting.

Author Contributions: Writing—Original Draft, X.L.; Writing—Review & Editing, S.H., H.L. and F.Y.; Data Curation, T.Z. and X.W. All authors have read and agreed to the published version of the manuscript.

Funding: This study was sponsored by the Research Project of Shanghai Investigation, Design & Research Institute Co., Ltd. (2021SZ(8)-003), Shanghai Action Plan for Science, Technology and Innovation (22dz1209204) and Research Project of YANGTZE Eco-Environment Engineering Research Center, China Three Gorges Corporation (NBWL202200482).

Data Availability Statement: The raw data supporting the conclusions of this article will be made available by the authors on request.

Conflicts of Interest: Authors Xi Lu, Song Huang, Haichen Liu, Fengwei Yang, Ting Zhang were employed by the company Shanghai Investigation, Design and Research Institute Co., Ltd. Author Xi Lu was employed by the company Three Gorges Smart Water Technology Co., Ltd. Author Xinyu Wan was employed by the company China Three Gorges Corporation. The remaining authors declare that the research was conducted in the absence of any commercial or financial relationships that could be construed as a potential conflict of interest.

References

1. Xu, H.; Vilanova, R. PI and Fuzzy Control for P-Removal in Wastewater Treatment Plant. *Int. J. Comput. Commun.* **2015**, *10*, 176. [CrossRef]
2. Bawiec, A. Efficiency of Nitrogen and Phosphorus Compounds Removal in Hydroponic Wastewater Treatment Plant. *Environ. Technol.* **2019**, *40*, 2062–2072. [CrossRef] [PubMed]
3. Chen, Y.; Lan, S.; Wang, L.; Dong, S.; Zhou, H.; Tan, Z.; Li, X. A Review: Driving Factors and Regulation Strategies of Microbial Community Structure and Dynamics in Wastewater Treatment Systems. *Chemosphere* **2017**, *174*, 173–182. [CrossRef] [PubMed]
4. Gutierrez, O.; Park, D.; Sharma, K.R.; Yuan, Z. Iron Salts Dosage for Sulfide Control in Sewers Induces Chemical Phosphorus Removal during Wastewater Treatment. *Water Res.* **2010**, *44*, 3467–3475. [CrossRef] [PubMed]
5. Huang, J.-X.; Cen, Y.-M.; Guan, Y.-T.; Zhang, W.-L. Application of Intelligent Control System for Che Mical Phosphorus Removal in Wastewater Treatment Process. *China Water Wastewater* **2022**, *38*, 104–107.
6. Ginige, M.P.; Kayaalp, A.S.; Cheng, K.Y.; Wylie, J.; Kaksonen, A.H. Biological Phosphorus and Nitrogen Removal in Sequencing Batch Reactors: Effects of Cycle Length, Dissolved Oxygen Concentration and Influent Particulate Matter. *Water Sci. Technol.* **2013**, *68*, 982–990. [CrossRef] [PubMed]
7. Gernaey, K.V.; Jørgensen, S.B. Benchmarking Combined Biological Phosphorus and Nitrogen Removal Wastewater Treatment Processes. *Control Eng. Pract.* **2004**, *12*, 357–373. [CrossRef]
8. Ji, B.; Yang, K.; Wang, H. Impacts of Poly-Aluminum Chloride Addition on Activated Sludge and the Treatment Efficiency of SBR. *Desalination Water Treat.* **2015**, *54*, 2376–2381. [CrossRef]
9. Zhang, J.; Tang, L.; Tang, W.; Zhong, Y.; Luo, K.; Duan, M.; Xing, W.; Liang, J. Removal and Recovery of Phosphorus from Low-Strength Wastewaters by Flow-Electrode Capacitive Deionization. *Sep. Purif. Technol.* **2020**, *237*, 116322. [CrossRef]
10. Takács, I.; Murthy, S.; Fairlamb, P.M. Chemical Phosphorus Removal Model Based on Equilibrium Chemistry. *Water Sci. Technol.* **2005**, *52*, 549–555. [CrossRef]
11. Kazadi Mbamba, C.; Lindblom, E.; Flores-Alsina, X.; Tait, S.; Anderson, S.; Saagi, R.; Batstone, D.J.; Gernaey, K.V.; Jeppsson, U. Plant-Wide Model-Based Analysis of Iron Dosage Strategies for Chemical Phosphorus Removal in Wastewater Treatment Systems. *Water Res.* **2019**, *155*, 12–25. [CrossRef] [PubMed]
12. Takács, I.; Murthy, S.; Smith, S.; McGrath, M. Chemical Phosphorus Removal to Extremely Low Levels: Experience of Two Plants in the Washington, DC Area. *Water Sci. Technol.* **2006**, *53*, 21–28. [CrossRef] [PubMed]
13. Xu, Y.; Zeng, X.; Bernard, S.; He, Z. Data-Driven Prediction of Neutralizer pH and Valve Position towards Precise Control of Chemical Dosage in a Wastewater Treatment Plant. *J. Clean. Prod.* **2022**, *348*, 131360. [CrossRef]
14. Hauduc, H.; Takács, I.; Smith, S.; Szabo, A.; Murthy, S.; Daigger, G.T.; Spérandio, M. A Dynamic Physicochemical Model for Chemical Phosphorus Removal. *Water Res.* **2015**, *73*, 157–170. [CrossRef] [PubMed]
15. Solon, K.; Flores-Alsina, X.; Kazadi Mbamba, C.; Ikumi, D.; Volcke, E.I.P.; Vaneeckhaute, C.; Ekama, G.; Vanrolleghem, P.A.; Batstone, D.J.; Gernaey, K.V.; et al. Plant-Wide Modelling of Phosphorus Transformations in Wastewater Treatment Systems: Impacts of Control and Operational Strategies. *Water Res.* **2017**, *113*, 97–110. [CrossRef] [PubMed]
16. Zhang, L.; Zhang, J.; Honggui, H.A.N.; Junfei, Q. FNN-Based Process Control for Biochemical Phosphorus in WWTP. *CIESC J.* **2020**, *71*, 1217.
17. Ruano, M.V.; Ribes, J.; Sin, G.; Seco, A.; Ferrer, J. A Systematic Approach for Fine-Tuning of Fuzzy Controllers Applied to WWTPs. *Environ. Model. Softw.* **2010**, *25*, 670–676. [CrossRef]
18. Sabahi, K.; Ghaemi, S.; Liu, J.; Badamchizadeh, M.A. Indirect Predictive Type-2 Fuzzy Neural Network Controller for a Class of Nonlinear Input-Delay Systems. *ISA Trans.* **2017**, *71*, 185–195. [CrossRef] [PubMed]
19. Cai, W.; Zhang, B.; Jin, Y.; Lei, Z.; Feng, C.; Ding, D.; Hu, W.; Chen, N.; Suemura, T. Behavior of Total Phosphorus Removal in an Intelligent Controlled Sequencing Batch Biofilm Reactor for Municipal Wastewater Treatment. *Bioresour. Technol.* **2013**, *132*, 190–196. [CrossRef]
20. Lochmatter, S.; Gonzalez-Gil, G.; Holliger, C. Optimized Aeration Strategies for Nitrogen and Phosphorus Removal with Aerobic Granular Sludge. *Water Res.* **2013**, *47*, 6187–6197. [CrossRef]
21. Tavakoli, A.R.; Seifi, A.R.; Arefi, M.M. Designing a Self-Constructing Fuzzy Neural Network Controller for Damping Power System Oscillations. *Fuzzy Sets Syst.* **2019**, *356*, 63–76. [CrossRef]
22. Sartorius, C.; Von Horn, J.; Tettenborn, F. Phosphorus Recovery from Wastewater—Expert Survey on Present Use and Future Potential. *Water Environ. Res.* **2012**, *84*, 313–322. [CrossRef]

23. Sha'aban, Y.A.; Tahir, F.; Masding, P.W.; Mack, J.; Lennox, B. Control Improvement Using MPC: A Case Study of pH Control for Brine Dechlorination. *IEEE Access* **2018**, *6*, 13418–13428. [CrossRef]
24. Wu, H.; Yan, F.; Wang, G.; Lv, C. A Predictive Control Based on Decentralized Fuzzy Inference for a pH Neutralization Process. *J. Process Control* **2022**, *110*, 76–83. [CrossRef]
25. Li, J.; Tang, Z.; Luan, H.; Liu, Z.; Xu, B.; Wang, Z.; He, W. An Improved Method of Model-Free Adaptive Predictive Control: A Case of pH Neutralization in WWTP. *Processes* **2023**, *11*, 1448. [CrossRef]
26. Song, Y.; Tadé, M.O.; Zhang, T. Stabilization and Algorithm of Integrator plus Dead-Time Process Using PID Controller. *J. Process Control* **2009**, *19*, 1529–1537. [CrossRef]
27. Wu, H.; Su, W.; Liu, Z. PID Controllers: Design and Tuning Methods. In Proceedings of the 2014 9th IEEE Conference on Industrial Electronics and Applications, Hangzhou, China, 9–11 June 2014; IEEE: Piscataway, NJ, USA; pp. 808–813.
28. Vilela, P.; Nam, K.; Yoo, C. Wastewater Treatment System Optimization for Sustainable Operation of the SHARON–Anammox Process under Varying Carbon/Nitrogen Loadings. *Water* **2023**, *15*, 4015. [CrossRef]
29. Barbu, M.; Vilanova, R.; Meneses, M.; Santin, I. On the Evaluation of the Global Impact of Control Strategies Applied to Wastewater Treatment Plants. *J. Clean. Prod.* **2017**, *149*, 396–405. [CrossRef]
30. Nikita, S.; Lee, M. Control of a Wastewater Treatment Plant Using Relay Auto-Tuning. *Korean J. Chem. Eng.* **2019**, *36*, 505–512. [CrossRef]
31. *GB 18918-2002*; Discharge Standard of Pollutants for Municipal Wastewater Treatment Plant. Ministry of Environmental Protection, General Administration of Quality Supervision, Inspection and Quarantine: Beijing, China, 2002.
32. *GB 11893-89*; Water Quality-Determination of Total Phosphorus-Ammonium Molybdate Spectrophotometric Method. Ministry of Environmental Protection: Beijing, China, 1989.
33. *HJ670-2013*; Water Quality-Determination of Orthophosphate and Total Phosphorus-Continuous Flow Analysis(CFA) and Ammonium Molybdate Spectrophotometry. Ministry of Environmental Protection: Beijing, China, 2013.
34. Liu, H.; Zhou, M.; Huang, S.; Lu, X.; Yang, F. Study and Control of Chemical Phosphorus Removal Process in Sewage Treatment Plant. *Appl. Chem. Industry* **2025**, *in process*.
35. Kim, D.W.; Yu, S.I.; Im, K.; Shin, J.; Shin, S.G. Responses of Coagulant Type, Dosage and Process Conditions to Phosphate Removal Efficiency from Anaerobic Sludge. *Int. J. Environ. Res. Public Health* **2022**, *19*, 1693. [CrossRef] [PubMed]

water

Review

Mechanisms, Applications, and Risk Analysis of Surfactant-Enhanced Remediation of Hydrophobic Organic Contaminated Soil

Lijun Wu [1,2,*], Jieru Zhang [3], Fenfei Chen [3], Junjie Li [3,*], Wen Wang [3], Shiyi Li [1] and Lifang Hu [4]

[1] Power China Huadong Engineering Corporation Limited, Hangzhou 311122, China; li_sy5@hdec.com
[2] Huadong Eco-Environmental Engineering Research Institute of Zhejiang Province, Hangzhou 311122, China
[3] Yangtze River Delta (Jiaxing) Ecological Development Corporation Limited, Jiaxing 314099, China; zhangjier1123@gmail.com (J.Z.); chen_ff@hdec.com (F.C.); wang_w3@hdec.com (W.W.)
[4] College of Quality and Safety Engineering, Institution of Industrial Carbon Metrology, China Jiliang University, Hangzhou 310018, China; lfhu@cjlu.edu.cn
* Correspondence: wu_lj2@hdec.com (L.W.); li_jj2@hdec.com (J.L.)

Abstract: Surfactant-Enhanced Remediation is increasingly being recognized for its exceptional effectiveness in eliminating non-aqueous phase liquids in soil. A comprehensive knowledge of the technique is essential for its field application. This paper provides a thorough examination of Surfactant-Enhanced Remediation incorporating insights based on the most recent advancements. Firstly, the fundamental process and major mechanisms that underpin the technology were summarized, including mobilization, solubilizing, and emulsifying. Secondly, the improvements achieved by using surfactants in soil remediation, through chemical, physical, and biological methods, have been elucidated through theoretical explanations and practical case studies. Thirdly, the risks and other limitations of Surfactant-Enhanced Remediation were discussed with an outlook for future development. This review aims to promote understanding of the effectiveness and risks holistically in field implementation of the technique.

Keywords: non-aqueous phase liquid; surfactants; mechanisms; soil remediation

1. Introduction

The contamination of soils by organic compounds is becoming an urgent global concern with the development of industrialization [1]. Organic pollutants are mostly soluble but non-aqueous phase liquids (NAPLs) are distinct due to their volatility, toxicity and insolubility in water [1–3]. Considering the relative densities to water, NAPLs can be categorized into light non-aqueous phase liquids (LNAPLs) and heavy non-aqueous phase liquids (DNAPLs). With a density lower than water, LNAPLs are primarily composed of hydrocarbon compounds such as gasoline, diesel, kerosene, aromatic hydrocarbons, and short-chain alkanes. DNAPLs, on the other hand, notably include Trichloroethylene, Perchloroethylene, Trichloroacetic acid, Chlorophenols, Chlorobenzenes, coal tar and other highly toxic chlorinated organic substances. Toxic and chemically stable, NAPLs can infiltrate, migrate, and interact with the soil matrix or become trapped within the soil's pore spaces acting as a persistent source of contamination [4,5]. Resistant to natural degradation, NAPLs tends to accumulate and disrupt soil functionality, posing a significant risk to the environment as well as to human health [6,7].

A variety of techniques [8] have been proposed to solve the contamination problem of soil and groundwater, including Permeable Reactive Barriers, bioremediation, Air Stripping, and the Pump and Treat (P&T) technique; of which, P&T is the most common approach. However, traditional P&T is not effective for NAPL remediation due to their low solubility and low mobility. As an improvement to P&T [9], Surfactant-Enhanced Remediation

(SER) was proposed, which involves the injection of water containing surfactants into the subsurface aquifer. With the aid of SER, the duration of P&T has been notably shortened while its effectiveness towards NAPLs has been amplified [10,11]. Surfactants are a class of amphiphilic substances renowned for their distinctive surface activity, which pose a unique dual-phase molecular structure, featuring a hydrophilic head and a lipophilic tail [12,13]. As shown in Figure 1, the hydrophilic head of surfactants integrates into the aqueous phase by interacting with water molecules, while their hydrophobic tails engage with nonpolar or weakly polar solvents, allowing them to be incorporated into the oil phase [14,15]. This dual interaction positions surfactants at the oil–water interface, displacing some water or oil molecules, reducing intermolecular forces, and thereby forming a stable monolayer and decreasing interfacial tension. As surfactant concentration in the solution rises, so does the adsorption at the interface, which in turn lowers the tension. Since capillary forces restrict the mobility of NAPLs, the mobilized contaminants can then be recovered in a P&T extraction well. Once the surfactant concentration surpasses the critical micelle concentration (CMC), the adsorption plateaus. Beyond CMC, hydrophobic tails of surfactant molecules self-assemble to form aggregates within the solution, known as micelles. Micelles are spherical or ellipsoidal structures that have their hydrophobic tails oriented inward and their hydrophilic heads facing outwards towards the water. This configuration endows great importance on hydrophilic heads which are often comprised of polar groups. Based on the hydrophilic head groups, surfactants can be classified into nonionic surfactants [16], anionic surfactants [17], cationic surfactants [18], gemini surfactants and special surfactants [19,20].

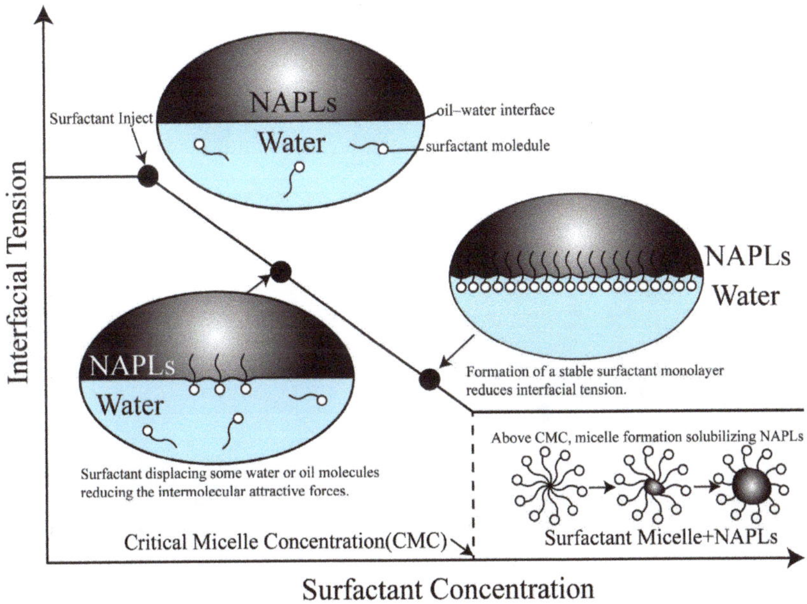

Figure 1. Schematic of Interfacial Tension Dynamics with Surfactant Concentration at the Molecular Level.

A variety of surfactants have been extensively investigated in SER, including sodium dodecyl benzene sulfonate (SDBS), Tween-80®, sodium dodecyl sulfate (SDS), hexadecyltrimethylammonium bromide (CTMAB), polyoxyethylene(10)octylphenyl ether(TX-100), cocamidopropyl hydroxysultane (CAHs) and polyethoxylate lauryl ether (Brij35) [21]. The mechanism underlying SER of NAPL contamination can be primarily categorized into solubilizing effect [22], mobilization effect [23] and emulsification [24]. The dominant mechanism varied with different types of NAPLs. The solubilization effect is often predominant in the remediation of DNAPLs, whereas the mobilization effect mostly plays the key role in the remediation of LNAPLs contamination. For example, the ratio of mobilized to solubilized oil in the porous rock was reported [25] to be 6:1 using n-Dodecyl β-D-maltoside as surfactant. A thin layer of surfactant formed and reached saturation relatively fast, which led to a reduction of the interfacial energy which favors the formation of microemulsions that promote the mobilization of NAPLs. However, the introduction of surfactants into an aquifer can also trigger complications and risks. Following the diminution of interfacial tension, unstable DNAPLs are subject to continued migration influenced by gravitational forces, hydrodynamic pressures, and capillary action, which may lead to an expansion of the contaminated area, thereby risking the contamination of previously unpolluted aquifer regions. Comprehending the mechanisms, risk, and state-of-the-art techniques is essential for the implementation of effective containment strategy. A systematic exposition of the mechanisms underpinning SER technology was reviewed followed by the examination of the synergistic applications of SER with other soil remediation methods. This paper then concluded with an analysis of the potential risks and other issues constraining the commercialization of SER in soil remediation.

2. Mechanisms of Surfactant-Enhanced Remediation Technologies

The mechanisms of Surfactant-Enhanced Remediation of NAPL-contaminated sites are primarily categorized into mobilization, emulsification, and solubilization, as depicted in Figure 2. Mobilization, which reduces the interfacial tension between NAPLs and water, thereby promoting the mobility and migration of NAPLs in porous media; emulsification, generating fine NAPL droplets stabilized by surfactant molecules, thus improving their dispersion in water; and solubilization, encapsulating hydrocarbon chains within micelles to increase the water solubility of non-aqueous solvents. The synergistic action of these mechanisms facilitates NAPLs elimination and biodegradation processes.

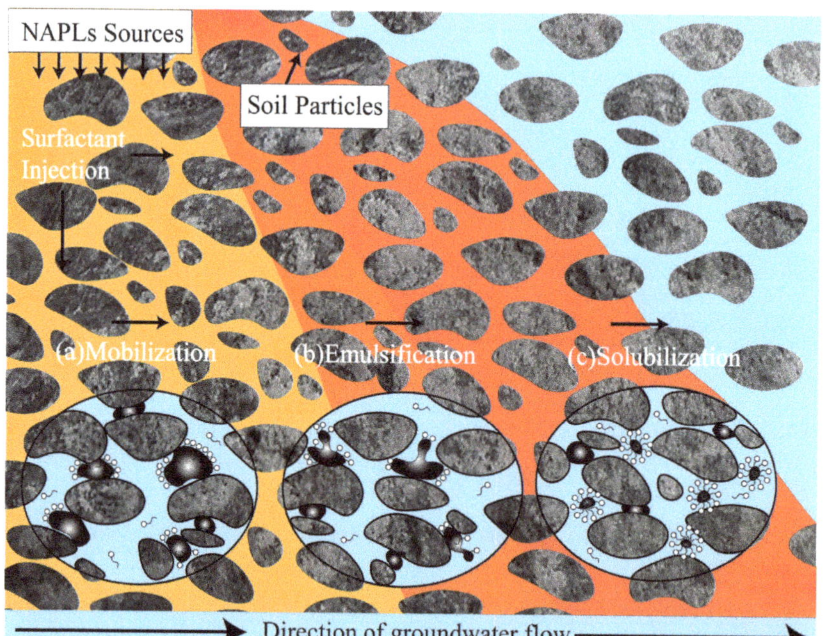

Figure 2. Surfactant-Enhanced NAPL Remediation Mechanisms: solubilization, emulsification, and flow enhancement.

2.1. Mobilization

The mechanism of the mobilization effect involves surfactant forming an adsorption layer at the water-NAPLs interface as shown in Figure 3. This reduces the interfacial tension between the water and NAPL phases, diminishing the capillary resistance within the porous media. Consequently, the stable DNAPLs are mobilized, migrating with the water flow in a liquid state. The ability of surfactant to reduce the oil–water interfacial tension determines the effectiveness of surfactant on the mobilization of NAPLs [26].

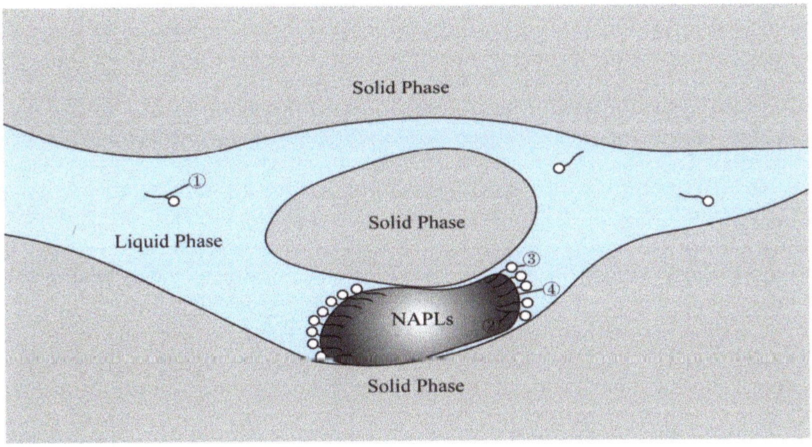

Figure 3. Schematic mobilization effect of surfactants on NAPLs (①: surfactant single molecule; ②: surfactant lipophilic group; ③: surfactant hydrophilic group; ④: oil–water interface).

To assess the critical conditions for the movement of NAPLs, Penell [27] proposed to use the total trapping number N_T to describe the state of NAPLs in porous media, as shown in the schematic diagram of the pore retention model in Figure 4 below.

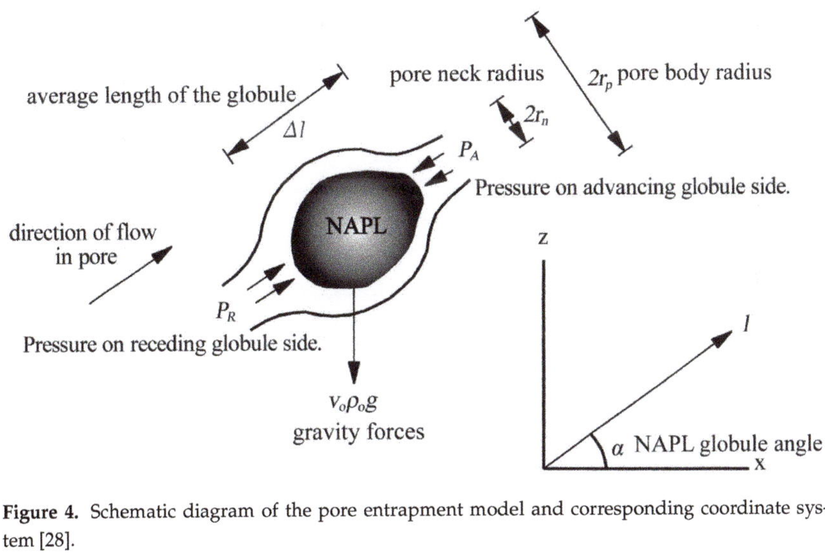

Figure 4. Schematic diagram of the pore entrapment model and corresponding coordinate system [28].

$$N_T = \sqrt{N_{CA}{}^2 + 2N_{CA}N_B \sin\alpha + N_B{}^2} \tag{1}$$

$$N_{CA} = \frac{q_{w_l} \mu_w}{\sigma_{ow} \cos \theta} \tag{2}$$

$$N_B = \frac{\Delta \rho g k k_{rw}}{\sigma_{ow} \cos \theta} \tag{3}$$

in which N_{CA} is the capillary number defined in terms of the aqueous flow component in the direction of the pore. N_B is the bond number representing the ratio of the buoyancy to capillary forces. σ_{ow} is the interfacial tension between the oil and water phases. q_{w_l} denotes the Darcy velocity of the water phase in the l direction. The angle α is measured between the flow and the positive x-axis (counterclockwise). The absolute permeability of the porous medium is characterized by k, while k_{rw} denotes the relative permeability to the aqueous phase. The dynamic viscosity of the aqueous phase is μ_w. $\Delta\rho$ signifies the difference between the density of water and the density of organic liquid, and θ is the contact angle.

The aforementioned equation quantitatively illustrated the mechanical equilibrium of gravity, viscous force, and capillary force on NAPLs in the pore space, while the generation of the mobilization effect is related to the capillary number (N_{CA}), capillary force, buoyancy force, and viscous force. When N_T exceeds a critical threshold, the NAPLs exhibit a mobilization effect [27]. The introduction of surfactants notably diminishes the interfacial tension between the oil–water phases. Concurrently, an increase in both N_B and N_{CA} facilitates the surpassing of the critical threshold of N_T. When N_{CA} is elevated, the viscous force becomes predominant, leading to a decrease in the interfacial tension within the fluid at the pore scale. In instances where the viscous force exceeds the capillary force, the mobility of NAPLs is significantly augmented [29,30]. Based on the total capture number N_T concept, Andrew et al. [31] produced migration potential maps showing how mixtures of composite multiple NAPLs are affected by viscous and interfacial tensions in both vertical and horizontal directions. Under a specified permeability condition, total trapping number influenced by surfactants that primarily operate through solubilization and emulsification mechanisms will be higher than that dominated by the mobilization mechanism.

Different types of surfactants exert varying impacts on the mobilization effect [32]. By blending multiple surfactants [30,33], the aqueous solubility of NAPLs can be significantly enhanced, thereby facilitating the occurrence of the mobilization mechanism. Increasing the concentration of surfactants can accelerate the decrease in interfacial tension [34] and low interfacial tension can help to enhance the mobilization mechanism [35], but higher surfactant concentration may also change the soil structure and flow pathway [36]. Apart from the nature of the surfactant, the nature of the porous medium, the pore water flow rate, and the environmental salinity may all affect the mobilization mechanism. For example, the alteration in the wettability of porous media leads to changes in the capillary pressure in the pores, which affects the mobilization effect to a great extend [37]. Certain surfactants have the capacity to promote the accumulation of negative charges on the surface of porous media, changing them from lipophilic to hydrophilic, which in turn intensify the mobilization effect of NAPLs [38–40]. The pore water flow rate exerts a limiting influence on the value of N_T. When the flow rate is low, N_T is diminished, making it difficult for the mobilization mechanism to manifest. Consequently, the removal efficiency of NAPLs is negligible [41]. To promote the mobilization of NAPLs, the addition of an appropriate amount of ions to the surfactant system to change the salinity is a promising strategy [25].

The mobilization effect of NAPLs offers a higher remediation rate for free-phase NAPLs, but there is a greater risk of secondary contamination due to the difficulty of controlling the movement of free-phase liquid [42], especially in the case of DNAPLs.

2.2. Solubilization

The solubilization effect involves the micellization process of surfactants, which distributes NAPLs into the hydrophobic core of the micelles. This increases the solubility of insoluble or slightly soluble NAPLs in the aqueous phase, allowing them to migrate from the porous medium to the aqueous phase through the formation of nanoscale agglomerates that encapsulate the contaminants [43,44]. The solubilizing effect of surfactants is mainly manifested in micellar solubilization, as shown in Figure 5.

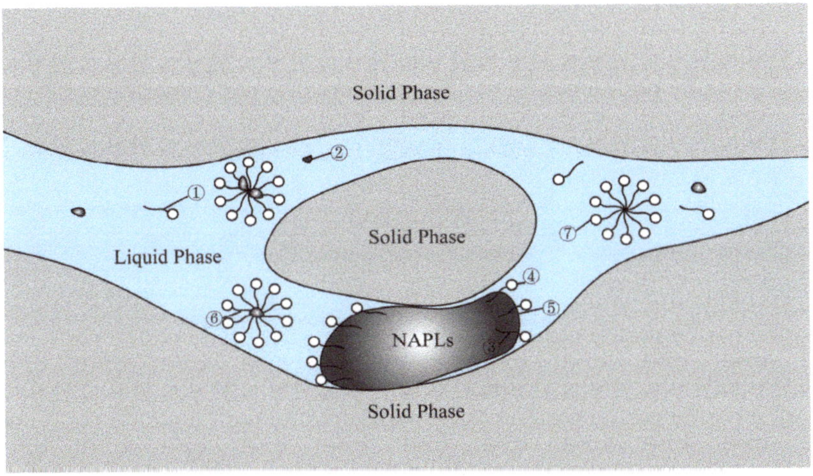

Figure 5. Schematic solubilization effect of surfactants on NAPLs (①: surfactant molecules, ②: NAPL droplets, ③: surfactant lipophilic groups, ④: surfactant hydrophilic groups, ⑤: oil–water interface, ⑥: micelles formed by surfactants and NAPLs, and ⑦: surfactant micelles).

The concentration at which a surfactant spontaneously forms micelles is called the critical micelle concentration (CMC). This pivotal concentration dictates the extent of the solubilization capacity. Surfactants exist solely as individual molecules below CMC. Once their concentrations surpass the CMC, surfactants are present both as individual molecules and as micelles, in a dynamic equilibrium between association and decomposition [45–47]. It was discovered that the CMC of nonionic surfactants in the aqueous phase decreases with an increase in the number of carbon atoms within the lipophilic group. Meanwhile, the higher the polarity of the hydrophilic group, the lower the tendency to form micelles, resulting in a higher CMC value [48].

Molar solubilization ratio (MSR) is a quantitative measure of the solubilizing ability of surfactants, which denotes the number of moles of compound solubilized per mole of surfactant [49]. It is expressed by the following formula:

$$\mathrm{MSR} = \frac{S - S_{\mathrm{CMC}}}{C_S - \mathrm{CMC}} \tag{4}$$

in which C_S is the concentration of the solution when the surfactant concentration is greater than CMC; S is the apparent solubility of the solute at a surfactant concentration of C_S; and S_{CMC} denotes the apparent solubility of the solute at a surfactant concentration of C_S as well as at the concentration of CMC.

In addition to the type and structure of surfactant, the ambient ionic strength and temperature had a significant effect on MSR [21,50]. Varied surfactants have different molar solubilization ratios. The solute partition coefficient between micellar and water phases K_{MC} can be calculated from the MSR [51] to find constant solubilizing capacity:

$$K_{MC} = \frac{\mathrm{MSR}/(1+\mathrm{MSR})}{S_{\mathrm{CMC}} V_w} = \frac{55.4 \times \mathrm{MSR}}{S_{\mathrm{CMC}}(1+\mathrm{MSR})} \tag{5}$$

On the basis of the above expression, the solubilizing effect of surfactants is related to the concentration of surfactant monomers and micelles in solution and their corresponding partition coefficients [50]:

$$S_w^*/S_w = 1 + X_{mn}K_{mn} + X_{mn}K_{MC} \tag{6}$$

where S_w^* is the apparent solubility of the solute at a total surfactant concentration of X; S_w is the solubility of the solute in pure water; X_{mn} is the surfactant monomer concentration; X_{mc} is the concentration of surfactant micelles; K_{mn} is the partition coefficient of the solute between the monomer and water phase; and K_{MC} is the solute partition coefficient between the micelle and water phase.

The solubilizing ability of a surfactant can be measured by the hydrophilic–lipophilic balance number (HLB) [23,52,53], whose value depends on the combined affinity of its hydrophilic and lipophilic groups for oil or water, respectively. High HLB values indicate strong hydrophilicity. When the HLB value exceeds 13, the solubilizing effect of the surfactant becomes even more pronounced, particularly in the case of nonionic surfactant solutions with high molecular weight and high HLB values [54].

Different surfactants have distinct CMCs. Surfactants with lower CMCs can produce stabilized polymers at low concentrations, thereby exerting a solubilizing effects [55]. It is advantageous for applications requiring a minimal surfactant dosage. Compared with single surfactants, complex surfactant systems often have more significant solubilizing effects, attributed to their reduced surface tension and CMC, coupled with the formation of more stable mixed micelles and lower adsorption and precipitation loss. Investigating the solubilizing effects of eight different types of surfactants and their complex system, Yang et al. [56] confirmed that complex systems of multiple surfactants had stronger solubilizing ability. The concentration of surfactant can also play an important role in the solubilizing effect of NAPLs [23]. Theoretically, the necessary condition for the solubilization mechanism to occur is that the concentration of surfactant is higher than CMC [23,53,57,58]. Nevertheless, even at sub-critical micelle concentrations (sub-CMC) [59,60], certain surfactants are capable of inducing solubilization. The work of Zhong [59] showed that at concentrations above CMC, the biosurfactant rhamnolipids formed micelles characterized by strong intermolecular interactions. Conversely, at concentrations below the CMC, the interactions between rhamnolipids and alkane molecules become predominant, resulting in a marked solubilizing effect. This effect is notably more pronounced than that observed at levels above the CMC, highlighting the unique behavior of rhamnolipids in facilitating the solubility of hydrocarbons.

Surfactants are easily adsorbed in soil and sensitive to the nature of porous media, and their adsorption in soil reduces the micellar solubilizing effect on NAPLs, which adversely affects remediation [61,62]. In addition, irregular soil pore structures restrict the passage of water and solute [63]. Moreover, flushing may lead to pore clogging due to the accumulation of surfactant micelles, which impede the effectiveness of remediation efforts [64].

The pore water flow rate during the aggregation process has considerable impact on surfactants' solubilization mechanism. A high flow rate can diminish the surfactants' interaction with NAPLs, leading to a reduction in micelle formation and consequently weakening the solubilization effect [27]. However, concurrently, this increased flow rate can enhance the transportation of the micellar aggregates, mitigating the occurrence of pore throat plugging [23].

As one main mechanism of SER of soil contamination by NAPLs, solubilization effectiveness depends on the type of surfactant used; hence, suitable surfactants should be carefully selected according to the specific contaminants present during the remediation process in order to achieve the optimal results.

2.3. *Emulsification*

Surfactants play an important role in the treatment of NAPL-contaminated soil, and their emulsification is one of the key mechanisms for enhanced remediation. By adsorbing at the "oil–water interface" to form stable nanoscale oil or water droplets, surfactants achieve an emulsifying effect, promoting the dispersion of NAPLs into micro-droplets [65, 66], enhancing mass transfer efficiency, and improving the mobility and recovery rate of NAPLs.

Emulsification products can be categorized into two types: microemulsions and emulsions. Microemulsions are formed through the micellar solubilization action and represent thermodynamically stable systems that are transparent or semi-transparent. On the other hand, emulsions are thermodynamically unstable systems, formed by the emulsification process that disperses the NAPL phase within an immiscible liquid phase. According to the difference between the dispersed and continuous phases, emulsion systems can be further classified into oil-in-water (O/W), water-in-oil (W/O), or multiple emulsions (W/O/W, O/W/O) [67], as illustrated in Figure 6. In porous media, the transport performance of emulsification products is lower than those of nanoscale aggregates produced by micellar solubilization [68], but moderate water-emulsion droplet size adjustments can improve the remediation efficiency [24]. Some studies indicate that enhanced emulsification of surfactants may be more advantageous than solubilization [69] in remediation applications [70].

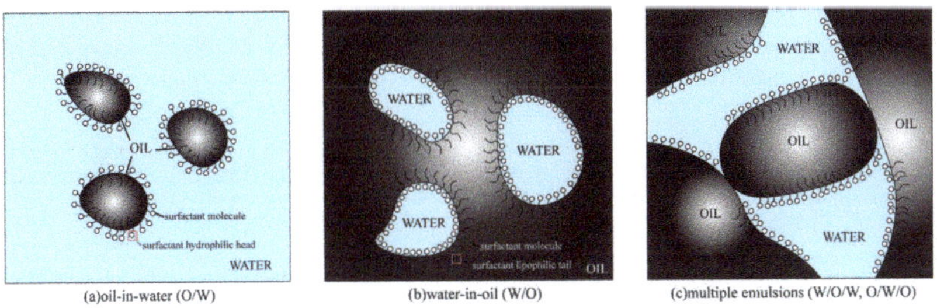

Figure 6. Varied types of emulsion systems.

Emulsification is caused by the density difference between the oil and water phases, resulting in the formation of emulsified droplets that move in accordance with gravitational fields, Brownian motion, or applied forces, and are in a state of continuous motion. The oil–water interfacial tension was rapidly reduced to mitigate the rupture and generate fine droplets in the emulsification. However, emulsified droplets are not sufficiently stable [71–73] to overcome collision, sedimentation, coagulation, and aggregation, resulting in remediation impediment. Therefore, this stability is pivotal in ensuring the effectiveness of surfactant-based remediation strategies.

Emulsification is a dynamic process in which surface-active molecules move rapidly to the interfacial region with the destruction of emulsified droplets. The emulsion stability is not only related to the nature of the surfactant solution [74], but also affected by the type of NAPLs [75], the ratio of NAPLs to water and the water content of the system [76]. Liu et al. found that surfactant AEOSHS derived from the modification of fatty alcohol ethoxylates yielded emulsions characterized by reduced droplet sizes, increased emulsification capacity, and enhanced emulsion stability. These attributes led to increases in the mobility and recycling efficiency of emulsified droplets in porous media [74]. In addition to the modification of surfactants, the addition of auxiliary substances such as polymers can also improve the stability of emulsions. For example, the addition of xanthan gum can form a 3D network of polymers, reducing the collision rate of droplets and improving the formation and stability of emulsions [77]. The introduction of sodium carbonate solution in the emulsion system can promote the adsorption at the oil–water interface and improve the mechanical strength of the emulsion film. In the application of foam-assisted oil recovery, high emulsion stability is more beneficial than the low interfacial tension for the flow of the emulsified oil [78]. The properties of emulsion in porous media are also affected by pore structure and pore water flow rate. Emulsions exhibit the shear thinning behavior as non-Newtonian fluids when passing through porous media. Different pore structures can alter the rheology of emulsions [79]. By increasing the pore water flow rate, the retention of emulsion in porous media can be reduced [80].

However, the formation of emulsions from surfactants during remediation can have negative effects. If the emulsion traps contaminants within a low mobile phase, increasing its volume will hinder the penetration of surfactants to the soil–oil interface due to its relatively static and highly viscous properties. It may pose a risk of secondary contamination, and present challenges for subsequent remediation [81].

2.4. Other Mechanisms

In addition to mobilization, solubilizing, and emulsifying effects, surfactants have the ability to increase the bioavailability of NAPLs, thereby enhancing the bioremediation process and promoting the biodegradation of NAPLs [82]. The degradation ability of NAPLs varies among different types of surfactants [83]. The micellar system formed by surfactants helps to increase the number of microorganisms and enhance the degradation efficiency of NAPLs [84]. The uptake of NAPLs by plant roots was promoted in the presence of surfactants, enhancing the phytoremediation effect, which shows promise in the remediation of organically contaminated soil and groundwater.

However, some of the metabolites produced by surfactants during the remediation process may be toxic and inhibit microbial activity [85,86]. Further investigation in this area holds promise and merits continued exploration in the future.

3. Surfactant-Enhanced Remediation Techniques

Widely distributed in the soil environment, NAPLs are not prone to be desorbed from soil pores, being characterized by limited mobility and degradation. As a result, the remediation effect of chemical, biological, and physical remediation techniques on NAPLs in soil is often unsatisfactory. Non-traditional approaches that leverage surfactants have the potential to enhance remediation efficiency significantly, offering the added benefits of reduced costs and expedited time.

3.1. Surfactant-Enhanced Chemical Oxidative Remediation Technology

In situ chemical oxidation (ISCO) is an advanced remediation technology that employs chemical oxidants and the potent oxidizing free radicals they generate to degrade organic pollutants in soil [87], converting them into small molecules, H_2O and CO_2, and NAPL contaminants within the soil matrix. Oxidizing agents of choice include persulfate, potassium permanganate, hydrogen peroxide and ozone, among which sodium persulfate is the most widely used in soil remediation [88]. Given the oxidation reaction usually occurs solely in the aqueous phase [89], the residual non-aqueous phase NAPLs that persist within in the soil are not susceptible to oxidization, thereby inducing a rebound effect [90] in which recalcitrant pollutions continue to be emitted.

Surfactants promote the dissolution of NAPLs into the aqueous phase, and synergistically amplify the chemical oxidation on NAPLs in the remediation process. Surfactant enhanced in situ chemical oxidation (S-ISCO) as a co-elution technique [91] has been extensively studied. This technology was first developed by VeruTEK (Bloomfield, CT, USA) and later acquired by EthicalChem LLC (South Windsor, CT, USA), which sells its VeruSOL surfactant to the oil production industry as a "green" product. In S-ISCO technology, the compatibility of surfactants and oxidizers is an important factor to be considered [92]. Although extensive research has shown that the addition of surfactant has an significant promotive effect on the chemical oxidation technology, the organic nature of surfactant can lead to interactions with oxidants, potentially inactivating the surfactants [93]. Additionally, the introduction of oxidants may escalate the non-productive consumption of surfactants [94] which could compromise the overall remediation efficacy.

Wei et al. [92] selected a binary mixture of SDBS/BS-12 to synergistically enhance the remediation of the oxidizing agent $KMnO_4$, using 1.73–23.07% of the commonly used surfactant in practical experiments, with a cost reduction of more than 50%. Demiray et al. [95] found that despite Tween 80 possibly affecting the kinetics of the oxidation reaction, its overall impact is to accelerate and facilitate the remediation process. The preferential adopting of surfactants that are more compatible with the oxidant system can maximize the remediation effect and have a positive impact on soil remediation.

3.2. *Surfactant-Enhanced Bioremediation Technologies*

Bioremediation encompasses two primary approaches: microbial remediation and phytoremediation. The efficiency of microbial remediation technology [96] is contingent upon the functionality and abundance of the microbial community in the environment. The degradation of NAPLs in soil is achieved under the combined action of organic nutrients and oxygen, and the specificity of the microorganisms and their susceptibility to external environmental factors significantly influences the remediation efficiency [97]. The combination of biosurfactant and microbial remediation technology can not only increase the degradation rate by more than 50% [98], but also substantially mitigate the secondary contamination effects associated with chemical surfactants; but, the biodegradation mechanism of surfactants remain elusive. Moreover, severe adverse effects on remediation were discovered relating to surfactants at high concentration [99].

Phytoremediation technology [100,101] utilizes plants to adsorb pollutants in soil or shallow groundwater through their roots. However, this method is characterized by a prolonged remediation time as well as limited remediation depth [102]. Surfactants can augment the combined plant-microorganism remediation technology by significantly increasing the abundance of bacterial flora, which, in return, elevates the removal rate of NAPLs. Non-ionic surfactants and biosurfactants demonstrate optimal performance as they mitigate the root toxicity associated with cationic surfactants [103–105].

3.3. *Surfactant-Enhanced Physical Remediation Technology*

Soil physical remediation technologies encompass a range of methods, including aeration remediation, electric remediation, and thermal treatment technologies. These are complemented by ex situ treatment techniques and land replacement strategies.

Aeration remediation technology is suited for soil environments characterized by high permeability and a loose structure [106]. This method expels NAPLs to the surface through air flow injection. Nevertheless, the method's remediation efficacy is constrained when addressing organic pollutants with attributes of low concentration and low volatility. To solve this problem, a technique referred to as surfactant-enhanced air sparging (SEAS) was proposed by adding surfactants to increase the mobility of organic pollutants and broaden the influence area of air in the soil matrix [107]. The efficiency of NAPAL's remediation is reported to be closely related to the airflow rate, surfactant concentration, aeration pressure, and the area of remediation [108]. Although this approach shows promise in low-permeability formations, additional research is warranted to elucidate the role of NAPLs in such environments [109].

Electric Remediation Technology [110] is another well practiced method in the field of soil remediation. The anode and cathode electrodes are inserted into the soil to generate an electric field where contaminants were extracted from the soil through electro-osmosis, electro-migration and electrophoresis [111–113]. However, the heat accumulated during the process will affect the soil properties in the long run, and it is more suitable for hypotonic soils with low acid buffer capacity. Nonionic surfactants are commonly used in conjunction with electrokinetic remediation techniques. Studies have demonstrated that the synergistic application of nonionic surfactants under a periodic voltage gradient can remove individual PAHs up to 69% [114]. Arumugam et al. [115] reported the integration of natural surfactants with electrokinetic remediation technology resulted in a 98% decomposition efficiency for organic pollutants and also increased subsequent bioavailability. In practical application, it is essential to consider the secondary contamination of surfactants and to identify the optimal operating conditions for electrokinetic remediation technology to ensure the most effective remediation outcomes [116].

Thermal desorption technology [117] in soil remediation refers to a process where heat is applied to contaminated soil to increase the temperature and volatilize organic compounds, thereby separating them from the soil matrix. Thermal desorption technology can regulate the temperature and residence time to achieve the best NAPL removal rate, and has the advantages of high removal efficiency, short remediation time, and minimal likelihood of inducing secondary pollution. However, the application of this technology faces limitations due to constraints posed by soil water content, high cost, and the potential for altering the physicochemical and biological properties of the soil [118]. Coupled with surfactant use, thermal desorption can implement a dual process approach, consisting of a cleaning phase followed by thermal desorption [119]. Surfactant based pretreatment diminishes the volume of soil to be treated by thermal desorption, thereby reducing the associated energy consumption costs. However, the limited number of cases of application of this technology necessitates additional research to substantiate its feasibility and effectiveness.

4. Risk Analysis of Surfactant-Enhanced Remediation

SER technology has the capacity to augment the solubility of pollutants, thereby facilitating their removal. However, it also presents challenges, such as the potential for residual concentrations to induce secondary contamination in remediation sites. The application of surfactants may also introduce heightened toxicity to the soil. Prolonged presence within the subsurface soil system could further lead to the contamination of groundwater resources.

Cationic surfactants have been observed [17,120] to interact with the negatively charged surfaces of porous media, potentially leading to adsorption and enrichment in the subsurface environment. This interaction can burden the soil medium, induce soil toxicity, exert adverse effects, reduce soil permeability, and impair soil function. On the other hand, anionic surfactants [76,121] are more susceptible to forming precipitates with cations in the soils. As for nonionic surfactants, it is often used as a common agent in SER technology [120] because of their stronger solubilizing effect, lower cost and lower toxicity to soil microorganisms [17]. However, some studies have proved that although the content of NAPLs in soil is significantly reduced post remediation, the residual surfactants can remain toxic to the plants in subsequent years [17].

To mitigate that risk, biosurfactants were proposed as an alternative in the remediation of soils contaminated with NAPLs [122]. Unlike traditional synthesized surfactants from petrochemical industrial processes, biosurfactants are generated by biological systems such as plants and microorganisms, representing a novel class of eco-friendly agents with lower toxicity and higher biodegradability [123,124]. Also, biosurfactants have a larger molecular structure and more ligand groups, endowing them with superior performance or additional properties that their synthetic counterparts often lack. For example, biosurfactants can be utilized as a carbon source by soil-inhabiting microbes to accelerate the pollutants' biodegradation [125]. Compared with traditional surfactants, the majority of biosurfactants are more efficient and effective in SER applications due to lower CMC, surface, and interfacial tension values. However, biosurfactants are constrained by limited production scales and high selectivity for target products, resulting in higher costs than synthetic surfactants [126], which poses challenges for their commercial application. Since the substrate alone accounts for almost half of the total cost of obtaining a biosurfactant, ongoing research in the field of biosurfactants is increasingly focusing on the utilization of cost-effective substrates, particularly agricultural waste [127].

5. Conclusions

Recent years saw growing research attention in SER technology thanks to its significant role in strengthening the efficacy of chemical, physical, and biological remediation of NAPL pollution in soil by leveraging mobilization, solubilization, emulsification and other mechanisms. In chemical remediation, surfactants promote the action of chemical oxidizers, while they can be used as carbon source for the activating of microorganisms in biodegradation methods. For physical remediation techniques, the presence of surfactants can broaden the influence zone of aeration or boost the electrokinetic process to accelerate NAPL removal. Detailed examination of the case studies concerning economic analysis, influencing factors, as well as the long term impact on the environment and human health is non-exhaustive and limited by relevant references. Further research and exploration is urgent in the following two areas:

1. Surfactants: The development of new surfactants, such as bilobal surfactants and switchable surfactants, is important in reducing the potential impact while improving the remediation efficiency of NAPLs [67,128]. Another strategy is to integrate various surfactants in the remediation process, leveraging their combined action towards NAPLs. Furthermore, surfactants and reaction intermediates warrant further investigations and ongoing monitoring to ensure SER was implemented with a minimum environmental risk.
2. Remediation technology: It is of great importance to further study the synergistic mechanism of SER coupled with different remediation technologies which may surpass the limitations of one single method while concurrently maximizing the outcome, such as with reduced environmental footprint, minimized surfactant usage, and enhanced NAPL removal.

Author Contributions: Conceptualization, L.W. and J.Z.; methodology, F.C.; validation, J.L., W.W. and S.L.; formal analysis, J.Z.; investigation, L.W.; resources, J.L.; data curation, F.C.; writing—original draft preparation, L.W.; writing—review and editing, F.C.; visualization, L.H.; supervision, S.L.; project administration, F.C All authors have read and agreed to the published version of the manuscript.

Funding: This research received no external funding.

Conflicts of Interest: Authors Lijun Wu and Shiyi Li were employed by the company Power China Huadong Engineering Corporation Limited. Authors Jiru Zhang, Fenfei Chen, Junjie Li and Wen Wang were employed by the company Yangtze River Delta (Jiaxing) Ecological Development Corporation Limited. The remaining authors declare that the research was conducted in the absence of any commercial or financial relationships that could be construed as a potential conflict of interest.

References

1. Essaid, H.I.; Bekins, B.A.; Cozzarelli, I.M. Organic contaminant transport and fate in the subsurface: Evolution of knowledge and understanding. *Water Resour. Res.* **2015**, *51*, 4861–4902. [CrossRef]
2. Du Fangzhou, S.X.; Kang, X. Improved Method and Software Development for Assessing NAPL Phase Presence in Contaminated Sites. *Saf. Environ. Eng.* **2022**, *29*, 175–182+195. [CrossRef]
3. Zhang, A.; Cai, W.; Wang, J.; Zhang, M.; Liu, X.; Geng, T. Comparison of Sampling Methods on Groundwater Petroleum Pollution. *Saf. Environ. Eng.* **2014**, *21*, 109–113+120. [CrossRef]
4. Council, N.R. *Contaminants in the Subsurface: Source Zone Assessment and Remediation*; The National Academies Press: Washington, DC, USA, 2005; p. 370.
5. Kavanaugh, M.C.; Abriola, L.M.; Newell, C.J. The DNAPL Remediation Challenge: Is There a Case for Source Depletion? United States Environmental Protection Agency: Washington, DC, USA, 2003.
6. Zhu, H.; Ye, S.; Wu, J.; Xu, H. Characteristics of soil lithology and pollutants in typical contamination sites in China. *Earth Sci. Front.* **2021**, *28*, 26–34. [CrossRef]
7. Ni, G. Research on the Soil/Groundwater Remediation Technologies for the Falling Oil Contaminated Sites in Daqing Oilfield. Ph.D. Thesis, Northeast Petroleum University, Heilongjiang, China, 2020. [CrossRef]
8. Liang, T.; Zhang, H. Review on Remediation Technology of Chloromethanes Contaminated Soil. In Proceedings of the Chinese Society of Environmental Science 2022 Annual Scientific and Technical Conference—Environmental Engineering Technology Innovation and Application Session, Jiang Xi, Nan Chang, China, 20 August 2022; pp. 769–773+953. [CrossRef]

9. Saxena, N.; Islam, M.M.; Baliyan, S.; Sharma, D. A comprehensive review on removal of environmental pollutants using a surfactant based remediation process. *RSC Sustain.* **2023**, *1*, 2148–2161. [CrossRef]
10. Peng, S.; Wu, W.; Chen, J. Removal of PAHs with surfactant-enhanced soil washing: Influencing factors and removal effectiveness. *Chemosphere* **2011**, *82*, 1173–1177. [CrossRef]
11. Befkadu, A.A.; Chen, Q. Surfactant-Enhanced Soil Washing for Removal of Petroleum Hydrocarbons from Contaminated Soils: A Review. *Pedosphere* **2018**, *28*, 383–410. [CrossRef]
12. Wang, F.; Chen, J.; Li, Y.; Lu, T.; Chen, W.; Qi, Z.; Wang, X.; Farooq, U. Anionic surfactant-mediated transport of tetracycline antibiotics with different molecular structures in saturated porous media. *J. Mol. Liq.* **2022**, *367*, 120402. [CrossRef]
13. Rosen, M.J.; Kunjappu, J.T. *Surfactants and Interfacial Phenomena*; John Wiley & Sons: Hoboken, NJ, USA, 2012.
14. Wei, W.; Ran, Z.; He, H.; Zhou, K.; Huangfu, Z.; Yu, J. Desorption process and morphological analysis of real polycyclic aromatic hydrocarbons contaminated soil by the heterogemini surfactant and its mixed systems. *Chemosphere* **2020**, *254*, 126854. [CrossRef]
15. Davin, M.; Starren, A.; Deleu, M.; Lognay, G.; Colinet, G.; Fauconnier, M.L. Could saponins be used to enhance bioremediation of polycyclic aromatic hydrocarbons in aged-contaminated soils? *Chemosphere* **2018**, *194*, 414–421. [CrossRef]
16. Okuda, I.; McBride, J.F.; Gleyzer, S.N.; Miller, C.T. Physicochemical Transport Processes Affecting the Removal of Residual DNAPL by Nonionic Surfactant Solutions. *Environ. Sci. Technol.* **1996**, *30*, 1852–1860. [CrossRef]
17. Di Trapani, D.; De Marines, F.; Greco Lucchina, P.; Viviani, G. Surfactant-enhanced mobilization of hydrocarbons from soil: Comparison between anionic and nonionic surfactants in terms of remediation efficiency and residual phytotoxicity. *Process Saf. Environ. Prot.* **2023**, *180*, 1–9. [CrossRef]
18. Isaac, O.T.; Pu, H.; Oni, B.A.; Samson, F.A. Surfactants employed in conventional and unconventional reservoirs for enhanced oil recovery—A review. *Energy Rep.* **2022**, *8*, 2806–2830. [CrossRef]
19. Liang, X.; Li, Y.; Bai, J.; Dong, J.; Li, W.; Mo, Y.; Jiang, D.; Zhang, W. Feasibility evaluation of novel anionic-nonionic gemini surfactants for surfactant-enhanced aquifer remediation. *J. Clean. Prod.* **2023**, *393*, 136338. [CrossRef]
20. Kurnia, I.; Fatchurrozi, M.; Anwary, R.G.; Zhang, G. Lessons learned from coreflood experiments with surfactant-polymer and alkali-surfactant-polymer for enhanced oil recovery. *Petroleum* **2022**, *9*, 487–498. [CrossRef]
21. Zhu, L.; Feng, S. Synergistic solubilization of polycyclic aromatic hydrocarbons by mixed anionic–nonionic surfactants. *Chemosphere* **2003**, *53*, 459–467. [CrossRef] [PubMed]
22. Zhong, L.; Mayer, A.S.; Pope, G.A. The effects of surfactant formulation on nonequilibrium NAPL solubilization. *J. Contam. Hydrol.* **2003**, *60*, 55–75. [CrossRef] [PubMed]
23. Huo, L.; Liu, G.; Li, Y.; Yang, X.; Zhong, H. Solubilization of residual dodecane by surfactants in porous media: The relation between surfactant partition and solubilization. *Colloids Surf. A Physicochem. Eng. Asp.* **2022**, *648*, 129421. [CrossRef]
24. Datta, P.; Tiwari, P.; Pandey, L.M. Oil washing proficiency of biosurfactant produced by isolated Bacillus tequilensis MK 729017 from Assam reservoir soil. *J. Pet. Sci. Eng.* **2020**, *195*, 107612. [CrossRef]
25. Javanbakht, G.; Goual, L. Mobilization and micellar solubilization of NAPL contaminants in aquifer rocks. *J. Contam. Hydrol.* **2016**, *185*, 61–73. [CrossRef]
26. Borkovec, M. From micelles to microemulsion droplets: Size distributions, shape fluctuations, and interfacial tensions. *J. Chem. Phys.* **1989**, *91*, 6268–6281. [CrossRef]
27. Pennell, K.D.; Abriola, L.M.; Weber, W.J. Surfactant-enhanced solubilization of residual dodecane in soil columns. 1. Experimental investigation. *Environ. Sci. Technol.* **1993**, *27*, 2332–2340. [CrossRef]
28. Pennell, K.D.; Pope, G.A.; Abriola, L.M. Influence of Viscous and Buoyancy Forces on the Mobilization of Residual Tetrachloroethylene during Surfactant Flushing. *Environ. Sci. Technol.* **1996**, *30*, 1328–1335. [CrossRef]
29. Das, A.; Nguyen, N.; Farajzadeh, R.; Southwick, J.G.; Vincent-Bonnieu, S.; Khaburi, S.; Al Kindi, A.; Nguyen, Q.P. Experimental study of injection strategy for Low-Tension-Gas flooding in low permeability, high salinity carbonate reservoirs. *J. Pet. Sci. Eng.* **2020**, *184*, 106564. [CrossRef]
30. Ramezanzadeh, M.; Aminnaji, M.; Rezanezhad, F.; Ghazanfari, M.H.; Babaei, M. Dissolution and remobilization of NAPL in surfactant-enhanced aquifer remediation from microscopic scale simulations. *Chemosphere* **2022**, *289*, 133177. [CrossRef]
31. Ramsburg, C.A.; Baniahmad, P.; Muller, K.A.; Robinson, A.D. Emulsion-based recovery of a multicomponent petroleum hydrocarbon NAPL using nonionic surfactant formulations. *J. Contam. Hydrol.* **2023**, *255*, 104144. [CrossRef] [PubMed]
32. Qi, Z.; Han, M.; Chen, S.; Wang, J. Surfactant enhanced imbibition in carbonate reservoirs: Effect of IFT reduction and surfactant partitioning. *JCIS Open* **2022**, *5*, 100045. [CrossRef]
33. Zhao, B.; Zhu, L.; Li, W.; Chen, B. Solubilization and biodegradation of phenanthrene in mixed anionic–nonionic surfactant solutions. *Chemosphere* **2005**, *58*, 33–40. [CrossRef]
34. Ogunmokun, F.A.; Wallach, R. Effect of surfactant surface and interfacial tension reduction on infiltration into hydrophobic porous media. *Geoderma* **2024**, *441*, 116735. [CrossRef]
35. Gardner, K.H.; Arias, M.S. Clay Swelling and Formation Permeability Reductions Induced by a Nonionic Surfactant. *Environ. Sci. Technol.* **1999**, *34*, 160–166. [CrossRef]
36. Zhang, W.; Tang, X.Y.; Weisbrod, N.; Zhao, P.; Reid, B.J. A coupled field study of subsurface fracture flow and colloid transport. *J. Hydrol.* **2015**, *524*, 476–488. [CrossRef]
37. Wang, D.M.; Butler, R.; Zhang, J.; Seright, R. Wettability Survey in Bakken Shale With Surfactant-Formulation Imbibition. *SPE Reserv. Eval. Eng.* **2012**, *15*, 695–705. [CrossRef]

38. Seyedabbasi, M.A.; Farthing, M.W.; Imhoff, P.T.; Miller, C.T. The influence of wettability on NAPL dissolution fingering. *Adv. Water Resour.* **2008**, *31*, 1687–1696. [CrossRef]
39. Alvarez, J.O.; Schechter, D.S. Altering Wettability in Bakken Shale by Surfactant Additives and Potential of Improving Oil Recovery during Injection of Completion Fluids. In Proceedings of the SPE Improved Oil Recovery Conference, Tulsa, OK, USA, 11–13 April 2016.
40. Li, L.; Chen, J.; Liu, J.; Xu, Z.; Wu, Y.; Zhao, M.; Zhao, G.; Dai, C. Anionic surfactant based on oil-solid interfacial interaction control for efficient residual oil development. *Colloids Surf. A Physicochem. Eng. Asp.* **2022**, *648*, 129396. [CrossRef]
41. Duffield, A.R.; Ramamurthy, R.S.; Campanelli, J.R. Surfactant Enhanced Mobilization of Mineral Oil within Porous Media. *Water Air Soil Pollut.* **2003**, *143*, 111–122. [CrossRef]
42. Bettahar, M.; Ducreux, J.; Schäfer, G.; Van Dorpe, F. Surfactant Enhanced In Situ Remediation of LNAPL Contaminated Aquifers: Large Scale Studies on a Controlled Experimental Site. *Transp. Porous Media* **1999**, *37*, 255–276. [CrossRef]
43. Lowe, D.F.; Oubre, C.L.; Ward, C.H. *Surfactants and Cosolvents for NAPL Remediation. A Technologies Practices Manual*; Lewis Publications: Boca Raton, FL, USA, 1999.
44. Harendra, S.; Vipulanandan, C. Effects of Surfactants on Solubilization of Perchloroethylene (PCE) and Trichloroethylene (TCE). *Ind. Eng. Chem. Res.* **2011**, *50*, 5831–5837. [CrossRef]
45. Liang, X.; Dong, J.; Zhang, W.; Mo, Y.; Li, Y.; Bai, J. Solubilization mechanism and mass-transfer model of anionic-nonionic gemini surfactants for chlorinated hydrocarbons. *Sep. Purif. Technol.* **2024**, *330*, 125534. [CrossRef]
46. Barbati, B.; Lorini, L.; Amanat, N.; Bellagamba, M.; Galantini, L.; Petrangeli Papini, M. Enhanced solubilization of strongly adsorbed organic pollutants using synthetic and natural surfactants in soil flushing: Column experiment simulation. *J. Environ. Chem. Eng.* **2023**, *11*, 110758. [CrossRef]
47. Wang, Z.; Yang, Z.; Chen, Y.F. Pore-scale investigation of surfactant-enhanced DNAPL mobilization and solubilization. *Chemosphere* **2023**, *341*, 140071. [CrossRef]
48. Iglesias, O.; Sanromán, M.A.; Pazos, M. Surfactant-Enhanced Solubilization and Simultaneous Degradation of Phenanthrene in Marine Sediment by Electro-Fenton Treatment. *Ind. Eng. Chem. Res.* **2014**, *53*, 2917–2923. [CrossRef]
49. Attwood, D.; Florence, A.T. *Surfactant Systems*; Springer: Berlin/Heidelberg, Germany, 1983.
50. Kile, D.E.; Chiou, C.T. Water solubility enhancements of DDT and trichlorobenzene by some surfactants below and above the critical micelle concentration. *Environ. Sci. Technol.* **2002**, *23*, 832–838. [CrossRef]
51. Edwards, D.A.; Luthy, R.G.; Liu, Z. Solubilization of polycyclic aromatic hydrocarbons in micellar nonionic surfactant solutions. *Environ. Sci. Technol.* **1991**, *25*, 127–133. [CrossRef]
52. Buzier, M.; Ravey, J.C. Solubilization properties of nonionic surfactants: I. Evolution of the ternary phase diagrams with temperature, salinity, HLB, and ACN. *J. Colloid Interface Sci.* **1983**, *91*, 20–33. [CrossRef]
53. Masrat, R.; Majid, K. Solubilization of pyrene by mixed polymer-cationic/nonionic surfactant systems: Effect of polymer concentration. *Colloids Surf. A Physicochem. Eng. Asp.* **2022**, *653*, 129974. [CrossRef]
54. Javanbakht, G.; Goual, L. Impact of Surfactant Structure on NAPL Mobilization and Solubilization in Porous Media. *Ind. Eng. Chem. Res.* **2016**, *55*, 11736–11746. [CrossRef]
55. Tick, G.; Slavic, D.R.; Akyol, N.H.; Zhang, Y. Enhanced-solubilization and dissolution of multicomponent DNAPL from homogeneous porous media. *J. Contam. Hydrol.* **2022**, *247*, 103967. [CrossRef]
56. Yang Siyue, S.Y.; Mao, M.; Wang, J.; Zhu, H.; Liu, H.; Yang, S. Experimental Study on Remediation of Petroleum Hydrocarbon Pollution in Subsurface Aquifers Based on SEAR Technology. *Res. Environ. Sci.* **2023**, *36*, 954–964. [CrossRef]
57. Feng, C.; Sun, L.; Liu, W.; Chen, C.; Li, B.; Sun, D. Effects of surfactant on the molecules of different polarity of solubilization: Based on the study of micellar microscopic morphology mechanism. *J. Pet. Sci. Eng.* **2022**, *208*, 109563. [CrossRef]
58. Zhao, X.; Gong, L.; Liao, G.; Luan, H.; Chen, Q.; Liu, D.; Feng, Y. Micellar solubilization of petroleum fractions by heavy alkylbenzene sulfonate surfactant. *J. Mol. Liq.* **2021**, *329*, 115519. [CrossRef]
59. Zhong, H.; Yang, X.; Tan, F.; Brusseau, M.L.; Yang, L.; Liu, Z.; Zeng, G.; Yuan, X. Aggregate-based sub-CMC Solubilization of n-Alkanes by Monorhamnolipid Biosurfactant. *New J. Chem.* **2016**, *40*, 2028–2035. [CrossRef] [PubMed]
60. Yang, X.; Tan, F.; Zhong, H.; Liu, G.; Ahmad, Z.; Liang, Q. Sub-CMC solubilization of n-alkanes by rhamnolipid biosurfactant: The Influence of rhamnolipid molecular structure. *Colloids Surf. B Biointerfaces* **2020**, *192*, 111049. [CrossRef] [PubMed]
61. Kang, S.; Jeong, H.Y. Sorption of a nonionic surfactant Tween 80 by minerals and soils. *J. Hazard. Mater.* **2015**, *284*, 143–150. [CrossRef] [PubMed]
62. Zhou, W.; Zhu, L. Influence of surfactant sorption on the removal of phenanthrene from contaminated soils. *Environ. Pollut.* **2008**, *152*, 99–105. [CrossRef] [PubMed]
63. Valvatne, P.H.; Blunt, M.J. Predictive pore-scale modeling of two-phase flow in mixed wet media. *Water Resour. Res.* **2004**, *40*, W07406. [CrossRef]
64. Guan, Z.; Tang, X.Y.; Nishimura, T.; Katou, H.; Liu, H.Y.; Qing, J. Surfactant-enhanced flushing enhances colloid transport and alters macroporosity in diesel-contaminated soil. *J. Environ. Sci.* **2018**, *64*, 197–206. [CrossRef] [PubMed]
65. Alexandridis, P.; Holzwarth, J.F.; Hatton, T.A. Thermodynamics of Droplet Clustering in Percolating AOT Water-in-Oil Microemulsions. *J. Phys. Chem.* **2002**, *99*, 8222–8232. [CrossRef]
66. Bodratti, A.M.; Sarkar, B.; Alexandridis, P. Adsorption of poly(ethylene oxide)-containing amphiphilic polymers on solid-liquid interfaces: Fundamentals and applications. *Adv. Colloid Interface Sci.* **2017**, *244*, 132–163. [CrossRef] [PubMed]

67. Pan, J.; Sun, L.; Liu, X.; Fang, Y. Precipitation-Dissolution switchable surfactants with the potential of simultaneous retrieving of surfactants and hydrophobic organic contaminants from emulsified and micellar eluents. *Chem. Eng. J.* **2023**, *458*, 141297. [CrossRef]
68. Yada, S.; Matsuoka, K.; Nagai Kanasaki, Y.; Gotoh, K.; Yoshimura, T. Emulsification, solubilization, and detergency behaviors of homogeneous polyoxypropylene-polyoxyethylene alkyl ether type nonionic surfactants. *Colloids Surf. A Physicochem. Eng. Asp.* **2019**, *564*, 51–58. [CrossRef]
69. Huang, C.W.; Chang, C.H. A laboratory study on foam-enhanced surfactant solution flooding in removing n-pentadecane from contaminated columns. *Colloids Surf. A Physicochem. Eng. Asp.* **2000**, *173*, 171–179. [CrossRef]
70. Mavaddat, M.; Abdollahi, A.; Mavaddat, Y.; Riahi, S. A New Approach to Use Mixture of Surfactants to Face Salinity Gradient in Microemulsion Flooding. In Proceedings of the 79th EAGE Conference and Exhibition, European Association of Geoscientists & Engineers, Paris, France, 12–15 June 2017.
71. Heeres, A.S.; Picone, C.S.F.; van der Wielen, L.A.M.; Cunha, R.L.; Cuellar, M.C. Microbial advanced biofuels production: Overcoming emulsification challenges for large-scale operation. *Trends Biotechnol.* **2014**, *32*, 221–229. [CrossRef] [PubMed]
72. McClements, D.J. *Food Emulsions*; CRC Press: Boca Raton, FL, USA, 2015.
73. Salehpour, M.; Sakhaei, Z.; Salehinezhad, R.; Mahani, H.; Riazi, M. Contribution of water-in-oil emulsion formation and pressure fluctuations to low salinity waterflooding of asphaltic oils: A pore-scale perspective. *J. Pet. Sci. Eng.* **2021**, *203*, 108597. [CrossRef]
74. Liu, J.; Zhong, L.; Zewen, Y.; Liu, Y.; Meng, X.; Zhang, W.; Zhang, H.; Yang, G.; Shaojie, W. High-efficiency emulsification anionic surfactant for enhancing heavy oil recovery. *Colloids Surf. A Physicochem. Eng. Asp.* **2022**, *642*, 128654. [CrossRef]
75. Ling, N.N.A.; Haber, A.; Graham, B.F.; Aman, Z.M.; May, E.F.; Fridjonsson, E.O.; Johns, M.L. Quantifying the Effect of Salinity on Oilfield Water-in-Oil Emulsion Stability. *Energy Fuels* **2018**, *32*, 10042–10049. [CrossRef]
76. Umar, A.A.; Saaid, I.B.M.; Sulaimon, A.A. Rheological and stability study of water-in-crude oil emulsions. *AIP Conf. Proc.* **2016**, *1774*, 040004. [CrossRef]
77. Sakhaei, Z.; Riazi, M. In-situ petroleum hydrocarbons contaminated soils remediation by polymer enhanced surfactant flushing: Mechanistic investigation. *Process Saf. Environ. Prot.* **2022**, *161*, 758–770. [CrossRef]
78. Zhao, J.; Torabi, F.; Yang, J. The role of emulsification and IFT reduction in recovering heavy oil during alkaline-surfactant-assisted CO_2 foam flooding: An experimental study. *Fuel* **2022**, *313*, 122942. [CrossRef]
79. Wang, K.; Pi, Y.; Wu, Y.; Jiao, G. Research on the Emulsification Performance of ASP Flooding Impact on Oil Displacement Effect. *Sci. Technol. Eng.* **2012**, *12*, 2428–2431.
80. She, Y.; Zhang, C.; Mahardika, M.A.; Patmonoaji, A.; Hu, Y.; Matsushita, S.; Suekane, T. Pore-scale study of in-situ surfactant flooding with strong oil emulsification in sandstone based on X-ray microtomography. *J. Ind. Eng. Chem.* **2021**, *98*, 247–261. [CrossRef]
81. Urum, K.; Pekdemir, T. Evaluation of biosurfactants for crude oil contaminated soil washing. *Chemosphere* **2004**, *57*, 1139–1150. [CrossRef] [PubMed]
82. Mrozik, A.; Piotrowska-Seget, Z. Bioaugmentation as a strategy for cleaning up of soils contaminated with aromatic compounds. *Microbiol. Res.* **2010**, *165*, 363–375. [CrossRef]
83. Billingsley, K.A.; Backus, S.M.; Wilson, S.; Singh, A.; Ward, O.P. Remediation of PCBs in soil by surfactant washing and biodegradation in the wash by *Pseudomonas* sp. LB400. *Biotechnol. Lett.* **2002**, *24*, 1827–1832. [CrossRef]
84. Teng Tingting, L.J. Research Progress on Identification of PAHs-Degrading Bacteria and Bioremediation of PAHs-Contaminated Soil. *J. Technol.* **2022**, *22*, 16–26.
85. Perini, B.L.B.; Bitencourt, R.L.; Daronch, N.A.; dos Santos Schneider, A.L.; De Oliveira, D. Surfactant-enhanced in-situ enzymatic oxidation: A bioremediation strategy for oxidation of polycyclic aromatic hydrocarbons in contaminated soils and aquifers. *J. Environ. Chem. Eng.* **2020**, *8*, 104013. [CrossRef]
86. Ghosh, I.; Mukherji, S. Diverse effect of surfactants on pyrene biodegradation by a Pseudomonas strain utilizing pyrene by cell surface hydrophobicity induction. *Int. Biodeterior. Biodegrad.* **2016**, *108*, 67–75. [CrossRef]
87. Wei, K.H.; Ma, J.; Xi, B.D.; Yu, M.D.; Cui, J.; Chen, B.L.; Li, Y.; Gu, Q.B.; He, X.S. Recent progress on in-situ chemical oxidation for the remediation of petroleum contaminated soil and groundwater. *J. Hazard. Mater.* **2022**, *432*, 128738. [CrossRef]
88. Xu, Y.; Zhang, L.; Wei, Z.; Zhang, X.; Zhao, C.; Li, H.; Hu, F.; Xu, L. Effects of Sulfate Radical Advanced Oxidation Technology on PAHs Remediation in Contaminated sites. *Soils* **2020**, *52*, 532–538. [CrossRef]
89. Pac, T.J.; Baldock, J.; Brodie, B.; Byrd, J.; Gil, B.; Morris, K.A.; Nelson, D.; Parikh, J.; Santos, P.; Singer, M.; et al. In situ chemical oxidation: Lessons learned at multiple sites. *Remediat. J.* **2019**, *29*, 75–91. [CrossRef]
90. O'Connor, D.; Hou, D.; Ok, Y.S.; Song, Y.; Sarmah, A.K.; Li, X.; Tack, F.M.G. Sustainable in situ remediation of recalcitrant organic pollutants in groundwater with controlled release materials: A review. *J. Control. Release* **2018**, *283*, 200–213. [CrossRef]
91. Besha, A.T.; Bekele, D.N.; Naidu, R.; Chadalavada, S. Recent advances in surfactant-enhanced In-Situ Chemical Oxidation for the remediation of non-aqueous phase liquid contaminated soils and aquifers. *Environ. Technol. Innov.* **2018**, *9*, 303–322. [CrossRef]
92. Wei, K.H.; Zheng, Y.M.; Sun, Y.; Zhao, Z.Q.; Xi, B.D.; He, X.S. Larger aggregate formed by self-assembly process of the mixture surfactants enhance the dissolution and oxidative removal of non-aqueous phase liquid contaminants in aquifer. *Sci. Total Environ.* **2024**, *912*, 169532. [CrossRef] [PubMed]
93. Garcia-Cervilla, R.; Santos, A.; Romero, A.; Lorenzo, D. Abatement of chlorobenzenes in aqueous phase by persulfate activated by alkali enhanced by surfactant addition. *J. Environ. Manag.* **2022**, *306*, 114475. [CrossRef]

94. García-Cervilla, R.; Santos, A.; Romero, A.; Lorenzo, D. Compatibility of nonionic and anionic surfactants with persulfate activated by alkali in the abatement of chlorinated organic compounds in aqueous phase. *Sci. Total Environ.* **2021**, *751*, 141782. [CrossRef]
95. Demiray, Z.; Akyol, N.H.; Akyol, G.; Copty, N.K. Surfactant-enhanced in-situ oxidation of DNAPL source zone: Experiments and numerical modeling. *J. Contam. Hydrol.* **2023**, *258*, 104233. [CrossRef] [PubMed]
96. Nwankwegu, A.S.; Onwosi, C.O. Bioremediation of gasoline contaminated agricultural soil by bioaugmentation. *Environ. Technol. Innov.* **2017**, *7*, 1–11. [CrossRef]
97. Ali, M.; Song, X.; Ding, D.; Wang, Q.; Zhang, Z.; Tang, Z. Bioremediation of PAHs and heavy metals co-contaminated soils: Challenges and enhancement strategies. *Environ. Pollut.* **2022**, *295*, 118686. [CrossRef]
98. Mnif, I.; Mnif, S.; Sahnoun, R.; Maktouf, S.; Ayedi, Y.; Ellouze-Chaabouni, S.; Ghribi, D. Biodegradation of diesel oil by a novel microbial consortium: Comparison between co-inoculation with biosurfactant-producing strain and exogenously added biosurfactants. *Environ. Sci. Pollut. Res.* **2015**, *22*, 14852–14861. [CrossRef]
99. Huizenga, J.M.; Schindler, J.; Simonich, M.T.; Truong, L.; Garcia-Jaramillo, M.; Tanguay, R.L.; Semprini, L. PAH bioremediation with Rhodococcus rhodochrous ATCC 21198: Impact of cell immobilization and surfactant use on PAH treatment and post-remediation toxicity. *J. Hazard. Mater.* **2024**, *470*, 134109. [CrossRef]
100. Gan, S.; Lau, E.V.; Ng, H.K. Remediation of soils contaminated with polycyclic aromatic hydrocarbons (PAHs). *J. Hazard. Mater.* **2009**, *172*, 532–549. [CrossRef]
101. Csutak, O.; Corbu, V.M. 17—Bioremediation of oil-contaminated soil by yeast bioaugmentation. In *Advances in Yeast Biotechnology for Biofuels and Sustainability*; Daverey, A., Dutta, K., Joshi, S., Gea, T., Eds.; Elsevier: Amsterdam, The Netherlands, 2023; pp. 395–447.
102. Li, X.; Tan, Q.; Zhou, Y.; Chen, Q.; Sun, P.; Shen, G.; Ma, L. Synergic remediation of polycyclic aromatic hydrocarbon-contaminated soil by a combined system of persulfate oxidation activated by biochar and phytoremediation with basil: A compatible, robust, and sustainable approach. *Chem. Eng. J.* **2023**, *452*, 139502. [CrossRef]
103. Lu, H.; Wang, W.; Li, F.; Zhu, L. Mixed-surfactant-enhanced phytoremediation of PAHs in soil: Bioavailability of PAHs and responses of microbial community structure. *Sci. Total Environ.* **2019**, *653*, 658–666. [CrossRef] [PubMed]
104. Liu, F.; Wang, C.; Liu, X.; Liang, X.; Wang, Q. Effects of Alkyl Polyglucoside (APG) on Phytoremediation of PAH-Contaminated Soil by an Aquatic Plant in the Yangtze Estuarine Wetland. *Water Air Soil Pollut.* **2013**, *224*, 1633. [CrossRef]
105. Xia, H.; Chi, X.; Yan, Z.; Cheng, W. Enhancing plant uptake of polychlorinated biphenyls and cadmium using tea saponin. *Bioresour. Technol.* **2009**, *100*, 4649–4653. [CrossRef]
106. Labianca, C.; De Gisi, S.; Picardi, F.; Todaro, F.; Notarnicola, M. Remediation of a Petroleum Hydrocarbon-Contaminated Site by Soil Vapor Extraction: A Full-Scale Case Study. *Appl. Sci.* **2020**, *10*, 4261. [CrossRef]
107. Chang YueHua, C.Y.; Yao Meng, Y.M.; Zhao YongSheng, Z.Y. Laboratory study of surfactant-enhanced air sparging remediation-The variation rule of the influence of zone and airflow distribution. *China Environ. Sci.* **2018**, *38*, 2585–2592. [CrossRef]
108. Xu, L.; Yan, L.; Zha, F.; Zhu, F.; Tan, X.; Kang, B.; Yang, C.; Lin, Z. Remediation characteristics of surfactant-enhanced air sparging (SEAS) technology on volatile organic compounds contaminated soil with low permeability. *J. Contam. Hydrol.* **2022**, *250*, 104049. [CrossRef] [PubMed]
109. Yao, M.; Yuan, Q.; Qu, D.; Liu, W.; Zhao, Y.; Wang, M. Effects of airflow rate distribution and nitrobenzene removal in an aquifer with a low-permeability lens during surfactant-enhanced air sparging. *J. Hazard. Mater.* **2022**, *437*, 129383. [CrossRef] [PubMed]
110. Roy, S.; Pandit, S. 1.2—Microbial Electrochemical System: Principles and Application. In *Microbial Electrochemical Technology*; Mohan, S.V., Varjani, S., Pandey, A., Eds.; Elsevier: Amsterdam, The Netherlands, 2019; pp. 19–48.
111. Zheng, F.; Gao, B.; Sun, Y.; Shi, X.; Xu, H.; Wu, J.; Gao, Y. Removal of tetrachloroethylene from homogeneous and heterogeneous porous media: Combined effects of surfactant solubilization and oxidant degradation. *Chem. Eng. J.* **2016**, *283*, 595–603. [CrossRef]
112. Risco, C.; López-Vizcaíno, R.; Sáez, C.; Yustres, A.; Cañizares, P.; Navarro, V.; Rodrigo, M.A. Remediation of soils polluted with 2,4-D by electrokinetic soil flushing with facing rows of electrodes: A case study in a pilot plant. *Chem. Eng. J.* **2016**, *285*, 128–136. [CrossRef]
113. Gebregiorgis Ambaye, T.; Vaccari, M.; Franzetti, A.; Prasad, S.; Formicola, F.; Rosatelli, A.; Hassani, A.; Aminabhavi, T.M.; Rtimi, S. Microbial electrochemical bioremediation of petroleum hydrocarbons (PHCs) pollution: Recent advances and outlook. *Chem. Eng. J.* **2023**, *452*, 139372. [CrossRef]
114. Hahladakis, J.N.; Latsos, A.; Gidarakos, E. Performance of electroremediation in real contaminated sediments using a big cell, periodic voltage and innovative surfactants. *J. Hazard. Mater.* **2016**, *320*, 376–385. [CrossRef] [PubMed]
115. Arumugam, A.; Fang, C.; Selvin, J.; Kuppusamy, S.; Ricky Devi, O.; Zhang, F.; Guo, X.; Kadaikunnan, S.; Balu, R.; Liu, X. Plant biomass extracted eco-friendly natural surfactant enhanced bio-electrokinetic remediation of crude oil contaminated soil. *Environ. Res.* **2024**, *245*, 117913. [CrossRef] [PubMed]
116. Hahladakis, J.N.; Calmano, W.; Gidarakos, E. Use and comparison of the non-ionic surfactants Poloxamer 407 and Nonidet P40 with HP-β-CD cyclodextrin, for the enhanced electroremediation of real contaminated sediments from PAHs. *Sep. Purif. Technol.* **2013**, *113*, 104–113. [CrossRef]
117. Denison, S.B.; Da Silva, P.D.; Koester, C.P.; Alvarez, P.J.J.; Zygourakis, K. Clays play a catalytic role in pyrolytic treatment of crude-oil contaminated soils that is enhanced by ion-exchanged transition metals. *J. Hazard. Mater.* **2022**, *437*, 129295. [CrossRef] [PubMed]

118. Wang, M.; Xie, X.; Wu, C. Ball milling enhances pyrolytic remediation of petroleum-contaminated soil and reuse as adsorptive/catalytic materials for wastewater treatment. *J. Water Process Eng.* **2024**, *58*, 104894. [CrossRef]
119. Fu, J.; Cai, P.; Zhan, M.; Xu, X.; Chen, T.; Li, X.; Jiao, W.; Yin, Y. Washing-thermal desorption remediation of paraffin and naphthenic based crude oil contaminated soil. *Environ. Eng.* **2022**, *40*, 167–172. [CrossRef]
120. Cheng, M.; Zeng, G.; Huang, D.; Yang, C.; Lai, C.; Zhang, C.; Liu, Y. Advantages and challenges of Tween 80 surfactant-enhanced technologies for the remediation of soils contaminated with hydrophobic organic compounds. *Chem. Eng. J.* **2017**, *314*, 98–113. [CrossRef]
121. Karthick, A.; Roy, B.; Chattopadhyay, P. A review on the application of chemical surfactant and surfactant foam for remediation of petroleum oil contaminated soil. *J. Environ. Manag.* **2019**, *243*, 187–205. [CrossRef]
122. Zhencheng, Y.; Yifan, S.; Yunfeng, Y. The application of molecular biology-based microbial remediation technologies in petroleum polluted environments. *Chin. J. Biotechnol.* **2024**, *40*, 739–757. [CrossRef]
123. Da Silva, A.F.; Banat, I.M.; Giachini, A.J.; Robl, D. Fungal biosurfactants, from nature to biotechnological product: Bioprospection, production and potential applications. *Bioprocess Biosyst. Eng.* **2021**, *44*, 2003–2034. [CrossRef] [PubMed]
124. Banat, I.M.; Franzetti, A.; Gandolfi, I.; Bestetti, G.; Martinotti, M.G.; Fracchia, L.; Smyth, T.J.; Marchant, R. Microbial biosurfactants production, applications and future potential. *Appl. Microbiol. Biotechnol.* **2010**, *87*, 427–444. [CrossRef] [PubMed]
125. Martienssen, M.; Schirmer, M. Use of Surfactants to Improve the Biological Degradation of Petroleum Hydrocarbons in a Field Site Study. *Environ. Technol.* **2007**, *28*, 573–582. [CrossRef] [PubMed]
126. Dolman, B.M.; Wang, F.; Winterburn, J.B. Integrated production and separation of biosurfactants. *Process Biochem.* **2019**, *83*, 1–8. [CrossRef]
127. Santos, B.L.P.; Vieira, I.M.M.; Ruzene, D.S.; Silva, D.P. Unlocking the potential of biosurfactants: Production, applications, market challenges, and opportunities for agro-industrial waste valorization. *Environ. Res.* **2024**, *244*, 117879. [CrossRef]
128. Dai, C.M.; Tong, W.K.; Hu, J.J.; Duan, Y.P.; Tu, Y.J.; Lai, X.Y.; Liu, S.G.; Li, J.X. Switchable Surfactant-Enhanced Remediation of Polycyclic Aromatic Hydrocarbons in Soil and Groundwater: A Review. *Res. Environ. Sci.* **2022**, *35*, 1925–1934. [CrossRef]

water

MDPI

Review

Occurrence, Risks, and Removal Methods of Antibiotics in Urban Wastewater Treatment Systems: A Review

Liping Zhu [1], Xiaohu Lin [2,*], Zichen Di [1], Fangqin Cheng [1,*] and Jingcheng Xu [3]

1 School of Environmental & Resource Science, Shanxi University, Taiyuan 030031, China; liberty_1120@126.com (L.Z.); dizichen@sxu.edu.cn (Z.D.)
2 Hangzhou Institute of Ecological and Environmental Sciences, Hangzhou 310014, China
3 College of Environmental Science and Engineering, Tongji University, Shanghai 200092, China; xujick@tongji.edu.cn
* Correspondence: tjhjxhlin@163.com (X.L.); cfangqin@sxu.edu.cn (F.C.); Tel.: +86-057188334112 (X.L.); +86-0351-7018533 (F.C.)

Abstract: Antibiotics, widely used pharmaceuticals, enter wastewater treatment systems and ultimately the aquatic environment through the discharge of wastewater from residential areas, hospitals, breeding farms, and pharmaceutical factories, posing potential ecological and health risks. Due to the misuse and discharge of antibiotics, the spread of antibiotic resistance genes (ARGs) in water bodies and significant changes in microbial community structure have direct toxic effects on aquatic ecosystems and human health. This paper summarizes the occurrence of antibiotics in wastewater treatment systems and their ecological and health risks, focusing on the impact of antibiotics on aquatic microorganisms, aquatic plants and animals, and human health. It points out that existing wastewater treatment processes have poor removal capabilities for antibiotics and even become an important pathway for the spread of some antibiotics. In terms of detection technology, the article discusses the application of immunoassays, instrumental analysis, and emerging sensor technologies in detecting antibiotics in sewage, each with its advantages and limitations. Future efforts should combine multiple technologies to improve detection accuracy. Regarding the removal methods of antibiotics, the paper categorizes physical, chemical, and biodegradation methods, introducing various advanced technologies including membrane separation, adsorption, electrochemical oxidation, photocatalytic oxidation, and membrane bioreactors. Although these methods have shown good removal effects in the laboratory, there are still many limitations in large-scale practical applications. This paper innovatively takes urban wastewater treatment systems as the entry point, systematically integrating the sources of antibiotics, environmental risks, detection technologies, and treatment methods, providing targeted and practical theoretical support and technical guidance, especially in the removal of antibiotics in wastewater treatment, on a scientific basis. Future efforts should strengthen the control of antibiotic sources, improve the efficiency of wastewater treatment, optimize detection technologies, and promote the formulation and implementation of relevant laws and standards to more effectively manage and control antibiotic pollution in the aquatic environment.

Keywords: antibiotics; wastewater treatment system; occurrence; environmental risk; detection; removal

1. Introduction

With the continuous development of organic chemical synthesis processes, an increasing number of compounds are being mass-produced and widely used in our daily lives. In recent years, many substances have uncontrollably entered the water environment, becoming new types of pollutants. Among them, pharmaceuticals and personal care products (PPCPs), persistent organic pollutants (POPs), endocrine disruptors (EDCs), and disinfection byproducts (DBPs) are some of the most prominent categories. These pollutants are characterized by their low concentrations, difficulty in terms of degradation, and high toxicity risks, which have led to widespread attention and research. Among them, antibiotics, which belong to PPCPs, have become a hot topic in scientific research due to their long-term and extensive use in treating bacterial infections in humans and animals. Since the advent of penicillin in 1929, hundreds of isolated or synthesized antibiotics have been utilized for the prevention and management of illnesses in both humans and animals [1]. Among the various categories, beta-lactam antibiotics (BLAs), fluoroquinolones (FQs), tetracyclines (TCs), macrolides (MLs), and sulfonamides (SAs) are the most commonly used antibiotics. Domestic life [2], hospitals [3,4], animal husbandry [5,6] and antibiotic manufacturing factories [7–9] are all significant sources of antibiotics in wastewater treatment systems, with medicinal antibiotics being of particular concern. For instance, in animal husbandry, to curb the spread of pathogens, uninfected animals are also compulsorily administered a certain dose of antibiotics for disease prevention. Medicinal antibiotics that enter living organisms are only partially effectively metabolized, with approximately 50–80% of the active antibiotic residues being excreted through feces and urine, and a large proportion of these residues enter the natural surroundings through urban wastewater treatment systems [10,11]. A plethora of studies have demonstrated the presence of antibiotics in surface water [12,13], groundwater [14], drinking water [13,15], and seawater [16,17] around the world.

Antibiotics are considered "pseudo-persistent" contaminants in the environment because they are not highly resistant to degradation, but the rate at which they enter the environment far exceeds their rate of degradation [18]. Additionally, although the concentration of antibiotics in aquatic environments is generally low (typically measured in ng/L [19–22]), their high biological activity [23] still poses a considerable risk to aquatic ecosystems and human health [24]. The increasing antibiotic resistance in bacteria has sparked much public discussion [2,20]. The residue of antibiotics in aquatic environments, once it reaches a certain level, can affect the composition and function of microbial communities, impacting microbial ecology by increasing mutation rates, facilitating the horizontal transfer of resistance genes, and driving the environmental selection of antibiotic-resistant bacteria [25,26]. This, in turn, gradually weakens humanity's ability to treat infectious diseases, perform surgery, and utilize immunosuppressive therapies, undermining the foundation of modern healthcare [27]. In addition, antibiotics can also have direct toxic effects on a range of aquatic plants and animals, altering species distribution and threatening the entire aquatic ecosystem [28,29]. The synergistic, additive, or antagonistic effects between other toxins in water and antibiotics are also not yet clear [30,31].

As mentioned earlier, urban wastewater treatment systems, as an essential part of the water resource cycle, contain a large amount of antibiotics from various sources. Currently, the treatment rate of antibiotics in wastewater treatment plants is generally low [29], and they have even become an important "source" for the spread of antibiotics and antibiotic-resistant bacteria in diverse aquatic environments [20,32,33]. How to effectively detect antibiotics in wastewater is the first question that needs to be studied. Compared with some conventional physicochemical parameters, the discharge of most antibiotics is not currently under effective regulation, largely due to the limitations of trace detection technology development. A variety of methods have been designed to ascertain antibiotics in wastewater, such as immunoassays [34,35], instrumental analysis methods [36], and various sensor detection methods. Different detection methods have their own advantages and disadvantages, and they each have applicable conditions or categories of antibiotics. A review of the enrichment and detection methods for antibiotics in water is beneficial for comparing their differences and sorting out the frontier directions of related research. Due to the increasing public concern about antibiotic pollution, research on antibiotic removal technologies is also emerging. In addition to the traditional activated sludge method, methods such as membrane separation [37,38], adsorption [39,40], advanced oxidation [41], and membrane bioreactors have also been developed for the removal of antibiotics from wastewater. However, the specific removal mechanisms and efficiencies of these methods are mostly still at the laboratory stage, and their practical applications may be limited by the conditions of wastewater treatment systems and treatment costs. We find that although there are already summaries of the environmental risks, detection technologies, and treatment methods for antibiotics, there are still few reviews focusing on antibiotics in wastewater treatment systems. Urban wastewater treatment systems are an essential part of the control of antibiotic pollution, and improving the summary and analysis in this area is of great significance and urgency for the in-depth research into and management of antibiotics.

Therefore, the main objectives of this study are as follows: (1) to summarize the influent and effluent concentrations of major categories of antibiotics in wastewater treatment systems in different regions, and to deeply analyze the potential impacts of antibiotics in current wastewater treatment systems on aquatic ecology and human health; (2) to systematically review the current detection technologies for antibiotics in wastewater, assess the accuracy and reliability of the various methods, and provide scientific guidance for actual detection work; and (3) to review the current effective treatment methods for antibiotics in wastewater, with the expectation of providing feasible operational plans to address the issue of antibiotic pollution. This paper innovatively focuses on the important link of urban wastewater treatment systems, not only effectively connecting the sources of antibiotics and the risks of their entry into the water environment in logical terms but also enhancing the specificity and practicality of the review of antibiotic detection and treatment methods. Through this study, we aim to furnish a scientific rationale and backing for the effective regulation and control of antibiotic pollution in the aquatic environment, at both the standard-setting and legal enforcement levels.

2. The Occurrence and Potential Risks of Antibiotics in Urban Wastewater Treatment Systems

2.1. *Antibiotic Consumption and Concentrations in Wastewater Treatment Systems*

Currently, the global consumption of antibiotics is staggering. A study by the National Academy of Sciences in the United States indicates that between 2000 and 2015, antibiotic consumption, measured in defined daily doses (DDDs), increased by 65% (from 21.1 to 34.8 billion DDDs), and the antibiotic consumption rate per 1000 inhabitants per day increased by 39% (from 11.3 to 15.7 DDDs). If the existing policies remain unchanged, forecasts indicate that global antibiotic consumption in 2030 could surge up to 200% compared to the estimated 42 billion DDDs (defined daily doses) in 2015 [42]. In 2021, among the 29 European Union/European Economic Area countries that provided data on human and food-producing animal consumption, the amounts of antibiotics consumed by humans and food-producing livestock were 3061 tons and 4994 tons, respectively [43]. Table 1 summarizes the categorization of certain antibiotics in the aforementioned European countries, as well as the range, median, and population-weighted mean of human and food-producing animal consumption, estimated in mg/kg of biomass.

Table 1. The classification of certain types of antibiotics in most European countries, as well as their range, median, and population-weighted mean of antimicrobial consumption in humans and food-producing animals [43].

	Antimicrobial Group	WHO Categorization [a]	AMEG Categorization [b]	Antimicrobial Consumption (mg/kg Estimated Biomass)					
				Humans			Food-Producing Animals		
				Range	Median	Mean	Range	Median	Mean
1	Third-and fourth-generation cephalosporins	Highest priority CIA	Category B	0.4–18.3	3.0	5.1	<0.01–0.5	0.2	0.2
2	Fluoroquinolones and other quinolones	Highest priority CIA	Category B	1.0–19.0	4.6	6.3	<0.01–14.8	0.9	2.9

Table 1. *Cont.*

	Antimicrobial Group	WHO Categorization [a]	AMEG Categorization [b]	Antimicrobial Consumption (mg/kg Estimated Biomass)					
				Humans			Food-Producing Animals		
				Range	Median	Mean	Range	Median	Mean
3	Polymyxins	Highest priority CIA	Category B	0–3.7	0.4	0.7	0–12.7	0.5	2.5
4	Aminopenicillins	HIA	Category C (with inhibitors) and D (without inhibitors)	6.5–101.0	47.2	64.1	0.05–59.6	8.8	25.8
5	Macrolides	CIA	Category C	0.5–11.1	5.0	6.2	0–22.6	5.0	7.8
6	Tetracyclines	HIA	Category D	0.3–6.0	1.7	1.9	0.04–113.4	16.2	23.6
	Total consumption			44.3–160.1	108.9	125.0	2.5–296.5	50.0	92.6

Notes: [a]: WHO, World Health Organization; CIA, critically important antimicrobial; HIA, highly important antimicrobial. [b]: AMEG, EMA's Antimicrobial Advice ad hoc Expert Group. Category A ('Avoid') encompasses antibiotics that are currently unauthorized for veterinary use in the EU. These medicines are of crucial importance in human medicine and may not be used in food-producing animals. Category B ('Restrict') refers to quinolones, third-and fourth-generation cephalosporins, and polymyxins. The use of these medicines in animals should be restricted. Category C ('Caution') covers antibiotics for which alternatives in human medicine generally exist in the EU. Their use should only be considered when no clinically effective antibiotics in Category D are available. Category D ("Prudence") comprises antibiotics that should be prioritized as first-line treatments whenever feasible. These antibiotics can be used in animals judiciously, meaning that unnecessary use and prolonged treatment durations should be avoided.

As shown in Table 1, despite the graded management of antibiotic use, in 2021, the population-weighted average consumption in the EU/EEA reached 125.0 mg/kg (range 44.3–160.1 mg/kg; median 108.9 mg/kg). The average consumption for food-producing animals reached 92.6 mg/kg (range 2.5–296.5 mg/kg; median 50.0 mg/kg).

These antibiotics have difficulty in being fully metabolized by humans and animals, and a substantial portion of them enter urban wastewater treatment systems. In addition to this, wastewater discharged from antibiotic-manufacturing factories, as well as improperly treated medical waste from hospitals, also deliver a significant amount of antibiotics to wastewater treatment systems. Since antibiotics are not strictly regulated in the wastewater discharge standards of most countries, traditional wastewater treatment plants generally do not have specialized processes for removing antibiotics. Most antibiotics can only be partially removed, displaying removal efficiencies spanning from negative percentages up to more than 90%. This means that some wastewater treatment plants may even release antibiotics into the wastewater, leading to higher concentrations in the effluent than in the influent. The removal effectiveness of different antibiotics in municipal wastewater treatment plants is also tightly related to their inherent physical and chemical characteristics [25]; hence, the removal efficiency of antibiotics can vary even within the same wastewater treatment plant. Figure 1 illustrates the concentrations of major categories of antibiotics in the influent and effluent of municipal wastewater treatment plants in different countries and regions.

The range of antibiotic concentrations present in the influent of wastewater treatment plants is approximately between 0.01 ng/L and 10 μg/L, and in the effluent, the concentration range is approximately between 0.01 ng/L and 1 μg/L. A red reference line is drawn at 100 ng/L, and by comparing the number of data points to the right of the reference line, it is evident that wastewater treatment plants have a certain removal effect on most high-concentration antibiotics. Additionally, different wastewater treatment plants and different types of antibiotics lead to noticeable differences in removal efficiency.

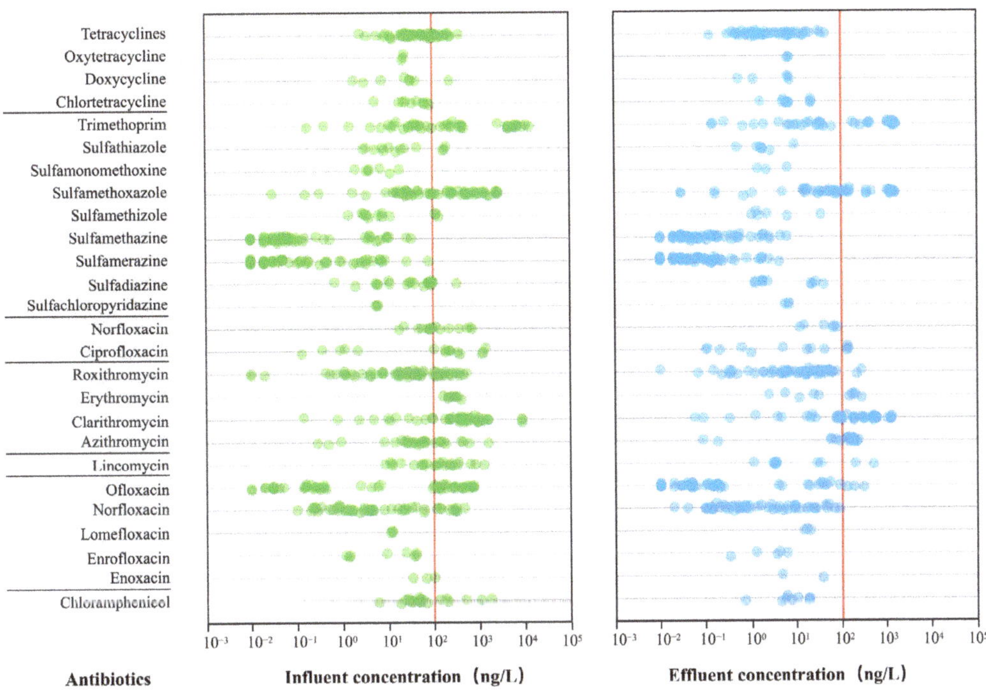

Figure 1. Concentrations of major classes of antibiotics in the influent and effluent of municipal wastewater treatment plants in different countries and regions (data from [20]).

2.2. Potential Ecological and Human Health Risks Posed by Antibiotics

Residual antibiotics eventually enter the receiving water bodies through the effluent of wastewater treatment systems, becoming a substantial source of antibiotics and their secondary metabolites in the aquatic environment [44]. Under these circumstances, the potential ecological and health risks posed by antibiotics in wastewater should be taken seriously. Figure 2 illustrates the process by which antibiotics enter the wastewater treatment system and, together with antibiotic resistance genes (ARGs), make their way into various water environments, causing environmental harm.

The occurrence of antibiotics in urban wastewater treatment systems initially impacts the dissemination of ARGs. ARGs are considered emerging micropollutants with environmental persistence [45]. As previously mentioned, a significant amount of antibiotics from various sources ultimately converge at wastewater treatment plants, exerting a substantial driving force on the emergence, evolution, and selection of ARGs [46]. Owing to the fact that ARGs can adhere to soil and sediment particles, the aquatic environment is more conducive to the widespread dissemination of ARGs among different geographical regions and diverse microbial species, including pathogenic bacteria [47]. Given that traditional wastewater treatment processes are nearly ineffective in removing DNA [26], residual antibiotics and ARGs enter surface water, drinking water, recreational water, and seawater with the effluent, further increasing the exposure of humans to antibiotics and the risk of ARG proliferation [48].

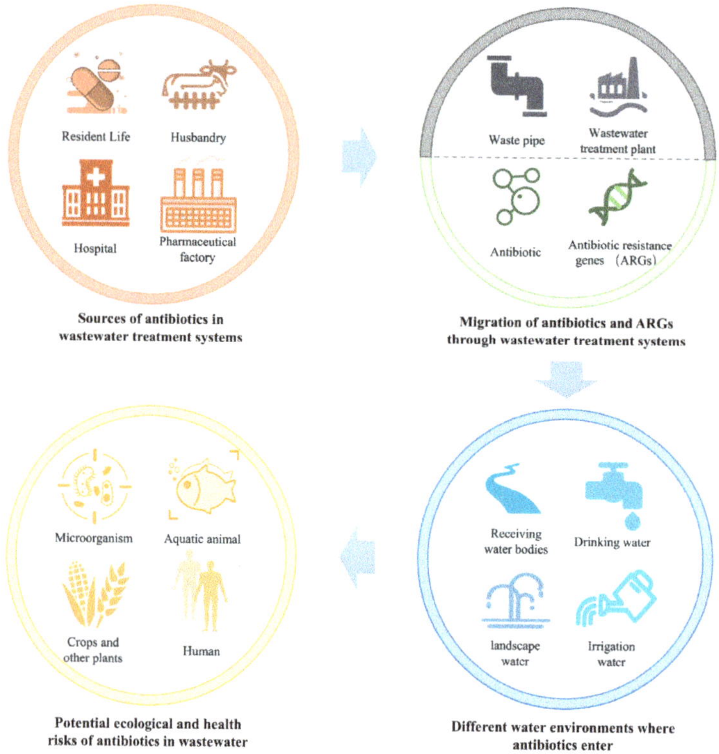

Figure 2. Environmental migration process of antibiotics and ARGs in municipal wastewater treatment systems.

In aquatic environments, microorganisms play crucial roles as producers, consumers, and decomposers, maintaining the stability of aquatic ecosystems [49]. Despite not reaching the minimum inhibitory concentration (MIC), antibiotics are significant drivers of evolutionary changes in aquatic microorganisms. Under long-term exposure to low concentrations, antibiotics are capable of modifying the composition and structure of microbial populations and communities in water, further inducing the emergence of antibiotic resistance and consequently altering the ecological functions of certain aquatic environments [50]. For general bacteria, studies have shown that fluoroquinolone antibiotics can induce the bacterial SOS response (a DNA damage repair mechanism), regulating the horizontal transfer of integrative and conjugative elements that encode various other traits such as bacterial virulence, antibiotic resistance, and bacterial metabolism [51,52]. In aquatic systems exposed to low levels of tetracycline, the abundance of tetracycline resistance genes increases compared to the 16S rRNA gene [53]. Research by Cairns et al. [54] indicates that antibiotics can affect the species richness of bacterial populations by increasing the differences in adaptability among taxa, reducing community diversity. Zhao et al. [55] have demonstrated that even at low levels, antibiotics can have a notable impact on the composition of freshwater microbial communities at the genus level without affecting the bacterial community's alpha diversity. From a macro perspective of aquatic ecological functions, it is known that tetracycline can inhibit the nitrification process in surface water to some extent [56], and some ammonium-oxidizing bacteria in experiments have shown sensitivity to antibiotics [57,58], significantly affecting the removal of nitrogen elements in water. Ofloxacin mildly inhibits two key steps in anaerobic digestion—methanogenesis and acetate kinetics [59]. Trace quantities of antibiotics in the aquatic environment might possibly affect the processes that promote carbonate precipitation and lead to an increase in atmospheric CO_2 concentrations.

Research has revealed that various antibiotics, such as sulfonamides, tetracyclines, and macrolides, exhibit potential detrimental impacts on the development and growth of cyanobacteria and other algal species [58]. Antibiotics can impact algal growth by inducing abscisic acid secretion, inhibiting cellular protein synthesis, and disrupting chloroplasts [60,61]. Since cyanobacteria are prokaryotes and structurally more similar to bacteria, they are more susceptible to the effects of antibiotics. In toxicity tests on cyanobacteria, the EC50 values are far below 1 mg/L [62]. Most green algae species also exhibit high sensitivity to macrolides such as clarithromycin and erythromycin, with EC50 values below 1 mg/L [58]. Additionally, low concentrations of antibiotics such as imipenem [63], tobramycin [64], and norfloxacin [65] can enhance the tolerance of Microcystis aeruginosa to antibiotics by altering its biofilm properties.

Antibiotics in wastewater have also garnered widespread concern for their toxicity to non-target organisms. For example, an environmental risk assessment encompassing 226 types of antibiotics revealed that a significant 44% of them possess high toxicity levels towards Daphnia magna [66]. Macrolides have also been found to be harmful to Daphnia, posing significant environmental risks [67,68]. Exposure to trace levels of β-ketoantibiotics (DKA) can affect various cellular and biological processes in zebrafish, including inducing severe histopathological changes in zebrafish heart tissue [69]. Sulfamethoxazole (SMX) affects the survival rate of zebrafish embryos and induces deformities in developing embryos [70]. Antibiotics are also harmful to plants. It has been proven that antibiotics can transfer between aquatic plants and poison them through metabolic disruption, oxidative damage, and damage to the photosynthetic system [71]. Irrigating crops with water contaminated by antibiotics can result in the accumulation of antibiotics in the edible portions of crops [72].

The human gut is home to approximately 800–1000 different species of bacteria [73]. Among these microorganisms, beneficial bacteria account for up to 95%. There exists a stable ecological balance among the gut microbiota, as well as between the microbiota and the human body [74]. Epidemiological, observational, and clinical reports have provided substantial evidence that antibiotic contaminants in water, when ingested by humans, can lead to an imbalance in the gut microbiome [75], resulting in the proliferation of harmful bacteria and opportunistic pathogens, causing intestinal diseases such as pseudomembranous colitis and colorectal cancer [74]. Prolonged exposure to antibiotics may gradually stimulate, enable the survival, and promote the proliferation of antibiotic-resistant bacteria within the human body. These bacteria may persist in the human gut for years, leading to immune alterations and metabolic disturbances [76]. However, due to the drug research process, the development of new antimicrobial drugs takes a long time—potentially over a decade before they become available to the public. Infections that are difficult to treat can lead to extended hospital stays, increased treatment frequency, and costly treatments, placing a significant burden on the healthcare system [77].

3. Detection Methods for Antibiotics in Urban Wastewater

3.1. Enrichment and Extraction Methods for Antibiotics in Water

Antibiotics in urban wastewater are generally present at low concentrations. To effectively measure the concentration of antibiotics in wastewater, the enrichment and extraction of antibiotics are required through pretreatment. Common pretreatment methods include solid-phase extraction (SPE), solid-phase microextraction (SPME), magnetic solid-phase extraction (MSPE), and dispersive liquid–liquid microextraction (DLLME). SPE primarily involves enriching, separating, and purifying target substances in water samples by utilizing solid-phase extraction columns, offering advantages such as a simple operation, strong selectivity, and good recovery rates [78]. The adsorbents can be single materials like ionic liquids [79], lignocellulosic materials [80], covalent organic frameworks [81], or composite materials [82]. SPME is a solvent-free pretreatment technique that enriches target analytes by directly immersing a coated fiber into the sample, utilizing the adsorption effect of the coating material. Many studies have achieved the efficient extraction of trace antibiotics in water samples by improving the fiber skeleton [83] and coating materials [84]. MSPE, based on SPE, uses magnetic nano-adsorbents to enhance its performance, thereby improving its adsorption capacity for antibiotics in water samples and increasing its detection sensitivity [85]. This method is simple, fast, does not require centrifugation or filtration, and the magnetic adsorbents can be reused, reducing contamination and loss during sample processing. Unlike the aforementioned pretreatment techniques, DLLME is a liquid-phase extraction technique that is widely employed due to its straightforward operation, cost-effectiveness, rapid extraction process, high recovery rates, and exceptional enrichment factors [86]. In addition, molecularly imprinted polymers (MIPs) and composite aerogels have also attracted considerable attention in the research community.

3.2. Immunoassay Methods

Immunoassay methods are traditional techniques for detecting antibiotics, mainly including enzyme-linked immunosorbent assay (ELISA), lateral flow immunoassay (LFIA), and fluorescence immunoassay. The principle behind these methods is the specific combination of antigens and antibodies [34]. ELISA is inherently cost-effective and user-friendly in terms of operation, and its application in the detection of environmental pollutants such as antibiotics can further enhance detection specificity and lower the detection limit. Hoffmann et al. [87] produced polyclonal antibodies against Sulfamethoxazole (SMX) and developed a direct competitive ELISA. This method can quantitatively detect SMX in the ng/L range in pre-concentrated environmental water samples, and it shows good consistency with the results obtained from LC-MS/MS instruments. LFIA represents a swift immunoassay technique that integrates immunoassay technology with chromatographic methods. A prevalent research focus currently lies in the development of composite nanomaterials as signal markers, aiming to elevate the efficacy and performance of LFIA [35,88]. Munirah et al. [89] conjugated streptomycin-specific monoclonal antibodies with gold nanoparticles (AuNPs) to prepare LFIA test strips for the concurrent quantitative and qualitative detection of streptomycin (STR) in pig serum and urine samples, effectively improving the sensitivity of LFIA for STR detection. Fluorescence immunoassay involves labeling antibodies or antigens with fluorescent substances and measuring the fluorescence to determine the presence of antibiotics. Chen et al. [90] combined fiber-embedded optofluidic nanochips with evanescent wave dual-color fluorescence technology to prepare evanescent wave dual-color fluorescence optofluidic nanochips (EDFON). By using the EDFON technique, a heterogeneous immunoassay was combined with a homogeneous hybridization chain reaction based on the time-resolved effect, enabling the highly sensitive and specific parallel quantitative detection of sulfamethazine (SMR) and the antibiotic resistance gene MCR-1.

3.3. Instrumental Analysis Methods

Instrumental analysis methods are among the most widely used techniques for detecting antibiotics, mainly divided into chromatographic methods, spectroscopic methods, and mass spectrometric methods. The most frequently utilized chromatographic method is high-performance liquid chromatography (HPLC), which separates individual compounds from a mixture through the interactions occurring between two phases (the stationary phase and the mobile phase) [36]. Numerous studies have improved the detection efficiency of HPLC for trace antibiotics in wastewater by optimizing sample pretreatment methods and injection conditions. Rabeea et al. [91] optimized a method for the quantitative determination of multiple antibiotics in wastewater samples using HPLC. The mobile phase consists of 1% formic acid and acetonitrile in a ratio of 84:16. A sample volume of 20 μL is injected into the HPLC column, and the flow rate through the column is maintained at 1.00 mL/min. By comparing the peak area of the real sample with the peak area of a standard solution, the quantification of multiple antibiotics can be achieved. Mahmoud et al. [92] established an HPLC–diode array detector (HPLC-DAD) method and a rapid HPLC method based on a core–shell stationary phase, coupled with the simplified and sensitive SPE procedure that they developed, effectively improving the sensitivity of antibiotic compound detection. Figure 3 illustrates the process flow of commonly used instrumental detection methods for antibiotics.

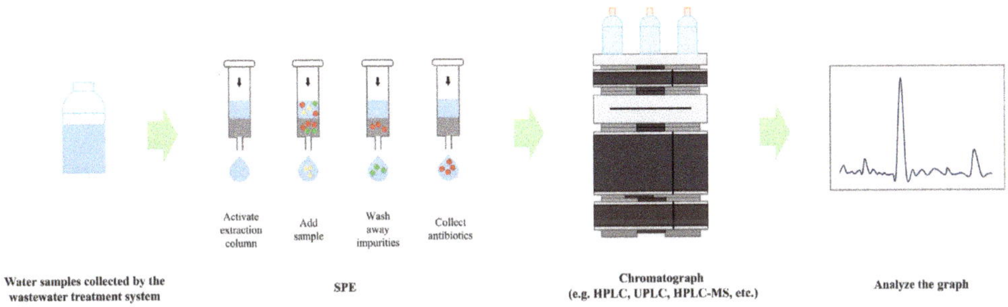

Figure 3. Workflow of common instrumental methods for antibiotic detection.

Spectroscopy primarily involves the analysis of the composition and concentration of compounds within a sample by quantifying the absorbance or emission of light at various wavelengths. Among the various spectroscopic techniques, ultraviolet–visible (UV–Vis) spectroscopy and surface-enhanced Raman spectroscopy (SERS) are widely employed for detecting antibiotics in wastewater. Notably, UV–Vis spectroscopy stands out as an efficient tool for the real-time monitoring of antibiotic levels in wastewater. Li et al. [93] used two submerged in situ UV–Vis sensors to explore the relationship between absorption spectra and antibiotics and studied the impact of optical path length on the limit of detection (LOD). They combined preprocessing algorithms, wavelength selection algorithms, and partial least squares (PLS) to measure the concentrations of components in a mixed water sample composed of ofloxacin, tetracycline, and chloramphenicol. The results demonstrated that this method effectively fulfills the monitoring requirements of specialized production wastewater facilities, including those in the medical and pharmaceutical industries. SERS is a technique that does not require labeling and is utilized for the analysis of trace chemicals. Currently, the research direction for detecting antibiotics using SERS mainly focuses on developing SERS substrates to enhance the detection of trace antibiotics. Pei et al. [94] developed a SERS substrate composed of a hybrid of gold nanoparticles/nanodiamantoids/carbon nitride (Au/ND/C_3N_4) with numerous functional groups and optical scattering phenomena, which can effectively capture target molecules and enhance Raman activity. It serves as a tool for the highly sensitive detection of antibiotic remnants in wastewater and has excellent self-cleaning capabilities, allowing for reuse.

Mass spectrometry (MS) is a method that separates ions based on their mass-to-charge ratio by utilizing electric and magnetic fields to achieve quantitative detection. It is generally not used alone but is often combined with chromatographic or spectroscopic methods [87]. David et al. [95] developed a direct injection analytical liquid chromatography–tandem mass spectrometry (LC-MS/MS) method for detecting trace antibiotics in wastewater, capable of quantifying 18 antibiotics in the influent and effluent of wastewater treatment plants at low ng/L levels. Bahar et al. [96] optimized parameters such as column temperature, eluent, mobile phase, and flow rate during the use of UPLC-MS/MS to detect 14 antibiotics in hospital and municipal wastewater, with detection limits varying between 0.07 and 2.72 μg/L. Félix et al. [97] explored the combined use of LC and GC with quadrupole time-of-flight mass spectrometry (QTOF MS) in their research, detecting 7 antibiotics in surface water and wastewater samples collected from Pasto, a town in the Andean highlands of Colombia (Nariño).

3.4. Sensor Detection Methods

The sensor-based detection of antibiotics is now one of the most researched and widely used emerging detection methods. Commonly used sensors include electrochemical sensors, optical sensors, and biosensors. Sensor detection methods offer high sensitivity, excellent selectivity, and good stability, but at the same time, some sensors may have relatively narrow application ranges and larger detection errors.

Electrochemical sensors are simple to prepare, cost-effective, and characterized by rapid analysis, high specificity, and good sensitivity for detecting target analytes, and they have been a popular choice for detecting antibiotics in wastewater [98]. The sensitivity of the sensors can be improved by optimizing the electrode materials. Gold nanomaterials [99], graphene, MOFs, MIPs [100], and others have received widespread attention. For instance, Adane et al. [101] integrated gold–silver alloy nanocoral clusters (Au-Ag-ANCCs) with a functionalized multi-walled carbon nanotubes–carbon paste electrode (f-MWCNT-CPE) and choline chloride (ChCl) nanocomposites for the simultaneous determination of rifampicin (RAMP) and norfloxacin (NFX) residues in water samples. Moreover, without resorting to intricate materials for modifying the electrode surface, the electrochemical performance of the sensor can also be optimized by selecting appropriate electrolyte solutions, setting the optimal pH, thoroughly polishing the electrode, and using methods such as differential pulse voltammetry and cyclic voltammetry in a three-electrode system [102].

Optical sensors also feature a high sensitivity, fast response times, and strong specificity, making them a popular research method currently [103]. In recent years, the field of optical sensors has seen significant advancements, with various recognition strategies being explored for detecting analytes. These include molecular imprinting, the utilization of nanomaterials with optical properties, and bio-interactions. The preparation and modification of certain special materials have emerged as key research areas, as these materials can offer an enhanced sensitivity, selectivity, and stability for optical sensors. Metal–Organic Frameworks (MOFs) are a promising type of fluorescent sensing material [104]. Lakshya et al. [105] used a dispersion of Mn-MOFs in an ethanol solution to directly detect tetracycline through fluorescence quenching. The sensor's significant detection limit was 66.39 nM, with a linear detection range for tetracycline from 0.0032 to 0.43 μm, and the Mn-MOF showed a remarkable selectivity for tetracycline, even in the presence of other antibiotics. A Zn-MOF [106], Cd-MOF [107], Zr-MOF [108], and others have also been widely used as fluorescent sensing materials for detecting various antibiotics in water.

Biosensors offer rapid and efficient detection without the need for complex pretreatment. Their molecular recognition components primarily consist of antibodies, microorganisms, aptamers, and enzymes [109], which are used for specific binding with the target analyte. Combining biosensors with other technologies can effectively enhance the accuracy of antibiotic detection in water. Janice et al. [110] developed a biosensor for detecting levofloxacin (LFX) using a combination of RNA Capture-SELEX and displacement chain detection. Wang et al. [111] created a group-targeted immunosensor utilizing evanescent wave fluorescence biosensor technology. By modifying the surface of a conical fiber optic with coated antigen (QN-BSA) as the sensing element, using fluorescently labeled QNs-specific antibodies as the recognition material, and utilizing a straightforward indirect competitive immunoassay approach, they achieved the highly sensitive recognition and quantification of QNs, meeting the needs for on-site detection.

In addition to the aforementioned methods, capillary electrophoresis (CE) [112] and diode array (DA) [34] are also used for the detection of antibiotics in water. Table 2 provides a brief summary of the typical detection methods for antibiotics in wastewater introduced in this article, based on the literature.

Combining Table 2 and the preceding analysis, it is evident that there are various methods for detecting antibiotics in wastewater, each with its own advantages and disadvantages. Immunoassays have relatively low detection limits but are more complex to operate, and the accuracy of the detection results can be readily compromised by external factors, potentially introducing errors in the analysis. Specific antibodies paired with new materials can further improve the sensitivity of immunoassays. The detection limits of different instrumental methods vary significantly, but they generally reach the μg/L level and can usually measure multiple antibiotics in one go. Many recent studies have integrated multiple instrumental detections methods to achieve sensitive and accurate results. The detection limits of sensor detection methods are highly related to their selectivity, and their repeatability and stability are relatively poor. Developing materials that can provide stable signals is a research focus, but reducing the cost of commercialization is an urgent task that goes hand in hand with it. In addition, the resistance of these detection technologies to complex components in wastewater, as well as the speed and convenience of on-site detection, still need further research and improvement.

Table 2. Summary of antibiotic detection by different methods (for analytical convenience, the units are unified to μg/L).

Detection Method		Metal	Detection of Antibiotics	LOD	Reference
Immunoassay	ELISA	—	Sulfamethoxazole	0.82	[87]
	LFIA	EuNPs	Nitrofuran	0.013–0.023	[88]
	LFIA	AuNPs	Streptomycin	5	[89]
	Fluorescence immunoassay	Evanescent wave dual-color fluorescence fiber-embedded optofluidic nanochip (EDFON)	Sulfamerazine	0.032	[90]
Instrumental analysis	HPLC	—	Ciprofloxacin, Levofloxacin, Ofloxacin, Ampicillin and Sulfamethoxazole	162–598	[91]
	UPLC-MS/MS	—	Quinolones	0.5×10^{-5}–0.5×10^{-4}	[113]
	UPLC-MS/MS	—	14 classes of antibiotics	0.07–2.72	[96]
	SERS	$Au/ND/C_3N_4$	Tetracycline	nanomolar level	[94]
	UV-Vis	—	Tetracycline, Ofloxacin, and Chloramphenicol	94–264	[93]
Sensor	Electrochemical sensor	Molecularly imprinted polymer (MIP)	Azithromycin	89.88	[100]
	Electrochemical sensor	Au–Ag-ANCCs/f-MWCNTs-CPE/ChCl	Rifampicin and Norfloxacin	0.0022–0.044	[101]
	Electrochemical sensor	Glassy carbon electrode	Sulfadiazine	1535	[102]
	Optical sensor	Mn-MOF	Tetracycline	1.4208–190.92	[105]
	Biosensor	RNA Aptamer	Levofloxacin	23,100	[110]
	Group-targeting biosensor	—	Quinolones	<0.15	[111]

4. Treatment Technologies for Antibiotics in Urban Wastewater

4.1. Physical Methods

Physical methods mainly include membrane separation technology and adsorption. The membrane separation process is a commonly used method for advanced wastewater treatment, characterized by a small footprint and good separation performance [37]. As membrane technology continues to advance rapidly, membrane separation processes have garnered increasing interest for the treatment of antibiotic-laden wastewater. Many experiments have studied processes such as reverse osmosis (RO), nanofiltration (NF), and ultrafiltration (UF) for removing tetracycline antibiotics from wastewater [38], with some RO/NF membranes achieving a rejection rate of up to 98.5% for the target antibiotics [114]. However, traditional membrane separation processes suffer from significant membrane fouling and poor selectivity issues. Cui et al. [115] designed an anti-fouling zwitterion PVDF-imprinted composite membrane (SPICM) for emulsion separation and selective tetracycline hydrochloride (TC) in wastewater. The results showed that, thanks to the synergistic effect between hydrophilicity/underwater superoleophobicity and active imprinted sites, the membrane's selective TC separation efficiency reached as high as 88.3%, even from oil-containing wastewater, effectively improving the shortcomings of traditional membrane separation processes.

Adsorption is another common physical technique used for the removal of antibiotics from water [116]. In conventional wastewater treatment plants, activated sludge serves as an important adsorbent. The adsorption process is a highly intricate one, being influenced by a multitude of factors including the physicochemical properties of both the activated sludge and the antibiotics, alongside the operational parameters of the biological treatment system [39,40]. Specifically, the ionization characteristics and hydrophilicity of the antibiotics themselves [117], the temperature, pH value, mixed liquor suspended solids (MLSS) concentration [118], and redox conditions [119] of the activated sludge system, among other factors, can all affect the adsorption behavior of antibiotics. In addition to activated sludge, materials with a higher specific surface area, porosity, and reactivity, such as clay minerals, carbon materials, metal composite materials, and nanomaterials, have become promising adsorbents for antibiotics in wastewater [120]. The main adsorption mechanisms involve site recognition, bridge enhancement, and site competition [121]. Zhao et al. [122] studied the adsorption and removal of antibiotics from swine wastewater using alkaline-modified biochar (KRBC). The well-fitted pseudo-second-order kinetics model and Freundlich isotherm model indicate that antibiotic adsorption is likely to be chemical adsorption and heterogeneous, with the –OH group playing a crucial role in the adsorption of antibiotics. Furthermore, the antibiotic removal effect was evaluated in a multi-pollutant system, and the results showed that the addition of Cu^{2+} and Zn^{2+} was beneficial for the removal of antibiotics.

Physical methods are widely applied in wastewater treatment, particularly membrane separation technology and adsorption techniques. In light of the strengths and weaknesses of membrane separation technology, future research should focus on developing membrane materials with higher anti-fouling properties, and enhancing selectivity can boost treatment efficiency while simultaneously reducing operational costs. For instance, the development of anti-fouling composite membranes has shown promising results in recent years, yet their long-term stability and cost-effectiveness in practical applications still need further validation. The performance of adsorption techniques is influenced by the physicochemical characteristics of the adsorbents and the composition of the wastewater. With the advancement in nanomaterials and novel composite materials, the efficiency of adsorption has significantly improved. Future efforts should further optimize the regeneration capabilities of adsorbents and their selective adsorption performance towards a variety of pollutants.

4.2. Chemical Methods

Chemical methods mainly include various advanced oxidation processes (AOPs), such as Fenton oxidation, ozonation, electrochemical oxidation (EO), photocatalytic oxidation, etc., all of which can be used for the degradation of different antibiotics in wastewater. Among them, the application effects of the first two methods are relatively poor. This is mainly because Fenton oxidation is limited by a narrow pH range, while ozonation is limited by the mass transfer process of ozone from the gas phase to the liquid phase [41].

Electrochemical oxidation (EO) is a process where organic matter is oxidized, transformed, or decomposed into non-toxic and harmless substances through the application of an electric current [123]. It has the advantages of being reagent-free, having a high efficiency in degrading pollutants, strong controllability, and minimal secondary pollution [124]. Electrochemical oxidation is divided into two modes: direct oxidation and indirect oxidation. Of the two, direct oxidation refers to the decomposition of antibiotics by directly interacting with the anode. Indirect oxidation refers to the reaction of strongly oxidative substances generated on the anode surface with antibiotics in the water under the influence of electric current, leading to their degradation [125]. A wealth of research indicates that traditional electrochemical systems are not very efficient in treating antibiotics and consume a significant amount of energy. To avoid anode loss during electrolysis and improve oxidation efficiency, an increasing number of new electrode materials have been developed, including boron-doped diamond (BDD) [126], carbon felt [127], Ti/IrO_2 [128], PbO_2 [129], and so on. These materials have a high oxygen evolution potential and can generate more hydroxyl radicals [130]. Current density, solution pH value, electrolyte concentration, and organic matter also affect the efficiency of redox reactions [126,131].

For wastewater treatment, photocatalytic oxidation stands as a green, eco-friendly, and cost-effective approach that refers to the photocatalytic reaction and redox process that occurs on the surface of a photocatalyst (such as H_2O_2, O_2) and target pollutants under light irradiation. The photocatalyst itself is crucial in this process [125]. A variety of new materials have been used as photocatalysts for the degradation of antibiotics, such as ZnO [132], TiO_2 [133], $MgTiO_3$ [134], and g-C_3N_4 [135]. The type and composition of the photocatalyst, initial substrate concentration, catalyst dosage, pH value of the reaction medium, ionic components in water, solvent type, and oxidants/electron acceptors all affect the photocatalytic degradation process of antibiotics [136]. Dimitrakopoulou et al. [137] used a UV-A/TiO_2 photocatalyst to degrade amoxicillin and found that there was no significant change in the degradation of amoxicillin at pH values of 5.0 and 7.5, but when the pH value increased from 5 to 7.5, the mineralization degree of amoxicillin decreased from 95% to 75%. Ahmadi et al. [138] studied the effect of the dose of MWCNT/TiO_2 photocatalyst on the degradation of tetracycline (TC) and found that when the catalyst dosage increased from 0.1 g/L to 0.2 g/L, the removal rate of tetracycline increased, but further increasing it to 0.4 g/L did not further improve the degradation efficiency of tetracycline.

These chemical methods have demonstrated good results in the degradation of antibiotics, but issues such as a high energy consumption and costs and complex operating conditions have limited their large-scale application. To address these challenges, future research directions should focus on developing low-energy, efficient catalyst materials, while optimizing reaction conditions to adapt to large-scale wastewater treatment. The capability of electrochemical oxidation in the degradation of antibiotics is particularly worth noting, especially the development of new electrode materials, which is expected to significantly enhance treatment efficiency and decrease energy usage. In addition, combining multiple oxidation technologies to enhance the degradation effect on different antibiotics is also a key focus for future research.

4.3. Biological Methods

For a long time, biological processes have been considered to be economical and environmentally friendly methods for removing antibiotics from wastewater, as they can degrade various antibiotics in situ under relatively mild conditions [139]. Biological methods mainly include conventional activated sludge (CAS) processes, membrane bioreactors (MBRs), and anaerobic reactor systems, among others.

CAS is the most prevalent method employed for biological wastewater treatment processes. Adsorption and biodegradation are the main pathways for the removal of antibiotics by activated sludge, but the treatment effect is not very satisfactory. In full-scale CAS, the removal rates of different antibiotics from the aqueous phase vary from −1% to 71% [140]. Microorganisms play an essential role in the biodegradation of antibiotics in the activated sludge process. Studies have shown that nitrifying bacteria are of great significance for the biodegradation of antibiotics, and the specific degradation process may mainly occur during the co-metabolic and endogenous respiration stages after nitrification [141]. Nguyen et al. [142] isolated a pure culture of denitrifying *Chromobacterium* sp. strain PR1 for the degradation of Sulfamethoxazole (SMX). The characteristics of antibiotics also affect their degradability. Antibiotics with a higher polarity and lower electronegativity of functional groups, and better hydrophilicity, tend to have higher bioavailability and are more easily degraded [143].

MBRs integrate the process of biodegradation utilizing activated sludge with immediate solid–liquid segregation via membrane filtration, offering a high removal efficiency for organic compounds and producing less sludge waste. Utilizing microfiltration or ultrafiltration membrane technology (with pore sizes ranging from 0.05 to 0.4 μm) in MBR systems can completely physically retain bacterial flocs and almost all suspended solids within the reactor [144]. The concentration of microorganisms in MBRs can reach up to 20 mg/L [145], and a high concentration of mixed liquor suspended solids (MLSSs) aids in the elimination of antibiotics [146]. Hamjinda et al. [147] studied the treatment effect of a two-stage membrane bioreactor (2S-MBR) on 10 types of antibiotics in the laboratory. The results indicated that the degree of antibiotic elimination depends on the type of antibiotic and the hydraulic retention time (HRT). Shi et al. [148] used a hollow-fiber MBR to treat wastewater containing low concentrations of sulfamethazine (SMZ). Over a 244-day operation, the overall removal efficiency of SMZ could reach 95.4 $\pm$ 4.5% under various SMZ concentrations and hydraulic retention times. It was also observed that the quantity of extracellular polymeric substances (EPSs) in the MBR diminished following prolonged operation under SMZ stress.

Anaerobic reactor systems are known for their low energy consumption, low sludge production, low maintenance costs, and the ability to produce methane as a byproduct [149]. They are typically used for treating high-concentration organic wastewater that is difficult to degrade, such as wastewater from antibiotic pharmaceutical plants and breeding wastewater containing substantial quantities of antibiotics, and are less commonly applied in the treatment of antibiotics in municipal wastewater.

Furthermore, enhancing the antibiotic removal capabilities of specific microbial species, such as photosynthetic bacteria, is also one of the hot topics. For instance, modulating the metabolic pathways of purple anoxygenic phototrophs can boost their uptake of photosynthetic electrons, and the optimized biofilm formed by *Rhodopseudomonas palustris* (*R. palustris*) achieves superior antibiotic degradation efficiency [150]. If these bacteria can be effectively combined with biofilm treatment technologies such as biofiltration, they will play a significant role in antibiotic removal.

It is also important to note that biological treatment processes may be affected by antibiotic-resistant bacteria [120]. For instance, the aged sludge in MBR systems is thought to harbor microorganisms with multiple drug resistances, posing potential ecological and health risks [151]. Furthermore, numerous mathematical models have been formulated to forecast the behavior and removal efficiency of antibiotics during biological wastewater treatment processes, such as the Activated Sludge Model for Xenobiotics (ASM-X). Polesel et al. [152] used the ASM-X framework to determine the impact of different factors on antibiotic removal during wastewater treatment, including solids retention time (SRT) as well as influent and effluent load dynamics.

Biological methods are relatively environmentally friendly and economical, and they have a high degradation efficiency for organic matter, but the removal effect of antibiotics still has uncertainties. The emergence of some antibiotic-resistant bacteria may even affect the overall treatment effect. Therefore, future research should focus on improving the removal capacity of antibiotics and their resistance genes in the biological treatment process. Membrane bioreactors combine the technology of biodegradation with membrane filtration, showing high pollutant removal efficiency, but the problem of membrane fouling is still severe. Therefore, the development of anti-fouling membrane materials and the optimization of reactor operation parameters are key directions for future development. Moreover, investigating the dynamic shifts in microbial communities throughout the antibiotic degradation process can aid in enhancing the overall stability and efficacy of the treatment system.

A summary of antibiotic treatment methods for urban wastewater indicates that, compared to physical and chemical methods, biological methods may offer better treatment efficacy and removal rates, particularly for wastewater containing low concentrations of antibiotics, while also generating less secondary pollution. However, they often require a more precise control of reaction conditions and have longer treatment cycles. Chemical methods may entail higher reagent costs than physical methods and pose a greater risk of potential secondary pollution. Combining physical, chemical, and biological approaches for antibiotic treatment leverages the strengths of each method, achieving efficient, economical, and environmentally friendly wastewater treatment. For instance, physical pretreatment methods can be effectively combined with advanced oxidation processes and biological filtration techniques. Physical pretreatment enhances the stability of subsequent treatments, advanced oxidation technologies can break down the molecular structure of antibiotics to facilitate biodegradation, and biological filtration technologies such as Biological Aerated Filters (BAFs) are high-rate aerobic biological systems [153,154].

Overall, the treatment of antibiotics in urban wastewater requires comprehensive consideration of treatment efficacy, cost, and environmental impact. Future research should focus on developing efficient, low-cost, and environmentally friendly treatment technologies, as well as optimizing the operational parameters of existing technologies to address the challenges posed by antibiotic pollution.

5. Conclusions

This article delves into the occurrence of antibiotics in municipal wastewater treatment systems, the ecological and human health risks they pose, detection technologies, and removal methods, exploring the current status and challenges. By analyzing the concentration ranges of major antibiotic categories in the influent and effluent of wastewater treatment plants, it is concluded that most countries currently lack effective regulatory measures for antibiotic pollution. Antibiotics enter the environment through wastewater treatment plants, posing potential threats to aquatic ecosystems (including microorganisms, aquatic plants, and animals) and human health. Furthermore, this article provides a comprehensive overview of techniques for detecting antibiotics in wastewater, from traditional enrichment techniques and immunoassays to advanced instrumental analysis methods and sensor detection methods. Reducing the release of antibiotics from wastewater treatment plants into the environment through advanced wastewater treatment technologies is a key aspect of mitigating the water pollution caused by antibiotics. This article introduces various techniques from three perspectives, physical, chemical, and biological, and provides a brief comparison of these three types of technologies. The detection and treatment methods discussed each have their own merits and demerits, and the specific choice should be made based on the actual situation, either by selecting a single technology or through a combined application.

In the future, strict control of antibiotic consumption at the source remains most critical, such as restricting the use of certain types of antibiotics in animal husbandry, strengthening the control of the prescription and sale of antibiotic drugs, and raising awareness of the threat of antibiotic resistance. At the same time, the monitoring and treatment of antibiotics in wastewater should further focus on the study of real wastewater components to enhance its practical application efficiency. Improving the practical application efficiency of sewage treatment technology and optimizing treatment processes to reduce the impact of antibiotics on the aquatic environment is an important direction for future research. In addition, the removal of ARGs and the assessment of the long-term impact of antibiotics on aquatic ecosystems should also become a focus of future research. It is hoped that through raising awareness, strengthening monitoring, and effective treatment, the regulation of antibiotic pollutants in urban wastewater will be strengthened, leading to the implementation of relevant standards and legislation.

Author Contributions: Conceptualization, L.Z. and X.L.; methodology, L.Z. and X.L.; software, L.Z.; formal analysis, L.Z.; investigation, L.Z.; resources, X.L., F.C. and J.X.; writing—original draft preparation, L.Z. and X.L.; writing—review and editing, L.Z., X.L. and Z.D.; visualization, L.Z.; supervision, X.L., Z.D., F.C. and J.X. All authors have read and agreed to the published version of the manuscript.

Funding: This research received no external funding.

Data Availability Statement: Data is contained within the article.

Conflicts of Interest: The authors declare no conflicts of interest.

References

1. Yang, Y.; Song, W.; Lin, H.; Wang, W.; Du, L.; Xing, W. Antibiotics and antibiotic resistance genes in global lakes: A review and meta-analysis. *Environ. Int.* **2018**, *116*, 60–73. [CrossRef] [PubMed]
2. Zhang, Q.; Ying, G.; Pan, C.; Liu, Y.; Zhao, J. Comprehensive evaluation of antibiotics emission and fate in the river basins of China: Source analysis, multimedia modeling, and linkage to bacterial resistance. *Environ. Sci. Technol.* **2015**, *49*, 6772–6782. [CrossRef]
3. Khan, F.A.; Söderquist, B.; Jass, J. Prevalence and diversity of antibiotic resistance genes in Swedish aquatic environments impacted by household and hospital wastewater. *Front. Microbiol.* **2019**, *10*, 688. [CrossRef]
4. Wang, Q.; Wang, P.; Yang, Q. Occurrence and diversity of antibiotic resistance in untreated hospital wastewater. *Sci. Total Environ.* **2018**, *621*, 990–999. [CrossRef]
5. Vidovic, N.; Vidovic, S. Antimicrobial resistance and food animals: Influence of livestock environment on the emergence and dissemination of antimicrobial resistance. *Antibiotics* **2020**, *9*, 52. [CrossRef] [PubMed]
6. Petrin, S.; Patuzzi, I.; Di Cesare, A.; Tiengo, A.; Sette, G.; Biancotto, G.; Corno, G.; Drigo, M.; Losasso, C.; Cibin, V. Evaluation and quantification of antimicrobial residues and antimicrobial resistance genes in two Italian swine farms. *Environ. Pollut.* **2019**, *255*, 113183. [CrossRef]
7. Saravanane, R.; Sundararaman, S. Effect of loading rate and HRT on the removal of cephalosporin and their intermediates during the operation of a membrane bioreactor treating pharmaceutical wastewater. *Environ. Technol.* **2009**, *30*, 1017–1022. [CrossRef]
8. Bielen, A.; Šimatović, A.; Kosić-Vukšić, J.; Senta, I.; Ahel, M.; Babić, S.; Jurina, T.; González Plaza, J.J.; Milaković, M.; Udiković-Kolić, N. Negative environmental impacts of antibiotic-contaminated effluents from pharmaceutical industries. *Water Res.* **2017**, *126*, 79–87. [CrossRef] [PubMed]
9. Larsson, D.G.J.; de Pedro, C.; Paxeus, N. Effluent from drug manufactures contains extremely high levels of pharmaceuticals. *J. Hazard. Mater.* **2007**, *148*, 751–755. [CrossRef]
10. Bilal, M.; Ashraf, S.S.; Barceló, D.; Iqbal, H.M.N. Biocatalytic degradation/redefining "removal" fate of pharmaceutically active compounds and antibiotics in the aquatic environment. *Sci. Total Environ.* **2019**, *691*, 1190–1211. [CrossRef]
11. Peng, X.; Tang, C.; Yu, Y.; Tan, J.; Huang, Q.; Wu, J.; Chen, S.; Mai, B. Concentrations, transport, fate, and releases of polybrominated diphenyl ethers in sewage treatment plants in the Pearl River Delta, South China. *Environ. Int.* **2009**, *35*, 303–309. [CrossRef] [PubMed]
12. Peng, X.; Yu, Y.; Tang, C.; Tan, J.; Huang, Q.; Wang, Z. Occurrence of steroid estrogens, endocrine-disrupting phenols, and acid pharmaceutical residues in urban riverine water of the Pearl River Delta, South China. *Sci. Total Environ.* **2008**, *397*, 158–166. [CrossRef] [PubMed]
13. Valcárcel, Y.; González Alonso, S.; Rodríguez-Gil, J.L.; Gil, A.; Catalá, M. Detection of pharmaceutically active compounds in the rivers and tap water of the Madrid Region (Spain) and potential ecotoxicological risk. *Chemosphere* **2011**, *84*, 1336–1348. [CrossRef]
14. López-Serna, R.; Jurado, A.; Vázquez-Suñé, E.; Carrera, J.; Petrović, M.; Barceló, D. Occurrence of 95 pharmaceuticals and transformation products in urban groundwaters underlying the metropolis of Barcelona, Spain. *Environ. Pollut.* **2013**, *174*, 305–315. [CrossRef]
15. Mahmood, A.R.; Hassan, F.M.; Al-Haideri, H.H.; Khubchandani, J. Detection of antibiotics in drinking water treatment plants in Baghdad City, Iraq. *Adv. Public. Health* **2019**, *2019*, 7851354. [CrossRef]
16. Zhao, H.; Zhou, J.L.; Zhang, J. Tidal impact on the dynamic behavior of dissolved pharmaceuticals in the Yangtze Estuary, China. *Sci. Total Environ.* **2015**, *536*, 946–954. [CrossRef]
17. Zou, S.; Xu, W.; Zhang, R.; Tang, J.; Chen, Y.; Zhang, G. Occurrence and distribution of antibiotics in coastal water of the Bohai Bay, China: Impacts of river discharge and aquaculture activities. *Environ. Pollut.* **2011**, *159*, 2913–2920. [CrossRef]
18. Polianciuc, S.I.; Gurzău, A.E.; Kiss, B.; Ștefan, M.G.; Loghin, F. Antibiotics in the environment: Causes and consequences. *Med. Pharm. Rep.* **2020**, *93*, 231–240. [CrossRef] [PubMed]
19. Saidulu, D.; Gupta, B.; Gupta, A.K.; Ghosal, P.S. A review on occurrences, eco-toxic effects, and remediation of emerging contaminants from wastewater: Special emphasis on biological treatment based hybrid systems. *J. Environ. Chem. Eng.* **2021**, *9*, 105282. [CrossRef]
20. Zhao, F.; Yu, Q.; Zhang, X. A Mini-Review of antibiotic resistance drivers in urban wastewater treatment plants: Environmental concentrations, mechanism and perspectives. *Water* **2023**, *15*, 3165. [CrossRef]
21. Kostich, M.S.; Batt, A.L.; Lazorchak, J.M. Concentrations of prioritized pharmaceuticals in effluents from 50 large wastewater treatment plants in the US and implications for risk estimation. *Environ. Pollut.* **2014**, *184*, 354–359. [CrossRef] [PubMed]
22. Luo, Y.; Guo, W.; Ngo, H.H.; Nghiem, L.D.; Hai, F.I.; Zhang, J.; Liang, S.; Wang, X.C. A review on the occurrence of micropollutants in the aquatic environment and their fate and removal during wastewater treatment. *Sci. Total Environ.* **2014**, *473–474*, 619–641. [CrossRef] [PubMed]

23. Liu, Y.; Gao, B.; Yue, Q.; Guan, Y.; Wang, Y.; Huang, L. Influences of two antibiotic contaminants on the production, release and toxicity of microcystins. *Ecotox Environ. Safe* **2012**, *77*, 79–87. [CrossRef]
24. Rathi, B.S.; Kumar, P.S.; Show, P. A review on effective removal of emerging contaminants from aquatic systems: Current trends and scope for further research. *J. Hazard. Mater.* **2021**, *409*, 124413. [CrossRef]
25. Kulik, K.; Lenart-Boroń, A.; Wyrzykowska, K. Impact of antibiotic pollution on the bacterial population within surface water with special focus on mountain Rivers. *Water* **2023**, *15*, 975. [CrossRef]
26. Wang, M.; Shen, W.; Yan, L.; Wang, X.; Xu, H. Stepwise impact of urban wastewater treatment on the bacterial community structure, antibiotic contents, and prevalence of antimicrobial resistance. *Environ. Pollut.* **2017**, *231*, 1578–1585. [CrossRef]
27. Bengtsson-Palme, J.; Milakovic, M.; Švecová, H.; Ganjto, M.; Jonsson, V.; Grabic, R.; Udikovic-Kolic, N. Industrial wastewater treatment plant enriches antibiotic resistance genes and alters the structure of microbial communities. *Water Res.* **2019**, *162*, 437–445. [CrossRef]
28. Harada, A.; Komori, K.; Nakada, N.; Kitamura, K.; Suzuki, Y. Biological effects of PPCPs on aquatic lives and evaluation of river waters affected by different wastewater treatment levels. *Water Sci. Technol.* **2008**, *58*, 1541–1546. [CrossRef] [PubMed]
29. Wang, H.; Che, B.; Duan, A.; Mao, J.; Dahlgren, R.A.; Zhang, M.; Zhang, H.; Zeng, A.; Wang, X. Toxicity evaluation of β-diketone antibiotics on the development of embryo-larval zebrafish (*Danio rerio*). *Environ. Toxicol.* **2014**, *29*, 1134–1146. [CrossRef]
30. Caldwell, D.J.; Mertens, B.; Kappler, K.; Senac, T.; Journel, R.; Wilson, P.; Meyerhoff, R.D.; Parke, N.J.; Mastrocco, F.; Mattson, B.; et al. risk-based approach to managing active pharmaceutical ingredients in manufacturing effluent. *Environ. Toxicol. Chem.* **2016**, *35*, 813–822. [CrossRef]
31. Spurgeon, D.J.; Jones, O.A.H.; Dorne, J.C.M.; Svendsen, C.; Swain, S.; Stürzenbaum, S.R. Systems toxicology approaches for understanding the joint effects of environmental chemical mixtures. *Sci. Total Environ.* **2010**, *408*, 3725–3734. [CrossRef] [PubMed]
32. Michael, I.; Rizzo, L.; McArdell, C.S.; Manaia, C.M.; Merlin, C.; Schwartz, T.; Dagot, C.; Fatta-Kassinos, D. Urban wastewater treatment plants as hotspots for the release of antibiotics in the environment: A review. *Water Res.* **2013**, *47*, 957–995. [CrossRef] [PubMed]
33. Rizzo, L.; Manaia, C.; Merlin, C.; Schwartz, T.; Dagot, C.; Ploy, M.C.; Michael, I.; Fatta-Kassinos, D. Urban wastewater treatment plants as hotspots for antibiotic resistant bacteria and genes spread into the environment: A review. *Sci. Total Environ.* **2013**, *447*, 345–360. [CrossRef] [PubMed]
34. Luo, Y.; Sun, Y.; Wei, X.; He, Y.; Wang, H.; Cui, Z.; Ma, J.; Liu, X.; Shu, R.; Lin, H.; et al. Detection methods for antibiotics in wastewater: A review. *Bioproc. Biosyst. Eng.* **2024**, *47*, 1433–1451. [CrossRef] [PubMed]
35. Prakashan, D.; Kolhe, P.; Gandhi, S. Design and fabrication of a competitive lateral flow assay using gold nanoparticle as capture probe for the rapid and on-site detection of penicillin antibiotic in food samples. *Food Chem.* **2024**, *439*, 138120. [CrossRef]
36. Kumar Mehata, A.; Lakshmi Suseela, M.N.; Gokul, P.; Kumar Malik, A.; Kasi Viswanadh, M.; Singh, C.; Selvin, J.; Muthu, M.S. Fast and highly efficient liquid chromatographic methods for qualification and quantification of antibiotic residues from environmental waste. *Microchem. J.* **2022**, *179*, 107573. [CrossRef]
37. Manjunath, S.V.; Kumar, M. Simultaneous removal of antibiotic and nutrients via Prosopis juliflora activated carbon column: Performance evaluation, effect of operational parameters and breakthrough modeling. *Chemosphere* **2021**, *262*, 127820. [CrossRef]
38. Pan, S.; Zhu, M.; Chen, J.P.; Yuan, Z.; Zhong, L.; Zheng, Y. Separation of tetracycline from wastewater using forward osmosis process with thin film composite membrane—Implications for antibiotics recovery. *Sep. Purif. Technol.* **2015**, *153*, 76–83. [CrossRef]
39. Kim, S.; Eichhorn, P.; Jensen, J.N.; Weber, A.S.; Aga, D.S. Removal of antibiotics in wastewater: Effect of hydraulic and solid retention times on the fate of tetracycline in the activated sludge process. *Environ. Sci. Technol.* **2005**, *39*, 5816–5823. [CrossRef]
40. Hyland, K.C.; Dickenson, E.R.; Drewes, J.E.; Higgins, C.P. Sorption of ionized and neutral emerging trace organic compounds onto activated sludge from different wastewater treatment configurations. *Water Res.* **2012**, *46*, 1958–1968. [CrossRef]
41. Oberoi, A.S.; Jia, Y.; Zhang, H.; Khanal, S.K.; Lu, H. Insights into the fate and removal of antibiotics in engineered biological treatment systems: A critical review. *Environ. Sci. Technol.* **2019**, *53*, 7234–7264. [CrossRef] [PubMed]
42. Klein, E.Y.; Van Boeckel, T.P.; Martinez, E.M.; Pant, S.; Gandra, S.; Levin, S.A.; Goossens, H.; Laxminarayan, R. Global increase and geographic convergence in antibiotic consumption between 2000 and 2015. *Pro. Natl. Acad. Sci. USA* **2018**, *115*, E3463–E3470. [CrossRef]
43. ECDC. Antimicrobial consumption and resistance in bacteria from humans and food-producing animals. *EFSA J.* **2024**, *22*, e8589.
44. Zeng, Y.; Chang, F.; Liu, Q.; Duan, L.; Li, D.; Zhang, H. Recent advances and perspectives on the sources and detection of antibiotics in aquatic environments. *J. Anal. Methods Chem.* **2022**, *2022*, 5091181. [CrossRef] [PubMed]
45. Hao, H.; Shi, D.; Yang, D.; Yang, Z.; Qiu, Z.; Liu, W.; Shen, Z.; Yin, J.; Wang, H.; Li, J.; et al. Profiling of intracellular and extracellular antibiotic resistance genes in tap water. *J. Hazard. Mater.* **2019**, *365*, 340–345. [CrossRef] [PubMed]
46. Chow, L.K.M.; Ghaly, T.M.; Gillings, M.R. A survey of sub-inhibitory concentrations of antibiotics in the environment. *J. Environ. Sci.* **2021**, *99*, 21–27. [CrossRef] [PubMed]
47. Zarei-Baygi, A.; Smith, A.L. Intracellular versus extracellular antibiotic resistance genes in the environment: Prevalence, horizontal transfer, and mitigation strategies. *Bioresour. Technol.* **2021**, *319*, 124181. [CrossRef]
48. Huijbers, P.M.C.; Blaak, H.; de Jong, M.C.M.; Graat, E.A.M.; Vandenbroucke-Grauls, C.M.J.E.; de Roda Husman, A.M. Role of the environment in the transmission of antimicrobial resistance to humans: A Review. *Environ. Sci. Technol.* **2015**, *49*, 11993–12004. [CrossRef]

49. Arora-Williams, K.; Olesen, S.W.; Scandella, B.P.; Delwiche, K.; Spencer, S.J.; Myers, E.M.; Abraham, S.; Sooklal, A.; Preheim, S.P. Dynamics of microbial populations mediating biogeochemical cycling in a freshwater lake. *Microbiome* **2018**, *6*, 165. [CrossRef]
50. Ding, C.; He, J. Effect of antibiotics in the environment on microbial populations. *Appl. Microbiol. Biotechnol.* **2010**, *87*, 925–941. [CrossRef]
51. Aminov, R.I. The role of antibiotics and antibiotic resistance in nature. *Environ. Microbiol.* **2009**, *11*, 2970–2988. [CrossRef] [PubMed]
52. Qin, T.T.; Kang, H.Q.; Ma, P.; Li, P.P.; Huang, L.Y.; Gu, B. SOS response and its regulation on the fluoroquinolone resistance. *Ann. Transl. Med.* **2015**, *3*, 358. [CrossRef] [PubMed]
53. Knapp, C.W.; Engemann, C.A.; Hanson, M.L.; Keen, P.L.; Hall, K.J.; Graham, D.W. Indirect evidence of transposon-mediated selection of antibiotic resistance genes in aquatic systems at low-level oxytetracycline exposures. *Environ. Sci. Technol.* **2008**, *42*, 5348–5353. [CrossRef]
54. Cairns, J.; Ruokolainen, L.; Hultman, J.; Tamminen, M.; Virta, M.; Hiltunen, T. Ecology determines how low antibiotic concentration impacts community composition and horizontal transfer of resistance genes. *Commun. Biol.* **2018**, *1*, 35. [CrossRef] [PubMed]
55. Zhou, Z.; Zhang, Z.; Feng, L.; Zhang, J.; Li, Y.; Lu, T.; Qian, H. Adverse effects of levofloxacin and oxytetracycline on aquatic microbial communities. *Sci. Total Environ.* **2020**, *734*, 139499. [CrossRef] [PubMed]
56. Klaver, A.L.; Matthews, R.A. Effects of oxytetracycline on nitrification in a model aquatic system. *Aquaculture* **1994**, *123*, 237–247. [CrossRef]
57. Magdaleno, A.; Saenz, M.E.; Juarez, A.B.; Moretton, J. Effects of six antibiotics and their binary mixtures on growth of *Pseudokirchneriella subcapitata*. *Ecotox Environ. Safe* **2015**, *113*, 72–78. [CrossRef]
58. Välitalo, P.; Kruglova, A.; Mikola, A.; Vahala, R. Toxicological impacts of antibiotics on aquatic micro-organisms: A mini-review. *Int. J. Hyg. Environ. Health* **2017**, *220*, 558–569. [CrossRef]
59. Fountoulakis, M.S.; Stamatelatou, K.; Lyberatos, G. The effect of pharmaceuticals on the kinetics of methanogenesis and acetogenesis. *Bioresour. Technol.* **2008**, *99*, 7083–7090. [CrossRef]
60. Halling-Sorensen, B. Algal toxicity of antibacterial agents used in intensive farming. *Chemosphere* **2000**, *40*, 731–739. [CrossRef]
61. Pomati, F.; Netting, A.G.; Calamari, D.; Neilan, B.A. Effects of erythromycin, tetracycline and ibuprofen on the growth of Synechocystis sp. and Lemna minor. *Aquat. Toxicol.* **2004**, *67*, 387–396. [CrossRef] [PubMed]
62. Ebert, I.; Bachmann, J.; Kuhnen, U.; Kuster, A.; Kussatz, C.; Maletzki, D.; Schluter, C. Toxicity of the fluoroquinolone antibiotics enrofloxacin and ciprofloxacin to photoautotrophic aquatic organisms. *Environ. Toxicol. Chem.* **2011**, *30*, 2786–2792. [CrossRef] [PubMed]
63. Bagge, N.; Schuster, M.; Hentzer, M.; Ciofu, O.; Givskov, M.; Greenberg, E.P.; Høiby, N. *Pseudomonas aeruginosa* biofilms exposed to imipenem exhibit changes in global gene expression and β-Lactamase and alginate production. *Antimicrob. Agents Chemother.* **2004**, *48*, 1175–1187. [CrossRef] [PubMed]
64. Hoffman, L.R.; D'Argenio, D.A.; MacCoss, M.J.; Zhang, Z.; Jones, R.A.; Miller, S.I. Aminoglycoside antibiotics induce bacterial biofilm formation. *Nature* **2005**, *436*, 1171–1175. [CrossRef] [PubMed]
65. Linares, J.F.; Gustafsson, I.; Baquero, F.; Martinez, J.L. Antibiotics as intermicrobial signaling agents instead of weapons. *Proc. Natl. Acad. Sci. USA* **2006**, *103*, 19484–19489. [CrossRef]
66. Sanderson, H.; Brain, R.A.; Johnson, D.J.; Wilson, C.J.; Solomon, K.R. Toxicity classification and evaluation of four pharmaceuticals classes: Antibiotics, antineoplastics, cardiovascular, and sex hormones. *Toxicology* **2004**, *203*, 27–40. [CrossRef]
67. Gros, M.; Petrović, M.; Ginebreda, A.; Barceló, D. Removal of pharmaceuticals during wastewater treatment and environmental risk assessment using hazard indexes. *Environ. Int.* **2010**, *36*, 15–26. [CrossRef]
68. Baumann, M.; Weiss, K.; Maletzki, D.; Schüssler, W.; Schudoma, D.; Kopf, W.; Kühnen, U. Aquatic toxicity of the macrolide antibiotic clarithromycin and its metabolites. *Chemosphere* **2015**, *120*, 192–198. [CrossRef]
69. Yin, X.; Wang, H.; Zhang, Y.; Dahlgren, R.A.; Zhang, H.; Shi, M.; Gao, M.; Wang, X. Toxicological assessment of trace beta-diketone antibiotic mixtures on zebrafish (*Danio rerio*) by proteomic analysis. *PLoS ONE* **2014**, *9*, e102731. [CrossRef]
70. Iftikhar, N.; Konig, I.; English, C.; Ivantsova, E.; Souders, C.L.; Hashmi, I.; Martyniuk, C.J. Sulfamethoxazole (SMX) Alters Immune and Apoptotic Endpoints in Developing Zebrafish (*Danio rerio*). *Toxics* **2023**, *11*, 178. [CrossRef]
71. Wei, H.; Hashmi, M.Z.; Wang, Z. The interactions between aquatic plants and antibiotics: Progress and prospects. *Environ. Pollut.* **2024**, *341*, 123004. [CrossRef] [PubMed]
72. Pan, M.; Chu, L.M. Fate of antibiotics in soil and their uptake by edible crops. *Sci. Total Environ.* **2017**, *599–600*, 500–512. [CrossRef] [PubMed]
73. Jernberg, C.; Lofmark, S.; Edlund, C.; Jansson, J.K. Long-term ecological impacts of antibiotic administration on the human intestinal microbiota. *ISME J.* **2007**, *1*, 56–66. [CrossRef]
74. Ben, Y.; Fu, C.; Hu, M.; Liu, L.; Wong, M.H.; Zheng, C. Human health risk assessment of antibiotic resistance associated with antibiotic residues in the environment: A review. *Environ. Res.* **2019**, *169*, 483–493. [CrossRef] [PubMed]
75. Bilal, M.; Mehmood, S.; Rasheed, T.; Iqbal, H.M.N. Antibiotics traces in the aquatic environment: Persistence and adverse environmental impact. *Curr. Opin. Environ. Sci. Health* **2020**, *13*, 68–74. [CrossRef]
76. Blaser, M.J. Antibiotic use and its consequences for the normal microbiome. *Science* **2016**, *352*, 544–545. [CrossRef]
77. EFSA. *Monitoring Antimicrobial Resistance*; EFSA: Parma, Italy, 2024.

78. Suseela, M.; Viswanadh, M.K.; Mehata, A.K.; Priya, V.; Vikas; Setia, A.; Malik, A.K.; Gokul, P.; Selvin, J.; Muthu, M.S. Advances in solid-phase extraction techniques: Role of nanosorbents for the enrichment of antibiotics for analytical quantification. *J. Chromatogr. A* **2023**, *1695*, 463937. [CrossRef]
79. Nguyen, T.T.; Huynh, T.T.T.; Nguyen, N.H.; Nguyen, T.H.; Tran, P.H. Recent advances in the application of ionic liquid-modified silica gel in solid-phase extraction. *J. Mol. Liq.* **2022**, *368*, 120623. [CrossRef]
80. Dias, F.D.S.; Meira, L.A.; Carneiro, C.N.; Dos Santos, L.F.M.; Guimarães, L.B.; Coelho, N.M.M.; Coelho, L.M.; Alves, V.N. Lignocellulosic materials as adsorbents in solid phase extraction for trace elements preconcentration. *TrAC Trends Anal. Chem.* **2023**, *158*, 116891. [CrossRef]
81. Liu, J.; Wang, J.; Guo, Y.; Yang, X.; Wu, Q.; Wang, Z. Effective solid-phase extraction of chlorophenols with covalent organic framework material as adsorbent. *J. Chromatogr. A* **2022**, *1673*, 463077. [CrossRef] [PubMed]
82. Xu, M.; Li, J.; Chang, Q.; Zang, X.; Zhang, S.; Wang, C.; Wang, Z. Molecularly imprinted conjugated microporous polymer composite as solid phase extraction adsorbent for the extraction of phenolic endocrine disrupting chemicals in beverages. *Microchem. J.* **2023**, *191*, 108752. [CrossRef]
83. Kardani, F.; Mirzajani, R. Electrospun polyacrylonitrile /MIL-53(Al) MOF@ SBA-15/ 4, 4′-bipyridine nanofibers for headspace solid-phase microextraction of benzene homologues in environmental water samples with GC-FID detection. *Microchem. J.* **2022**, *180*, 107591. [CrossRef]
84. Gong, X.; Xu, L.; Kou, X.; Zheng, J.; Kuang, Y.; Zhou, S.; Huang, S.; Zheng, Y.; Ke, W.; Chen, G.; et al. Amino-functionalized metal–organic frameworks for efficient solid-phase microextraction of perfluoroalkyl acids in environmental water. *Microchem. J.* **2022**, *179*, 107661. [CrossRef]
85. Fu, Q.; Xia, Z.; Sun, X.; Jiang, H.; Wang, L.; Ai, S.; Zhao, R. Recent advance and applications of covalent organic frameworks based on magnetic solid-phase extraction technology for food safety analysis. *TrAC Trends Anal. Chem.* **2023**, *162*, 117054. [CrossRef]
86. Sereshti, H.; Karami, F.; Nouri, N. A green dispersive liquid-liquid microextraction based on deep eutectic solvents doped with β-cyclodextrin: Application for determination of tetracyclines in water samples. *Microchem. J.* **2021**, *163*, 105914. [CrossRef]
87. Hoffmann, H.; Baldofski, S.; Hoffmann, K.; Flemig, S.; Silva, C.P.; Esteves, V.I.; Emmerling, F.; Panne, U.; Schneider, R.J. Structural considerations on the selectivity of an immunoassay for sulfamethoxazole. *Talanta* **2016**, *158*, 198–207. [CrossRef]
88. Mei, Q.; Ma, B.; Li, J.; Deng, X.; Shuai, J.; Zhou, Y.; Zhang, M. Simultaneous detection of three nitrofuran antibiotics by the lateral flow immunoassay based on europium nanoparticles in aquatic products. *Food Chem.* **2024**, *439*, 138171. [CrossRef]
89. Alhammadi, M.; Aliya, S.; Umapathi, R.; Oh, M.; Huh, Y.S. A simultaneous qualitative and quantitative lateral flow immunoassay for on-site and rapid detection of streptomycin in pig blood serum and urine. *Microchem. J.* **2023**, *195*, 109427. [CrossRef]
90. Chen, D.; Xu, W.; Lu, Y.; Zhuo, Y.; Ji, T.; Long, F. Rapid and sensitive parallel on-site detection of antibiotics and resistance genes in aquatic environments using evanescent wave dual-color fluorescence fiber-embedded optofluidic nanochip. *Biosens. Bioelectron.* **2024**, *257*, 116281. [CrossRef] [PubMed]
91. Zafar, R.; Bashir, S.; Nabi, D.; Arshad, M. Occurrence and quantification of prevalent antibiotics in wastewater samples from Rawalpindi and Islamabad, Pakistan. *Sci. Total Environ.* **2021**, *764*, 142596. [CrossRef]
92. Mahmoud, R.A.; Hadad, G.M.; Abdel Salam, R.A.; Mokhtar, H.I. Optimization of a solid-phase extraction coupled with a high-performance liquid chromatography and diode array ultraviolet detection method for monitoring of different antibiotic class residues in water samples. *J. AOAC Int.* **2024**, *107*, 52–60. [CrossRef] [PubMed]
93. Li, F.; Wang, X.; Yang, M.; Zhu, M.; Chen, W.; Li, Q.; Sun, D.; Bi, X.; Maletskyi, Z.; Ratnaweera, H. Detection Limits of Antibiotics in Wastewater by Real-Time UV–VIS Spectrometry at Different Optical Path Length. *Processes* **2022**, *10*, 2614. [CrossRef]
94. Pei, J.; Tian, Z.; Yu, X.; Zhang, S.; Ma, S.; Sun, Y.; Boukherroub, R. Highly-sensitive SERS detection of tetracycline: Sub-enhancement brought by light scattering of nano-diamond. *Appl. Surf. Sci.* **2023**, *608*, 155270. [CrossRef]
95. Fabregat-Safont, D.; Gracia-Marín, E.; Ibáñez, M.; Pitarch, E.; Hernández, F. Analytical key issues and challenges in the LC-MS/MS determination of antibiotics in wastewater. *Anal. Chim. Acta* **2023**, *1239*, 340739. [CrossRef] [PubMed]
96. Ikizoglu, B.; Turkdogan, F.I.; Kanat, G.; Aydiner, C. Seasonal analysis of commonly prescribed antibiotics in Istanbul city. *Environ. Monit. Assess.* **2023**, *195*, 566. [CrossRef] [PubMed]
97. Hernandez, F.; Ibanez, M.; Portoles, T.; Hidalgo-Troya, A.; Ramirez, J.D.; Paredes, M.A.; Hidalgo, A.F.; Garcia, A.M.; Galeano, L.A. High resolution mass spectrometry-based screening for the comprehensive investigation of organic micropollutants in surface water and wastewater from Pasto city, Colombian Andean highlands. *Sci. Total Environ.* **2024**, *922*, 171293. [CrossRef] [PubMed]
98. Silva, L.R.G.; Carvalho, J.H.S.; Stefano, J.S.; Oliveira, G.G.; Prakash, J.; Janegitz, B.C. Electrochemical sensors and biosensors based on nanodiamonds: A review. *Mater. Today Commun.* **2023**, *35*, 106142. [CrossRef]
99. Zhou, Y.; Wang, J. Detection and removal technologies for ammonium and antibiotics in agricultural wastewater: Recent advances and prospective. *Chemosphere* **2023**, *334*, 139027. [CrossRef]
100. Pan, Y.; Shan, D.; Ding, L.L.; Yang, X.D.; Xu, K.; Huang, H.; Wang, J.F.; Ren, H.Q. Developing a generally applicable electrochemical sensor for detecting macrolides in water with thiophene-based molecularly imprinted polymers. *Water Res.* **2021**, *205*, 117670. [CrossRef]
101. Adane, W.D.; Chandravanshi, B.S.; Getachew, N.; Tessema, M. A cutting-edge electrochemical sensing platform for the simultaneous determination of the residues of antimicrobial drugs, rifampicin and norfloxacin, in water samples. *Anal. Chim. Acta* **2024**, *1312*, 342746. [CrossRef]

102. Liu, Y.; Chen, J.; Hu, H.; Qu, K.; Cui, Z. A low-cost electrochemical method for the determination of sulfadiazine in aquaculture wastewater. *Int. J. Environ. Res. Public. Health* **2022**, *19*, 16945. [CrossRef] [PubMed]
103. Zhang, Z.; Zhang, H.; Tian, D.; Phan, A.; Seididamyeh, M.; Alanazi, M.; Ping Xu, Z.; Sultanbawa, Y.; Zhang, R. Luminescent sensors for residual antibiotics detection in food: Recent advances and perspectives. *Coordin Chem. Rev.* **2024**, *498*, 215455. [CrossRef]
104. Raja Lakshmi, P.; Nanjan, P.; Kannan, S.; Shanmugaraju, S. Recent advances in luminescent metal–organic frameworks (LMOFs) based fluorescent sensors for antibiotics. *Coord. Chem. Rev.* **2021**, *435*, 213793. [CrossRef]
105. Sankhla, L.; Kushwaha, H.S. Development of optical sensor for detection of tetracycline using manganese Metal–Organic Framework (Mn-MOF). *J. Electron. Mater.* **2024**, *53*, 1896–1902. [CrossRef]
106. Zhao, Y.; Wang, Y.J.; Wang, N.; Zheng, P.; Fu, H.R.; Han, M.L.; Ma, L.F.; Wang, L.Y. Tetraphenylethylene-Decorated Metal-Organic Frameworks as Energy-Transfer Platform for the Detection of Nitro-Antibiotics and White-Light Emission. *Inorg. Chem.* **2019**, *58*, 12700–12706. [CrossRef]
107. Lei, M.; Ge, F.; Ren, S.; Gao, X.; Zheng, H. A water-stable Cd-MOF and corresponding MOF@melamine foam composite for detection and removal of antibiotics, explosives, and anions. *Sep. Purif. Technol.* **2022**, *286*, 120433. [CrossRef]
108. Yang, Q.; Hong, H.; Luo, Y. Heterogeneous nucleation and synthesis of carbon dots hybrid Zr-based MOFs for simultaneous recognition and effective removal of tetracycline. *Chem. Eng. J.* **2020**, *392*, 123680. [CrossRef]
109. Mao, K.; Zhang, H.; Pan, Y.; Yang, Z. Biosensors for wastewater-based epidemiology for monitoring public health. *Water Res.* **2021**, *191*, 116787. [CrossRef] [PubMed]
110. Kramat, J.; Kraus, L.; Gunawan, V.J.; Smyej, E.; Froehlich, P.; Weber, T.E.; Spiehl, D.; Koeppl, H.; Blaeser, A.; Suess, B. Sensing Levofloxacin with an RNA Aptamer as a Bioreceptor. *Biosensors* **2024**, *14*, 56. [CrossRef] [PubMed]
111. Wang, B.; Liu, L.; Zhang, H.; Wang, Z.; Chen, K.; Wu, B.; Hu, L.; Zhou, X.; Liu, L. A group-targeting biosensor for sensitive and rapid detection of quinolones in water samples. *Anal. Chim. Acta* **2024**, *1301*, 342475. [CrossRef]
112. Vera-Candioti, L.; Olivieri, A.C.; Goicoechea, H.C. Development of a novel strategy for preconcentration of antibiotic residues in milk and their quantitation by capillary electrophoresis. *Talanta* **2010**, *82*, 213–221. [CrossRef] [PubMed]
113. Zhu, Y.; He, P.; Hu, H.; Qi, M.; Li, T.; Zhang, X.; Guo, Y.; Wu, W.; Lan, Q.; Yang, C.; et al. Determination of quinolone antibiotics in environmental water using automatic solid-phase extraction and isotope dilution ultra-performance liquid chromatography tandem mass spectrometry. *J. Chromatogr. B Anal. Technol. Biomed. Life Sci.* **2022**, *1208*, 123390. [CrossRef] [PubMed]
114. Košutić, K.; Dolar, D.; Ašperger, D.; Kunst, B. Removal of antibiotics from a model wastewater by RO/NF membranes. *Sep. Purif. Technol.* **2007**, *53*, 244–249. [CrossRef]
115. Cui, J.; Zhang, Y.; Pan, Y.; Li, J.; Xie, A.; Xue, C.; Pan, J. Preparation of antifouling zwitterion PVDF-imprinted composite membranes for selective antibiotic and oil/water emulsion separation. *React. Funct. Polym.* **2023**, *187*, 105580. [CrossRef]
116. Cheng, N.; Wang, B.; Wu, P.; Lee, X.; Xing, Y.; Chen, M.; Gao, B. Adsorption of emerging contaminants from water and wastewater by modified biochar: A review. *Environ. Pollut.* **2021**, *273*, 116448. [CrossRef]
117. Yang, S.; Lin, C.; Wu, C.; Ng, K.; Yu-Chen Lin, A.; Andy Hong, P. Fate of sulfonamide antibiotics in contact with activated sludge—Sorption and biodegradation. *Water Res.* **2012**, *46*, 1301–1308. [CrossRef]
118. Ben, W.; Qiang, Z.; Yin, X.; Qu, J.; Pan, X. Adsorption behavior of sulfamethazine in an activated sludge process treating swine wastewater. *J. Environ. Sci.* **2014**, *26*, 1623–1629. [CrossRef]
119. Lakshminarasimman, N.; Quinones, O.; Vanderford, B.J.; Campo-Moreno, P.; Dickenson, E.V.; McAvoy, D.C. Biotransformation and sorption of trace organic compounds in biological nutrient removal treatment systems. *Sci. Total Environ.* **2018**, *640–641*, 62–72. [CrossRef]
120. Gupta, A.; Vyas, R.K.; Vyas, S. A review on antibiotics pervasiveness in the environment and their removal from wastewater. *Sep. Sci. Technol.* **2023**, *58*, 326–344. [CrossRef]
121. Wang, J.; Guo, X.; Xue, J. Biofilm-developed microplastics as vectors of pollutants in aquatic environments. *Environ. Sci. Technol.* **2021**, *55*, 12780–12790. [CrossRef]
122. Zhao, H.; Wang, Z.; Liang, Y.; Wu, T.; Chen, Y.; Yan, J.; Zhu, Y.; Ding, D. Adsorptive decontamination of antibiotics from livestock wastewater by using alkaline-modified biochar. *Environ. Res.* **2023**, *226*, 115676. [CrossRef] [PubMed]
123. Feng, Y.; Yang, L.; Liu, J.; Logan, B.E. Electrochemical technologies for wastewater treatment and resource reclamation. *Environ. Sci. Water Res.* **2016**, *2*, 800–831. [CrossRef]
124. Yuan, Q.; Qu, S.; Li, R.; Huo, Z.; Gao, Y.; Luo, Y. Degradation of antibiotics by electrochemical advanced oxidation processes (EAOPs): Performance, mechanisms, and perspectives. *Sci. Total Environ.* **2023**, *856*, 159092. [CrossRef] [PubMed]
125. Wang, J.; Zhuan, R. Degradation of antibiotics by advanced oxidation processes: An overview. *Sci. Total Environ.* **2020**, *701*, 135023. [CrossRef] [PubMed]
126. Frontistis, Z.; Mantzavinos, D.; Meriç, S. Degradation of antibiotic ampicillin on boron-doped diamond anode using the combined electrochemical oxidation—Sodium persulfate process. *J. Environ. Manag.* **2018**, *223*, 878–887. [CrossRef]
127. Yao, B.; Luo, Z.; Yang, J.; Zhi, D.; Zhou, Y. Fe(II)Fe(III) layered double hydroxide modified carbon felt cathode for removal of ciprofloxacin in electro-Fenton process. *Environ. Res.* **2021**, *197*, 111144. [CrossRef]
128. Miyata, M.; Ihara, I.; Yoshid, G.; Toyod, K.; Umetsu, K. Electrochemical oxidation of tetracycline antibiotics using a Ti/IrO_2 anode for wastewater treatment of animal husbandry. *Water Sci. Technol.* **2011**, *63*, 456–461. [CrossRef]

129. Hu, J.; Bian, X.; Xia, Y.; Weng, M.; Zhou, W.; Dai, Q. Application of response surface methodology in electrochemical degradation of amoxicillin with Cu-PbO_2 electrode: Optimization and mechanism. *Sep. Purif. Technol.* **2020**, *250*, 117109. [CrossRef]
130. Nabgan, W.; Saeed, M.; Jalil, A.A.; Nabgan, B.; Gambo, Y.; Ali, M.W.; Ikram, M.; Fauzi, A.A.; Owgi, A.; Hussain, I.; et al. A state of the art review on electrochemical technique for the remediation of pharmaceuticals containing wastewater. *Environ. Res.* **2022**, *210*, 112975. [CrossRef]
131. Ma, J.; Wang, X.; Sun, H.; Tang, W.; Wang, Q. A review on three-dimensional electrochemical technology for the antibiotic wastewater treatment. *Environ. Sci. Pollut. Res.* **2023**, *30*, 73150–73173. [CrossRef]
132. Vignati, D.; Lofrano, G.; Libralato, G.; Guida, M.; Siciliano, A.; Carraturo, F.; Carotenuto, M. Photocatalytic ZnO-Assisted degradation of spiramycin in urban wastewater: Degradation kinetics and toxicity. *Water* **2021**, *13*, 1051. [CrossRef]
133. Nasuhoglu, D.; Rodayan, A.; Berk, D.; Yargeau, V. Removal of the antibiotic levofloxacin (LEVO) in water by ozonation and TiO2 photocatalysis. *Chem. Eng. J.* **2012**, *189–190*, 41–48. [CrossRef]
134. Sneha, Y.; Yashas, S.R.; Thinley, T.; Prabagar, J.S.; Puttaiah, S.H. Photocatalytic degradation of lomefloxacin antibiotics using hydrothermally synthesized magnesium titanate under visible light-driven energy sources. *Environ. Sci. Pollut. Res. Int.* **2022**, *29*, 67969–67980. [CrossRef]
135. Singh, M.; Rugma, T.P.; Golda, A.S.; Neppolian, B.; Naushad, M.; Lakhera, S.K. Selective vanadium etching and in-situ formation of δ-Bi_2O_3 on m-BiVO4 with g-C3N4 nanosheets for photocatalytic degradation of antibiotic tetracycline. *J. Clean. Prod.* **2024**, *442*, 140921. [CrossRef]
136. Saadati, F.; Keramati, N.; Ghazi, M.M. Influence of parameters on the photocatalytic degradation of tetracycline in wastewater: A review. *Crit. Rev. Environ. Sci. Technol.* **2016**, *46*, 757–782. [CrossRef]
137. Dimitrakopoulou, D.; Rethemiotaki, I.; Frontistis, Z.; Xekoukoulotakis, N.P.; Venieri, D.; Mantzavinos, D. Degradation, mineralization and antibiotic inactivation of amoxicillin by UV-A/TiO_2 photocatalysis. *J. Environ. Manag.* **2012**, *98*, 168–174. [CrossRef]
138. Ahmadi, M.; Ramezani Motlagh, H.; Jaafarzadeh, N.; Mostoufi, A.; Saeedi, R.; Barzegar, G.; Jorfi, S. Enhanced photocatalytic degradation of tetracycline and real pharmaceutical wastewater using MWCNT/TiO_2 nano-composite. *J. Environ. Manag.* **2017**, *186*, 55–63. [CrossRef]
139. Wang, J.; Wang, S. Microbial degradation of sulfamethoxazole in the environment. *Appl. Microbiol. Biotechnol.* **2018**, *102*, 3573–3582. [CrossRef]
140. Verlicchi, P.; Galletti, A.; Petrovic, M.; Barceló, D.; Al Aukidy, M.; Zambello, E. Removal of selected pharmaceuticals from domestic wastewater in an activated sludge system followed by a horizontal subsurface flow bed—Analysis of their respective contributions. *Sci. Total Environ.* **2013**, *454–455*, 411–425. [CrossRef]
141. Alvarino, T.; Suarez, S.; Lema, J.M.; Omil, F. Understanding the removal mechanisms of PPCPs and the influence of main technological parameters in anaerobic UASB and aerobic CAS reactors. *J. Hazard. Mater.* **2014**, *278*, 506–513. [CrossRef]
142. Nguyen, P.Y.; Carvalho, G.; Reis, A.C.; Nunes, O.C.; Reis, M.A.M.; Oehmen, A. Impact of biogenic substrates on sulfamethoxazole biodegradation kinetics by Achromobacter denitrificans strain PR1. *Biodegradation* **2017**, *28*, 205–217. [CrossRef] [PubMed]
143. Chen, C.X.; Aris, A.; Yong, E.L.; Noor, Z.Z. A review of antibiotic removal from domestic wastewater using the activated sludge process: Removal routes, kinetics and operational parameters. *Environ. Sci. Pollut. Res.* **2022**, *29*, 4787–4802. [CrossRef] [PubMed]
144. Tambosi, J.L.; de Sena, R.F.; Favier, M.; Gebhardt, W.; José, H.J.; Schröder, H.F.; Moreira, R.D.F.P. Removal of pharmaceutical compounds in membrane bioreactors (MBR) applying submerged membranes. *Desalination* **2010**, *261*, 148–156. [CrossRef]
145. Radjenovic, J.; Petrovic, M.; Barceló, D. Analysis of pharmaceuticals in wastewater and removal using a membrane bioreactor. *Anal. Bioanal. Chem.* **2007**, *387*, 1365–1377. [CrossRef] [PubMed]
146. Sahar, E.; Ernst, M.; Godehardt, M.; Hein, A.; Herr, J.; Kazner, C.; Melin, T.; Cikurel, H.; Aharoni, A.; Messalem, R.; et al. Comparison of two treatments for the removal of selected organic micropollutants and bulk organic matter: Conventional activated sludge followed by ultrafiltration versus membrane bioreactor. *Water Sci. Technol.* **2011**, *63*, 733–740. [CrossRef] [PubMed]
147. Hamjinda, N.S.; Chiemchaisri, W.; Chiemchaisri, C. Upgrading two-stage membrane bioreactor by bioaugmentation of Pseudomonas putida entrapment in PVA/SA gel beads in treatment of ciprofloxacin. *Int. Biodeter. Biodegr.* **2017**, *119*, 595–604. [CrossRef]
148. Shi, B.; Wang, Y.; Geng, Y.; Liu, R.; Pan, X.; Li, W.; Sheng, G. Application of membrane bioreactor for sulfamethazine-contained wastewater treatment. *Chemosphere* **2018**, *193*, 840–846. [CrossRef]
149. Balu, S.; Chuaicham, C.; Balakumar, V.; Rajendran, S.; Sasaki, K.; Sekar, K.; Maruthapillai, A. Recent development on core-shell photo(electro)catalysts for elimination of organic compounds from pharmaceutical wastewater. *Chemosphere* **2022**, *298*, 134311. [CrossRef]
150. Sun, J.; Yang, P.; Huang, S.; Li, N.; Zhang, Y.; Yuan, Y.; Lu, X. Enhanced removal of veterinary antibiotic from wastewater by photoelectroactive biofilm of purple anoxygenic phototroph through photosynthetic electron uptake. *Sci. Total Environ.* **2020**, *713*, 136605. [CrossRef] [PubMed]
151. Chiemchaisri, W.; Chiemchaisri, C.; Witthayaphirom, C.; Saengam, C.; Mahavee, K. Reduction of antibiotic-resistant-*E. coli, -K. pneumoniae, -A. baumannii* in aged-sludge of membrane bioreactor treating hospital wastewater. *Sci. Total Environ.* **2022**, *812*, 152470. [CrossRef]

152. Polesel, F.; Andersen, H.R.; Trapp, S.; Plosz, B.G. Removal of antibiotics in biological wastewater treatment systems-A critical assessment using the activated sludge modeling framework for Xenobiotics (ASM-X). *Environ. Sci. Technol.* **2016**, *50*, 10316–10334. [CrossRef] [PubMed]
153. Wu, C.; Zhou, Y.; Sun, X.; Fu, L. The recent development of advanced wastewater treatment by ozone and biological aerated filter. *Environ. Sci. Pollut. Res.* **2018**, *25*, 8315–8329. [CrossRef] [PubMed]
154. Jin, L.; Sun, X.; Ren, H.; Huang, H. Biological filtration for wastewater treatment in the 21st century: A data-driven analysis of hotspots, challenges and prospects. *Sci. Total Environ.* **2023**, *855*, 158951. [CrossRef] [PubMed]

water

MDPI

Article

Determination of the Occurrence of Trihalomethanes in the Drinking Water Supply of the City of Cuenca, Ecuador

Bolívar Hernández [1], Paola Duque-Sarango [1,*], María Dolores Tonón [2], Mónica Abril-González [2], Verónica Pinos-Vélez [2,3], Cristian R. García-Sánchez [4] and Manuel J. Rodríguez [4]

[1] Grupo de Investigación sobre Recursos Hídricos (GIRH-UPS), Universidad Politécnica Salesiana, El Vecino Campus, Calle Vieja 12-30 y Elia Liut, Cuenca 010203, Ecuador; jhernandezs2@est.ups.edu.ec

[2] Department of Water Resources and Environmental Sciences, Universidad de Cuenca, Eco-Campus Balzay, Av. Victor Manuel Albornoz, Cuenca 010202, Ecuador; maria.tonon@ucuenca.edu.ec (M.D.T.); monica.abrilg@ucuenca.edu.ec (M.A.-G.); veronica.pinos@ucuenca.edu.ec (V.P.-V.)

[3] Department of Biosciences, Ecocampus Balzay, Universidad de Cuenca, Cuenca 010202, Ecuador

[4] Graduate School of Land Planning and Regional Development, Faculty of Planning, Architecture, Art and Design, Université Laval, Québec City, QC G1V 0A6, Canada; crgas1@ulaval.ca (C.R.G.-S.); manuel.rodriguez@esad.ulaval.ca (M.J.R.)

* Correspondence: pduque@ups.edu.ec; Tel.: +593-0958923036

Abstract: Water chlorination, fundamental for its microbiological safety, generates by-products, such as trihalomethanes (THMs), potentially associated with carcinogenic and reproductive risks. This study determined the levels of chloroform ($CHCl_3$) in drinking water in Cuenca, Ecuador, a topic that has been little explored in the region. During five months, water samples were collected from three water treatment systems (Cebollar, Tixan, and Sustag), and in situ measurements of physicochemical parameters such as free chlorine, pH, temperature, electrical conductivity, and turbidity were performed in the storage and distribution area. The determination of $CHCl_3$ was performed following the Hach protocol. For data analysis, the Kruskal–Wallis test was employed, followed by Dunn's post hoc method and Spearman's correlation coefficient. The results revealed a progressive decrease in free residual chlorine throughout the distribution systems. $CHCl_3$ concentrations ranged from 11.75 μg/L to 21.88 μg/L, remaining below the Ecuadorian regulatory limit of 300 μg/L. There was no consistent correlation between $CHCl_3$ and physicochemical parameters. These findings align with previous research, suggesting that the variability in $CHCl_3$ formation is associated with different water treatment conditions and environmental variables. This study highlights the importance of monitoring disinfection processes to minimize THMs and other DBPs, ensure public health, and contribute to sustainable drinking water management in Ecuador.

Keywords: trihalomethanes; chloroform; chlorination; drinking water quality; Cuenca; disinfection by-products; water treatment systems

1. Introduction

Water scarcity and insecurity represent critical challenges in today's world, putting the health and safety of the population at risk in the short and long term [1]. In this context, ensuring the microbiological safety of drinking water is fundamental in water treatment systems [2], with chlorine disinfection being a common practice to inactivate microorganisms and prevent their development during water storage and distribution [3]. This process aims to eliminate pathogenic organisms present in water to make it suitable for human consumption and other domestic activities [4,5]. Access to water in adequate quantity, which is safe, of acceptable quality, and economically accessible, is recognized as a fundamental human right and constitutes a key element in the Sustainable Development Goals [6].

Chemical methods to disinfect water mainly include the use of chlorine, chlorine dioxide, ozone, and chloramines, which have been widely applied worldwide for several decades [7,8]. However, the generation of numerous disinfection by-products (DBPs) represents a significant concern, especially in chlorinated drinking water, because chlorination byproducts, such as THMs, are frequently used as indicators of other DBPs [9]. THMs are usually the most abundant type of DBPs in chlorinated water. The formation of these by-products depends mainly on the number of precursors (organic and inorganic materials present in the untreated water), the characteristics of the treatment and disinfection processes [10], environmental conditions (such as water temperature), and distribution conditions (especially the water residence time). Worldwide, more than 700 types of DBPs have been detected in drinking water, from which the most studied groups are THMs and haloacetic acids (HAAs) [11,12]. The species present in the highest concentrations in chlorinated drinking water is commonly chloroform ($CHCl_3$) [13], especially when raw water contains little levels of bromide.

Chlorine doses and free residual chlorine are key factors in the formation of THMs. The primary sources of chlorine in drinking water include direct chlorination during water treatment and residual chlorine from distribution networks. Additionally, industrial and agricultural activities may contribute to chlorine-based compounds in source waters. Therefore, having monitoring data for residual chlorine and a thorough understanding of the mechanisms of its decay, as well as the processes leading to the formation of THMs, is essential to effectively manage these compounds in water supply systems [11,14]. Primarily, the formation of THMs occurs through the reaction of chlorine with natural organic matter (NOM) over time, a process that depends not only on the amount but also on the specific type of organic matter [15,16]. In addition, the physicochemical properties of water, such as temperature, pH, and presence of chlorophyll and nitrogen content, significantly influence chlorine demand and THM formation. Also, since water quality parameters can vary considerably over time and space (within the distribution system), these fluctuations also affect chlorine demand and, consequently, DBP management [16].

The issue of potential human health effects from exposure to DBPs is a matter of significant concern, as well as their potential reproductive and developmental implications [17]. The main route of exposure to THMs is ingestion, although dermal and inhalation exposure is also relevant, considering that these compounds are volatile at room temperature [18]. Several epidemiological studies have established associations between chlorination byproducts and a variety of diseases, such as musculoskeletal congenital disabilities [19], kidney disease [20], low birth weight [21], effects on male reproductive health, impaired ovarian function in women [22,23], increased risk of bladder cancer [24], and risk of colorectal cancer [25].

Several techniques have been reported for the determination of THMs in water, including advanced methods such as gas chromatography–negative chemical ionization–mass spectrometry (GC-NCI-MS), gas chromatography with electron capture detection (GC-ECD), and the Purge and Trap technique coupled with GC-ECD, which offer high precision and sensitivity [26–28]. Other approaches include the head-space technique coupled with gas chromatography–mass spectrometry (HS-GC-MS) and solid phase microextraction (SPME) or liquid phase microextraction (LPME) techniques, valuable for their simplicity and low solvent consumption when combined with GC-ECD or GC-MS [29,30]. In addition, modern artificial intelligence-based methods, such as artificial neural networks and support vector machines, have been explored to predict the presence of THMs using Python® and MATLAB® [31].

Additionally, more accessible methods have been investigated, such as spectrophotometric and colorimetric methods, known for their ease of implementation and low cost. These techniques have proven to be effective for monitoring THMs trends in the field [32,33]. In this context, the Hach THM Plus™ colorimetric method (method 10,132) is included among the available options for THMs evaluation, being recognized in recent studies for its ability to generate reliable results under specific conditions [34,35].

International agencies have set standards and guidelines for the presence of THMs in drinking water. The U.S. Environmental Protection Agency [36] set a limit of 0.08 mg/L for total THMs, while the World Health Organization [37] sets specific guideline levels for the various species: 0.3 mg/L for chloroform, 0.1 mg/L for bromoform, 0.1 mg/L for dibromochloromethane, and 0.06 mg/L for bromodichloromethane. In the European Union, the regulation establishes a maximum limit of 0.1 mg/L for total THMs [38]. Ecuadorian regulations [39] establish maximum permissible limits for some compounds: 0.3 mg/L for chloroform, 3.0 mg/L for monochloramine, and 0.06 mg/L for bromodichloromethane. In Ecuador, although there are studies on water quality, few have focused on DBPs, such as the study by Salazar-Flores et al. [40]. While these studies have been valuable, their scope has been limited in terms of geographical coverage and the number of compounds analyzed. Furthermore, advanced analytical techniques that could enable more precise detection have not been explored. This lack of research on THMs hinders the assessment of regulatory compliance and the control of public health risks. In addition, to mitigate THM formation, alternative disinfection methods such as chloramination and advanced oxidation processes (AOPs) can be considered. On the other hand, optimizing chlorine dosing and applying precursor removal strategies (e.g., activated carbon filtration) can significantly reduce THM formation while maintaining adequate disinfection levels [37].

In this context, this study in Ecuador represents a crucial advance in understanding the spatio-temporal occurrence of $CHCl_3$, one of the most common THMs in drinking water. In Cuenca canton, there is an aggravated scenario due to the limited surveillance of DBPs, which generates unawareness of the problem and hinders the implementation of adequate measures. The purpose of this research is to evaluate the presence of $CHCl_3$ in the drinking water supply of the city of Cuenca, Ecuador, a topic that has been little explored in the country. The innovative contribution of this study lies in the application of field photometric techniques for the detection of $CHCl_3$, an approach that seeks to facilitate the future development of water quality control and monitoring strategies. In addition, the research responds to the lack of data on DBP in the region, providing valuable information on its occurrence and possible implications on public health and drinking water quality.

2. Materials and Methods

2.1. Description of the Study Area

This study was conducted in the canton of Cuenca, located in the province of Azuay in the south-central region of Ecuador (Figure 1). This territory extends from the western cordillera to the inter-Andean valley of the Andes. Its geography includes high mountain landscapes, such as the paramo, as well as valley floor areas, where the city of Cuenca, the main urban settlement, is located at an altitude of approximately 2500 masl [41]. Cuenca's drinking water system is organized into four subsystems, named after the rivers where the water comes from: Tomebamba, Machangara, Yanuncay, and Culebrillas. In this study, the subsystems corresponding to the Tomebamba, Machangara, and Yanuncay rivers were considered, each with its own catchment, treatment, and distribution infrastructure, whose waters are processed in the Cebollar, Tixan, and Sustag water treatment plants, respectively [42,43].

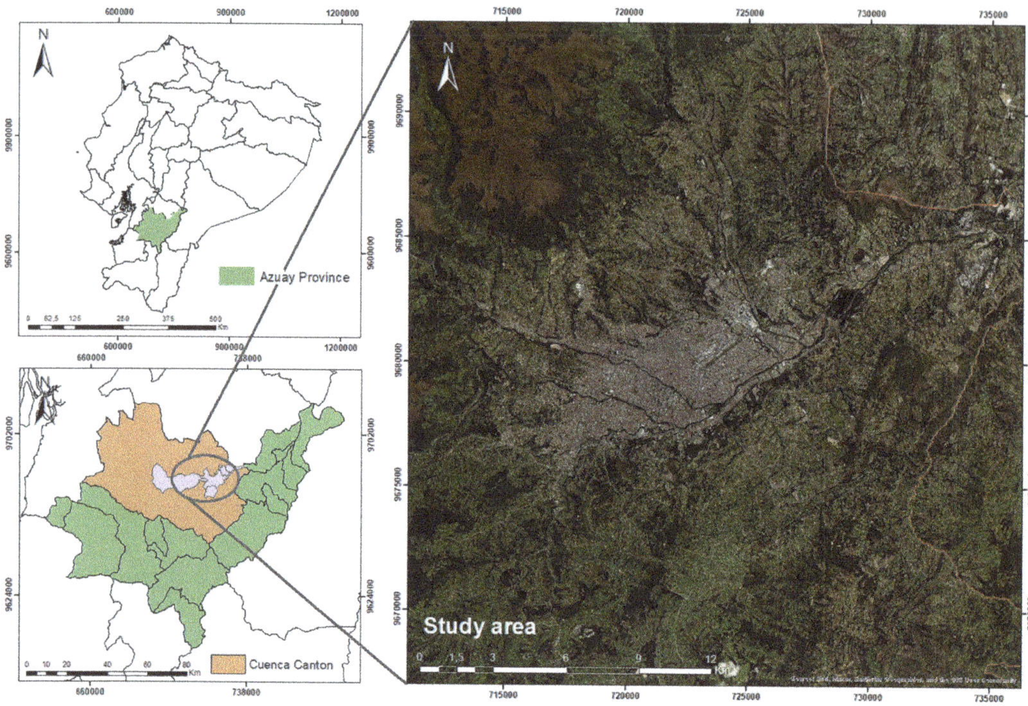

Figure 1. Study area.

2.2. Sampling

Four sampling zones were identified in the three drinking water treatment systems: Cebollar (C), Tixan (T), and Sustag (S). In each system, sampling was conducted in the treated water storage area (CS, TS, SS) and at three additional points along the distribution network (C1–C3, T1–T3, S1–S3). These points were selected in residences near the treatment plant, at an intermediate and end point of the distribution network (Figure 2).

Sampling was carried out during five months in 2023 and 2024, covering the periods from December and March to June, with eight sampling events. Two types of samples were collected at each point: the first, in 40 mL vials, for the determination of chloroform ($CHCl_3$), and the second, in 710 mL sterile bags, intended for laboratory turbidity measurement using HANNA® HI98703 equipment.

Additionally, in situ measurements of physicochemical parameters were performed, including free chlorine (free Cl) with the DR 300 colorimeter from Hach®, pH with the pHtestr30 from Oakton®, temperature and electrical conductivity with the Multi 340i from WTW®. In total, 40 samples were analyzed.

The samples were kept in a container on ice during the sampling process. Thereafter, the samples were transferred to the laboratory and stored at a temperature of 4 °C until analysis.

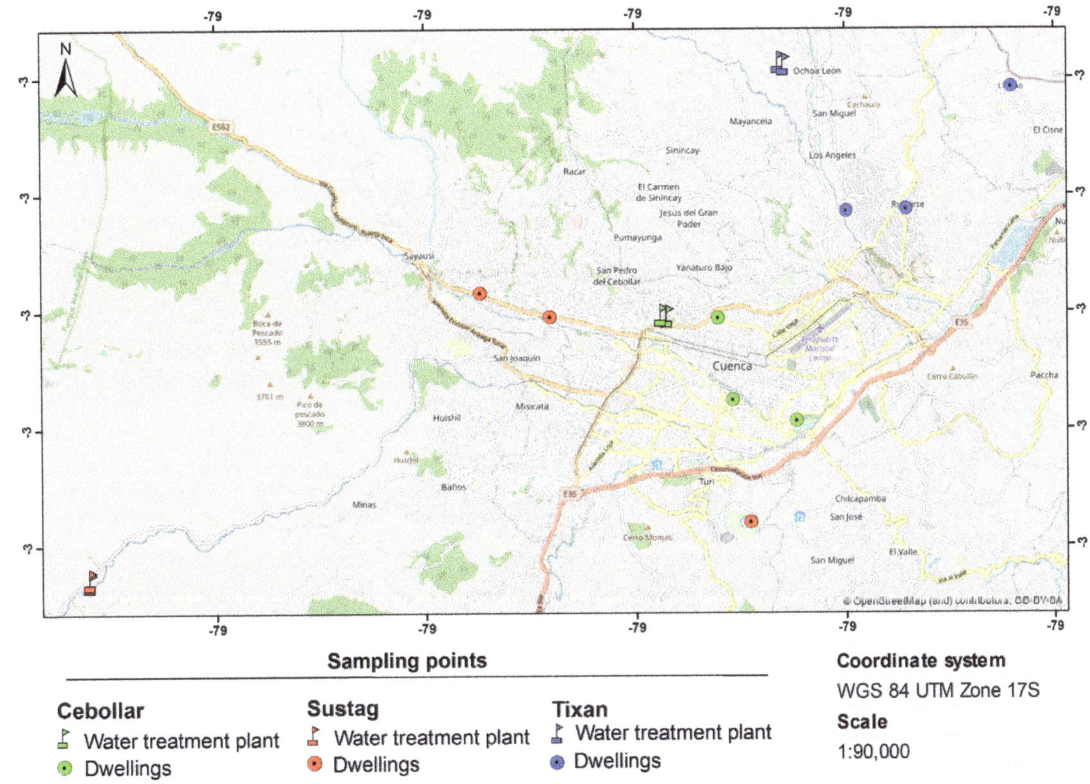

Figure 2. Location of sampling points.

2.3. Determination of $CHCl_3$

The determination of $CHCl_3$ was determined using the THM Plus method, according to Hach® method 10,132, with a measuring range of 10 to 600 µg/L $CHCl_3$ surveyed. The reagent set includes THM Plus reagent solutions 1, 2, and 3, as well as sachets of THM Plus 4 powder [44]. The process for the determination of $CHCl_3$ was determined by the protocol proposed by Hach® [45], using the DR 1900 kit.

Prior to analysis, it was necessary to add three drops of THM Plus Reagent 1 to the freshly collected samples in the 40 mL vials, following the protocol specifications [45]. As part of the procedure, initially, two baths were prepared: one with hot water (500 mL) and one with cold water (18–25 °C, 500 mL). Water samples were transferred to 10 mL vials labeled for correct identification. Additionally, a blank was prepared using deionized water to ensure analysis accuracy. To each cell, 3 mL of THM Plus Reagent 2 was added, avoiding shaking until the cells were closed entirely. Subsequently, the samples were mixed to ensure homogeneity of the reagent and placed in a hot water bath for 5 min. After this time, the cells were transferred to the cooling bath for another 5 min. They were then removed and inverted three times to homogenize the temperature. A total of 1 mL of THM Plus Reagent 3 was added to each cell, and the cells were returned to the cooling bath for another 5 min. At the end of the cooling time, one sachet of THM Plus Reagent 4 powder was added to each cell, and the cells were shaken until the powder was completely dissolved. After dissolution, 15 min were waited before proceeding with the measurement. For the final analysis, the prepared samples and blank were transferred to DR 1900 square cells and allowed to stand for 30 s to enable the turbidity to settle. Finally, each sample was measured using the prepared blank as a reference.

2.4. Statistical Analysis

A descriptive analysis of the data was performed, involving the calculation of measures of central tendency and dispersion to summarize the main characteristics of the data. To evaluate the assumptions of normality, the Shapiro–Wilk test was applied, and for homoscedasticity, the Levene test was used. Most of the data groups do not follow a normal distribution and do not present homogeneity of variance. Consequently, we chose to use nonparametric tests. For the analysis of variance, the Kruskal–Wallis test was used. Subsequently, a post hoc test was performed using Dunn's test for the parameters that showed significant differences in the analysis of variance. In addition, a correlation analysis was performed using Spearman's correlation coefficient for the three water treatment systems.

3. Results

3.1. Physicochemical Characteristics of Water Quality

The results obtained from the physicochemical analysis of the water samples at the different water treatment systems under study, C, S, and T, show notable differences in the values of pH, temperature, electrical conductivity (EC), turbidity, and free chlorine concentration (free Cl) (Table 1). Cebollar has the highest electrical conductivity, turbidity, and free chlorine levels (Figure S1). Sustag has the highest temperature and the lowest levels of turbidity and electrical conductivity (Figure S2). Tixan has similar characteristics to those previously described for Cebollar and Sustag, although it shows higher pH levels in water (Figure S3).

Table 1. Average values of the physicochemical parameters of water (standard deviations into parenthesis).

Treatment Plant	Code	pH	Temperature (°C)	CE (µS/cm)	Turbidity (NTU)	Free Cl (mg/L)
Cebollar	CS	7.20 ± 0.31	15.01 ± 0.66	114.48 ± 17.88	0.71 ± 0.68	1.20 ± 0.17
	C1	7.34 ± 0.24	20.23 ± 2.17	123.25 ± 17.64	1.07 ± 0.58	1.01 ± 0.31
	C2	7.26 ± 0.48	20.36 ± 1.93	115.50 ± 21.16	1.04 ± 0.32	0.88 ± 0.31
	C3	7.33 ± 0.15	20.64 ± 1.70	123.08 ± 14.26	1.57 ± 1.35	0.77 ± 0.33
Sustag	SS	7.06 ± 0.50	15.18 ± 2.11	77.14 ± 8.05	0.46 ± 0.24	1.24 ± 0.30
	S1	6.76 ± 0.65	22.61 ± 4.02	82.38 ± 13.26	0.53 ± 0.39	0.88 ± 0.28
	S2	6.81 ± 0.65	21.50 ± 2.28	77.77 ± 9.68	0.53 ± 0.18	0.73 ± 0.23
	S3	7.01 ± 0.32	19.98 ± 2.80	83.63 ± 11.77	0.62 ± 0.33	0.34 ± 0.19
Tixan	TS	7.54 ± 0.49	15.15 ± 1.58	110.50 ± 11.29	0.54 ± 0.48	1.05 ± 0.37
	T1	7.44 ± 0.25	19.55 ± 2.73	103.75 ± 7.92	0.44 ± 0.25	0.87 ± 0.35
	T2	7.46 ± 0.25	20.16 ± 1.87	106.13 ± 7.20	0.51 ± 0.26	0.79 ± 0.29
	T3	7.70 ± 0.21	20.01 ± 2.52	118.13 ± 12.29	0.65 ± 0.41	0.29 ± 0.16

3.2. Free Chlorine Levels

The Kruskal–Wallis test applied to the free Cl concentrations in the three water treatment systems results in a p-value of 1.114×10^{-6} (Table S1), indicating that there are statistically significant differences between the various sampling points within each water system. Dunn's test shows that, in the Cebollar plant, there is a significant difference between sampling points CS and C3; in the Sustag plant, between points SS and S2, SS and S3, and S1 and S3; and in the Tixan plant, between points TS and T2, TS and T3, and T1 and T3 ($p < 0.05$, in all cases).

The box plot (Figure 3) compares the variability of free Cl concentration (mg/L) at different sampling points along the three water systems. Each sampling point on the X-axis represents a specific site within the distribution network, starting from the initial storage of treated water (CS, SS, TS) and progressing along the network to the extremity (C3, S3, T3). Cebollar shows lower variability at the initial sampling points (CS, C1), but increases towards the intermediate and end points (C2, C3). Sustag shows higher initial chlorine concentrations in SS, with a pronounced decrease towards points S2 and S3. Tixan shows a greater dispersion in free Cl values at its first points (TS and T2), and stabilization is observed towards points T1 and T3. The differences in chlorine variability among the three plants could be associated with the specific conditions of each system, such as the type of source water, the treatment applied, the design of the distribution network, and the water residence time.

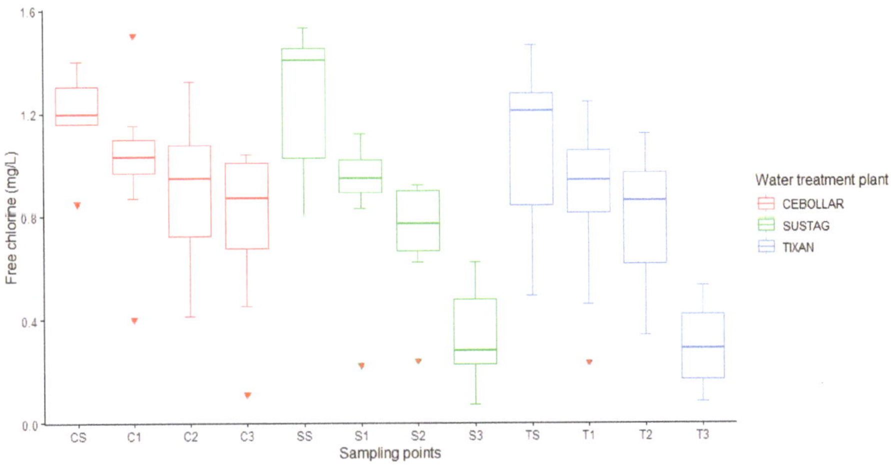

Figure 3. Comparison of the variability of free chlorine concentrations in the three drinking water systems.

Figure 4 shows a decreasing trend in the average free Cl concentration as a function of the sampling points. This progressive decrease in the three plants suggests a reduced free Cl throughout the treatment process, probably due to the chlorine demand by organic matter and other compounds in the water. In addition, the graphs on the right (Figure 4) show the concentration of free Cl at each sampling point over time, differentiated by groups. Free chlorine concentrations show temporal variations at each point, with noticeable fluctuations at the initial points and relative stability at the endpoints, although with occasional peaks. These variations could be associated with changes in the quality of the raw water, adjustments in the doses of chlorine applied or variations in the operating conditions of each plant.

3.3. $CHCl_3$ Concentrations

The concentrations of $CHCl_3$ in the drinking water treatment systems analyzed show a relatively high variability, as detailed in Table 2. At Cebollar, concentrations fluctuate between 12.25 μg/L and 20.88 μg/L, with a slight decrease at sampling point C3, where 17.13 μg/L was recorded. At Sustag, concentrations range between 11.75 μg/L and 21.88 μg/L. Finally, at Tixan, $CHCl_3$ concentrations range between 13.00 μg/L and 19.88 μg/L.

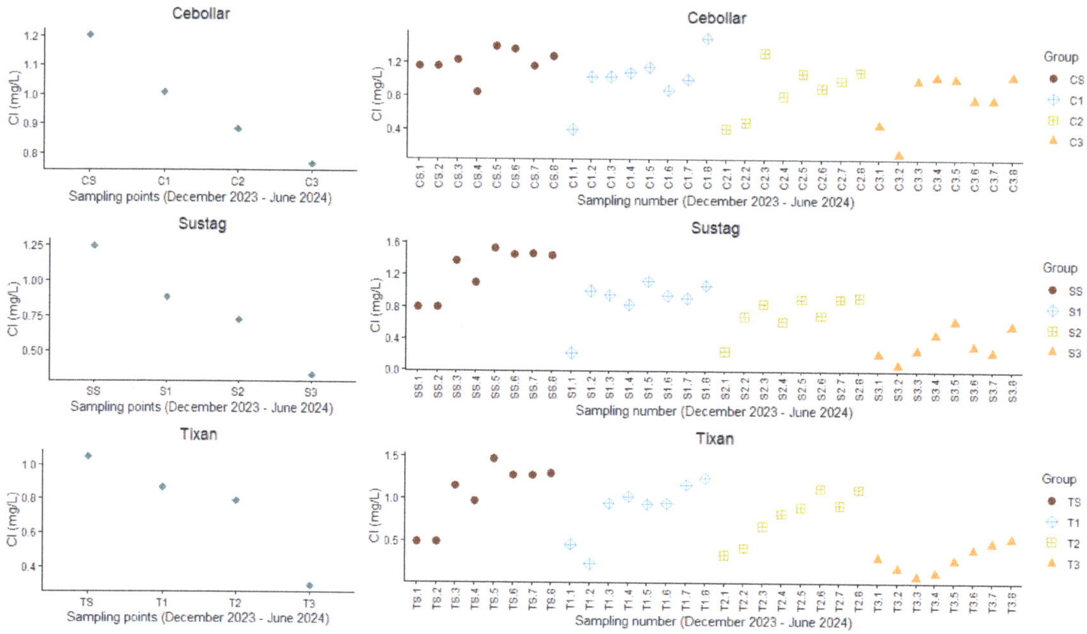

Figure 4. Variability of free chlorine concentrations at the different sampling locations.

Table 2. Average concentrations of $CHCl_3$ at the different sampling locations.

PTA	Code	$CHCl_3$ (μg/L)
Cebollar	CS	12.25 ± 5.07
	C1	25.75 ± 6.82
	C2	20.88 ± 5.54
	C3	17.13 ± 3.69
Sustag	SS	21.88 ± 3.98
	S1	14.25 ± 5.73
	S2	11.75 ± 4.87
	S3	17.75 ± 6.74
Tixan	TS	14.25 ± 6.23
	T1	15.75 ± 6.18
	T2	13.00 ± 5.66
	T3	19.88 ± 6.44

Figure 5 shows the spatial variations of $CHCl_3$. In Cebollar, it is evident that the values start low and reach a peak around sampling point C1, before dropping at point C3. At Sustag, they show a downward trend from the initial sampling point SS, get a minimum at S2, and then increase again at point S3. At Tixan, the levels also have an undulating behavior, reaching a maximum at point T1, decreasing at T2, and rising again at T3. The graphs on the right (Figure 5) show the variability of $CHCl_3$ in each sampling location group. Here, significant variability is observed in each group, indicating fluctuations across samples. At each location, the initial group has a higher concentration in some samples, while at other points, the concentrations appear to stabilize or fluctuate.

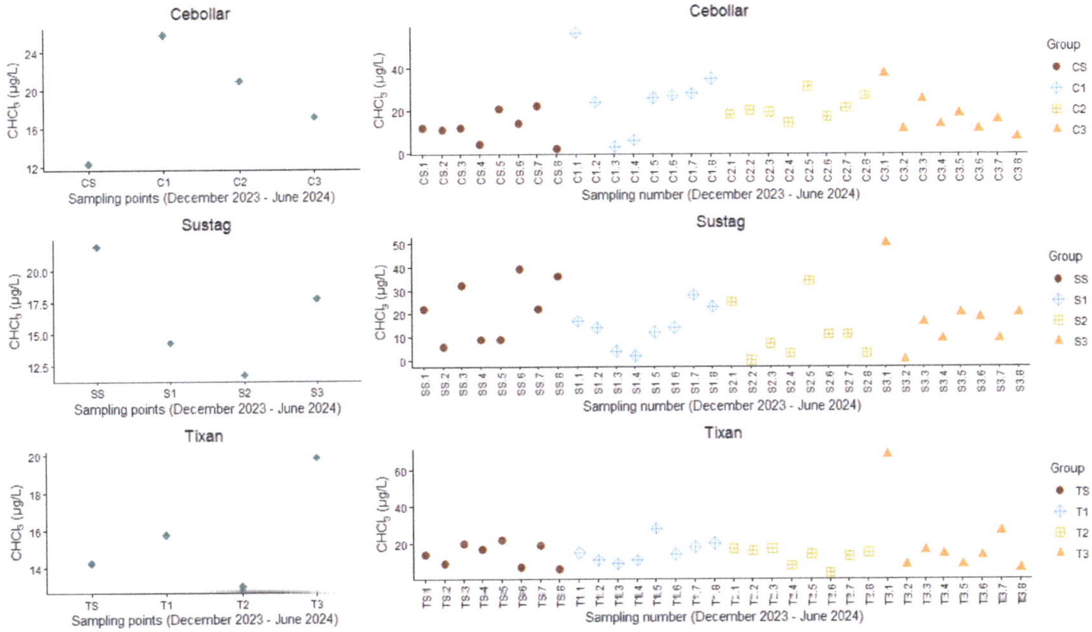

Figure 5. Variability of $CHCl_3$ levels at the different sampling locations.

In general, Cebollar seems to have higher $CHCl_3$ values compared to Sustag and Tixan. In Sustag, fluctuations are more considerable compared to Tixan, where variations are smoother, which could indicate differences in treatment conditions or water quality in each area.

3.4. Spearman's Correlation Analysis

The variables analyzed in this section include pH, Temp (temperature), EC (electrical conductivity), Turb (turbidity), FC (free chlorine), and $CHCl_3$.

Free chlorine presents both positive and negative correlations with $CHCl_3$ at the different sampling points. For example, at the Cebollar plant points, the correlation coefficients are 0.32 at CS, −0.29 at C1, 0.50 at C2, and −0.28 at C3 (Table S2). In the Sustag plant, the values are 0.30 in SS, −0.05 in S1, 0.07 in S2, and 0.39 in S3 (Table S3). Finally, in the Tixan plant, correlations of 0.16 in TS, 0.24 in T1, −0.74 in T2, and −0.18 in T3 are observed (Table S4). These results indicate that the relationship between free chlorine and chloroform does not follow a consistent pattern among plants or sampling points. In addition, other variables such as pH, temperature, electrical conductivity, and turbidity also do not show a uniform trend of correlation with $CHCl_3$, which could reflect local differences in treatment conditions and water characteristics (Figure 6).

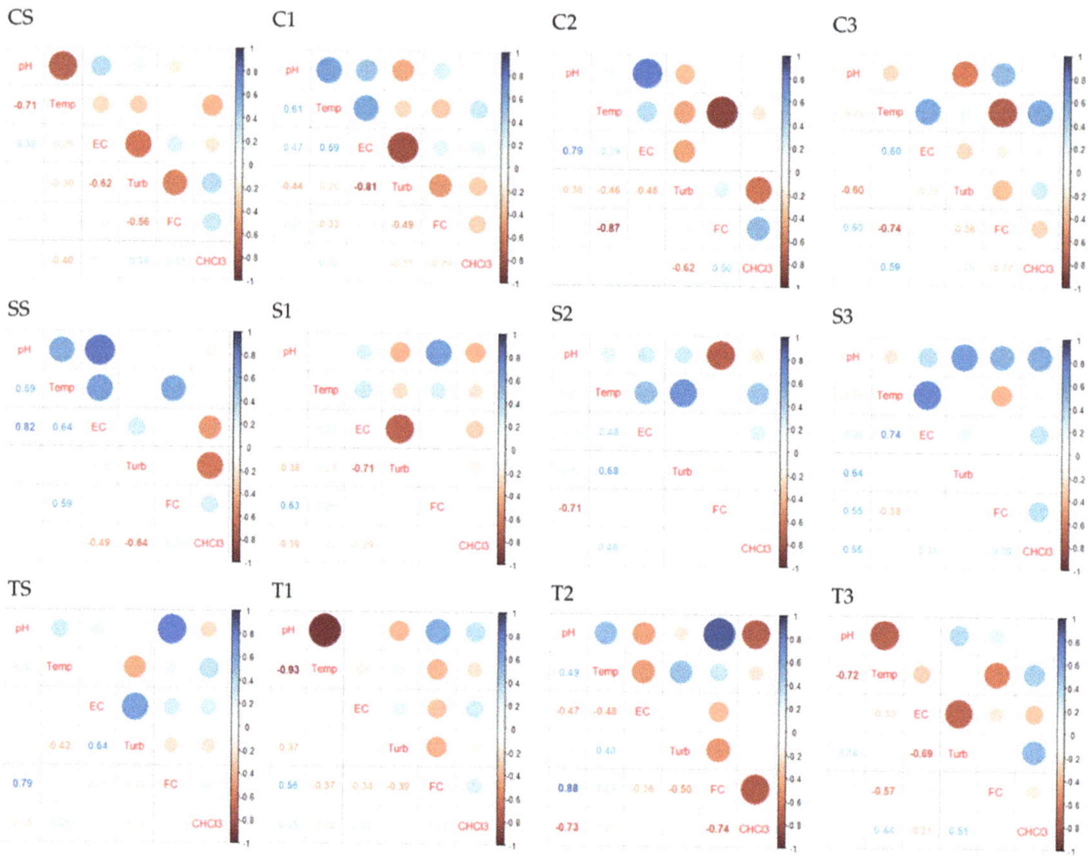

Figure 6. Spearman correlation analysis for pH, temperature, electrical conductivity, turbidity, free chlorine, and chloroform.

4. Discussion

The present study evaluated the presence of $CHCl_3$ as an indicator of THMs in the drinking water supply of Cuenca, Ecuador, considering three different drinking water treatment systems (Cebollar, Sustag, and Tixan). A fundamental aspect of this analysis was the monitoring of free chlorine, given its critical role in contributing to DBP formation. In addition, key parameters such as temperature, pH, and electrical conductivity were studied because, according to Padhi et al. [16], these parameters directly influence the chemical reactions that lead to the generation of THMs.

Water pH ranged from 6.76 to 7.70, which is within the optimal range for THM formation. According to previous studies, THMs concentration decreases, and HAAs increase as pH decreases. Furthermore, pH also plays a vital role in determining the type and amount of DBPs formed, as lower and acidic pHs ($pH \leq 7$) result in the formation of less $CHCl_3$ [46,47]. As for temperature, the observed variations (15.01 °C to 22.61 °C) could significantly influence the reaction kinetics of free chlorine with natural organic matter since higher temperatures usually increase the rate of DBP formation [48,49]. Electrical conductivity (77.77 and 123.25 µS/cm), although the relationship is not fully established, plays an indirect role in THMs formation and would be associated with the availability of inorganic compounds that modulate chlorine demand in the system, as suggested by Amarasooriya et al. [50]. Also, turbidity, which ranged from 0.46 to 1.57 NTU, reflected the number of suspended particles, which may interfere with the efficiency of the disinfection process by demanding available chlorine [51]. In this context, despite the theoretical influence of these parameters on chlorine demand and THMs formation, especially $CHCl_3$, the statistical analysis of this study failed to establish a clear correlation between them. This can be explained by the complexity of chemical interactions in the treatment system, where multiple reactions occur simultaneously, making it difficult to identify individual factors with a direct bearing on THMs formation, as reported by Padhi et al. [16].

Free chlorine concentrations ranged from 0.29 to 1.24 mg/L, showing a progressively decreasing pattern during the water travel within the distribution network. This can be explained by the chlorine demand induced by the organic matter present in the water, as well as by other compounds that interact with chlorine in the disinfection stages. Previous studies [10,14–16] have pointed out that natural organic matter (NOM) is a key factor in reducing the concentration of free residual chlorine. In addition, aspects such as hydraulic residence time, pipe length, diameter, roughness, material type, and age, as well as water quality conditions, including pH, electrical conductivity, temperature, and turbidity, have a considerable impact on residual chlorine decay [52]. These factors also contribute to the observed fluctuations in free chlorine concentrations, underscoring the need for continuous monitoring of this parameter and for operational adjustments of treatment processes (e.g., organic matter removal and chlorine doses) to minimize DBP formation and ensure the quality of the drinking water supply.

Chloroform occurrence in all the analyzed points shows fluctuations from 11.75 μg/L to 21.88 μg/L. These values are below the maximum permissible limit of 300 μg/L for chloroform according to Ecuadorian regulations [39]. These results are consistent with previous studies in Ecuador, such as that of Salazar-Flores et al. [40], who reported that $CHCl_3$ concentrations in drinking water in the cities of Pedro Vicente Maldonado and Latacunga during 2018 and 2019 ranged between 18 μg/L and 20 μg/L, and between 12 μg/L and 16 μg/L, respectively.

Studies conducted in the region and other countries have shown significant variability in THMs concentrations in drinking water. In Panama, for example, total THMs concentrations ranged from 0.01 to 4.15 μg/L, with $CHCl_3$ being the predominant compound (52.1%) [53]. In Venezuela, according to the study by Sarmiento et al. [54], total THMs concentrations fluctuated between 47.84 and 93.23 μg/L, where $CHCl_3$ was the main compound, representing 83% of total THMs. In other Latin American countries, variable levels of THMs have also been recorded. To mention a few, in Brazil, the average concentrations were 58.5 μg/L, in Mexico 47.4 μg/L, in Colombia 31.3 μg/L, in Peru 31.7 μg/L, in Argentina 31.7 μg/L, and in Chile 16.5 μg/L, while in countries outside the region such as the United States (33.6 μg/L) and Spain (85 μg/L) a high variability was also evident [10].

5. Conclusions

Monitoring and evaluating the formation of THMs, specifically chloroform, in drinking water supplies is crucial to ensure public health and compliance with water quality standards. The results obtained in this study underscore the importance of understanding the factors that influence the formation of these compounds, such as the presence of natural organic matter, the physicochemical conditions of the water, the disinfection process, and the behavior of free residual chlorine during the distribution network. Although the chloroform levels found in Cuenca's drinking water treatment systems were below the maximum regulatory limit, the need for rigorous monitoring and operational adjustments in the disinfection processes is highlighted. The variability of THM concentrations in different contexts highlights the importance of adopting efficient disinfection practices tailored to the specific characteristics of each water source to minimize long-term public health risks.

This study provides a solid basis for future efforts to improve water treatment systems to benefit the population.

Supplementary Materials: The following supporting information can be downloaded at https://www.mdpi.com/article/10.3390/w17040591/s1, Figure S1: Physicochemical parameters measured at the sampling points of the Cebollar Plant; Figure S2: Physicochemical parameters measured at the sampling points of the Sustag Plant; Figure S3: Physicochemical parameters measured at the sampling points of the Tixan Plant; Table S1: Kruskal-Wallis test of the Free Chlorine values measured at the three sampling zones (Cebollar, Sustag, and Tixan); Table S2: Results of the Spearman correlation test in the Cebollar sampling system; Table S3: Results of the Spearman correlation test in the Sustag sampling system; Table S4: Results of the Spearman correlation test in the Tixan sampling system.

Author Contributions: Conceptualization, B.H. and P.D.-S.; methodology, M.J.R. and C.R.G.-S.; validation, P.D.-S. and V.P.-V.; formal analysis, B.H. and M.A.-G.; research, B.H. and P.D.-S.; data curation, B.H.; writing-original draft preparation, B.H.; writing-review and editing, P.D.-S.; supervision, P.D.-S., V.P.-V. and M.D.T.; project administration, P.D.-S. and M.D.T.; funding acquisition, P.D.-S.; project administration, P.D.-S. and M.D.T.; supervision, P.D.-S., V.P.-V. and M.D.T.; project administration, P.D.-S.; funding acquisition, P.D.-S. and M.J.R. All authors have read and agreed to the published version of the manuscript.

Funding: This research was funded by Salesian Polytechnic University, project number 006-001-2024-01-18.

Data Availability Statement: The raw data supporting the conclusions of this article will be available upon request from the authors.

Acknowledgments: The authors would like to thank the following institutions for funding the project on the detection of trihalomethanes in water: the VIUC of the University of Cuenca, the Salesian Polytechnic University for the approval of project 006-001-2024-01-18, Research on Drinking water of Université Laval for support in logistics, in particular Cristian García for field and laboratory help, and ETAPA EP for the facilities provided during the sampling process.

Conflicts of Interest: The authors declare no conflicts of interest.

References

1. Duque-Sarango, P.; Romero-Martínez, L.; Pinos-Vélez, V.; Sánchez-Cordero, E.; Samaniego, E. Comparative Study of UV Radiation Resistance and Reactivation Characteristics of *E. coli* ATCC 8739 and Native Strains: Implications for Water Disinfection. *Sustainability* **2023**, *15*, 9559. [CrossRef]
2. Duque-Sarango, P.; Delgado-Armijos, N.; Romero-Martínez, L.; Pinos-Vélez, V. Assessing the potential of ultraviolet irradiation for inactivating waterborne fungal spores: Kinetics and photoreactivation studies. *Front. Environ. Sci.* **2023**, *11*, 1212807. [CrossRef]
3. Cheswick, R.; Moore, G.; Nocker, A.; Hassard, F.; Jefferson, B.; Jarvis, P. Chlorine disinfection of drinking water assessed by flow cytometry: New insights. *Environ. Technol. Innov.* **2020**, *19*, 101032. [CrossRef]
4. Srivastav, A.L.; Patel, N.; Chaudhary, V.K. Disinfection by-products in drinking water: Occurrence, toxicity and abatement. *Environ. Pollut.* **2020**, *267*, 115474. [CrossRef]
5. Romero-Martínez, L.; Duque-Sarango, P.; González-Martín, C.; Moreno-Andrés, J.; Acevedo-Merino, A.; Nebot, E. Inactivation efficacy and reactivation of fecal bacteria with a flow-through LED ultraviolet reactor: Intraspecific response prevails over interspecific differences. *J. Water Process Eng.* **2023**, *52*, 103497. [CrossRef]
6. WHO. "Drinking-Water", World Health Organization. Available online: https://lc.cx/wNxWH5 (accessed on 29 September 2024).
7. Chawla, H.; Chandra, A.; Ingole, P.P.; Garg, S. Recent advancements in enhancement of photocatalytic activity using bismuth-based metal oxides Bi_2MO_6 (M = W, Mo, Cr) for environmental remediation and clean energy production. *J. Ind. Eng. Chem.* **2021**, *95*, 1–15. [CrossRef]
8. Tsitsifli, S.; Kanakoudis, V. Disinfection Impacts to Drinking Water Safety—A Review. In *EWaS3 2018*; MDPI: Basel Switzerland, 2018; p. 603. [CrossRef]
9. Dubey, S.; Gusain, D.; Sharma, Y.C.; Bux, F. The occurrence of various types of disinfectant by-products (trihalomethanes, haloacetic acids, haloacetonitrile) in drinking water. In *Disinfection By-Products in Drinking Water*; Elsevier: Amsterdam, The Netherlands, 2020; pp. 371–391. [CrossRef]

10. Villanueva, C.M.; Evlampidou, I.; Ibrahim, F.; Donat-Vargas, C.; Valentin, A.; Tugulea, A.M.; Echigo, S.; Jovanovic, D.; Lebedev, A.T.; Lemus-Pérez, M.; et al. Global assessment of chemical quality of drinking water: The case of trihalomethanes. *Water Res.* **2023**, *230*, 119568. [CrossRef] [PubMed]
11. Brown, D.; Bridgeman, J.; West, J.R. Predicting chlorine decay and THM formation in water supply systems. *Rev. Environ. Sci. Biotechnol.* **2011**, *10*, 79–99. [CrossRef]
12. Hu, G.; Mian, H.R.; Mohammadiun, S.; Rodriguez, M.J.; Hewage, K.; Sadiq, R. Appraisal of machine learning techniques for predicting emerging disinfection byproducts in small water distribution networks. *J. Hazard. Mater.* **2023**, *446*, 130633. [CrossRef] [PubMed]
13. Sathasivan, A.; Kastl, G.; Korotta-Gamage, S.; Gunasekera, V. Trihalomethane species model for drinking water supply systems. *Water Res.* **2020**, *184*, 116189. [CrossRef]
14. Hua, P.; Gao, Q.; Wang, Z.; Jiang, S.; de Oliveira, K.R.F.; Macedo, D.O. Modeling and elucidation the effects of iron deposits on chlorine decay and trihalomethane formation in drinking water distribution system. *Water Res.* **2021**, *207*, 117804. [CrossRef] [PubMed]
15. Clayton, G.E.; Thorn, R.M.S.; Reynolds, D.M. Comparison of Trihalomethane Formation Using Chlorine-Based Disinfectants Within a Model System; Applications Within Point-of-Use Drinking Water Treatment. *Front. Environ. Sci.* **2019**, *7*, 35. [CrossRef]
16. Padhi, R.K.; Subramanian, S.; Mohanty, A.K.; Satpathy, K.K. Comparative assessment of chlorine reactivity and trihalomethanes formation potential of three different water sources. *J. Water Process Eng.* **2019**, *29*, 100769. [CrossRef]
17. Kumari, M.; Gupta, S.K. Occurrence and Exposure to Trihalomethanes in Drinking Water: A Systematic Review and Meta-analysis. *Expo. Health* **2022**, *14*, 915–939. [CrossRef]
18. Tovar, S.S.T.; Susa, M.R. Cancer risk assessment from exposure to trihalomethanes in showers by inhalation. *Environ. Res.* **2021**, *196*, 110401. [CrossRef] [PubMed]
19. Kaufman, J.A.; Wright, J.M.; Evans, A.; Rivera-Núñez, Z.; Meyer, A.; Narotsky, M.G. Disinfection by-product exposures and the risk of musculoskeletal birth defects. *Environ. Epidemiol.* **2020**, *4*, e081. [CrossRef] [PubMed]
20. Medgyesi, D.N.; Mohan, S.; Bangia, K.; Spielfogel, E.S.; Fisher, J.A.; Jones, R.R.; Ward, M.H.; Lacey, J.V., Jr.; Sanchez, T.R. Trihalomethanes from residential community water supplies and chronic kidney disease risk among women in California. In Proceedings of the ISEE 2024: 36th Annual Conference of the International Society of Environmental Epidemiology, Santiago, Chile, 25–28 August 2024. [CrossRef]
21. An, S.L.; Xiong, S.M.; Shen, X.B.; Ni, Y.Q.; Chen, W.; He, C.D.; Zhou, Y.Z. The associations between exposure to trihalomethanes during pregnancy and adverse birth outcomes: A systematic review and meta-analysis. *Chemosphere* **2022**, *293*, 133524. [CrossRef] [PubMed]
22. Zhang, M.; Deng, Y.-L.; Liu, C.; Lu, W.-Q.; Zeng, Q. Impacts of disinfection byproduct exposures on male reproductive health: Current evidence, possible mechanisms and future needs. *Chemosphere* **2023**, *331*, 138808. [CrossRef] [PubMed]
23. Deng, Y.L.; Luo, Q.; Liu, C.; Zeng, J.Y.; Lu, T.T.; Shi, T.; Cui, F.P.; Yuan, X.Q.; Miao, Y.; Zhang, M.; et al. Urinary biomarkers of exposure to drinking water disinfection byproducts and ovarian reserve: A cross-sectional study in China. *J. Hazard. Mater.* **2022**, *421*, 126683. [CrossRef]
24. Evlampidou, I.; Font-Ribera, L.; Rojas-Rueda, D.; Gracia-Lavedan, E.; Costet, N.; Pearce, N.; Vineis, P.; Jaakkola, J.J.; Delloye, F.; Makris, K.C.; et al. Trihalomethanes in Drinking Water and Bladder Cancer Burden in the European Union. *Environ. Health Perspect.* **2020**, *128*, 017001. [CrossRef]
25. Helte, E.; Säve-Söderbergh, M.; Larsson, S.C.; Martling, A.; Åkesson, A. Disinfection by-products in drinking water and risk of colorectal cancer: A population-based cohort study. *JNCI J. Natl. Cancer Inst.* **2023**, *115*, 1597–1604. [CrossRef] [PubMed]
26. Hu, G.; Wang, H.; Yu, K.; Shen, W.; Hou, Y.; Ji, M.; Zhu, Y.; Tian, W.; Li, X. Determination of four trihalomethanes in ship ballast water by gas chromatography-negative chemical ionization-mass spectrometry. *Chin. J. Chromatogr.* **2022**, *40*, 584–589. [CrossRef] [PubMed]
27. Tafesse, N.; Porcelli, M.; Hirpessa, B.B.; Gasana, J.; Padhi, R.K.; Robele, S.; Ambelu, A. Trihalomethanes and physicochemical quality of drinking water in Addis Ababa, Ethiopia. *Heliyon* **2023**, *9*, e19446. [CrossRef]
28. Sánchez-Duque, G.; Lozada-Castro, J.J.; Hara, E.L.Y.; Grassi, M.T.; Rosero-Moreano, M.; Ríos-Acevedo, J.J. Alternative Ecosorbent for the Determination of Trihalomethanes in Aqueous Samples in SPME Mode. *Molecules* **2022**, *27*, 8653. [CrossRef] [PubMed]
29. Momeniha, F.; Oskouie, A.A.; Esrafili, A.; Janani, L.; Jafari, A.J. Trihalomethanes in exhaled air, indoor air and water: A parallel design trial in chlorine and ozone-chlorine disinfected swimming pools. *Build. Environ.* **2021**, *205*, 108316. [CrossRef]
30. Jin, M.; Wen, Z.F.; Liu, Y.J.; Qian, M.; Zhou, Y.; Bian, Y.; Zhang, Y.; Feng, X.S. Trihalomethanes in water samples: Recent update on pretreatment and detection methods. *Chemosphere* **2023**, *341*, 140005. [CrossRef]
31. Mahato, J.K.; Gupta, S.K. Exploring applicability of artificial intelligence and multivariate linear regression model for prediction of trihalomethanes in drinking water. *Int. J. Environ. Sci. Technol.* **2022**, *19*, 5275–5288. [CrossRef]

32. Cheshmekhezr, S.; Alimoradi, S.; Torabian, A.; Pardakhti, A.; Babaei, L. Investigation of the formation and effects of upstream trihalomethanes in Tehran's raw and drinking water using the spectrophotometric method. *J. Water Process Eng.* **2021**, *44*, 102426. [CrossRef]
33. Shariati-Rad, M.; Fattahi, F. A simple equipment and colorimetric method for determination of chloroform in water. *Anal. Chim. Acta* **2020**, *1100*, 208–214. [CrossRef] [PubMed]
34. Rasheduzzaman, M.; O'Connell, B.; Krometis, L.-A.; Brown, T.; Cohen, A. Point-of-use chlorine residuals and disinfection byproduct occurrences in rural households served by public water utilities in Appalachian Virginia. *J. Water Health* **2024**, *22*, 1064–1074. [CrossRef]
35. Ali, S.I.; Arnold, M.; Liesner, F.; Fesselet, J.-F. Characterization of Disinfection By-Products Levels at an Emergency Surface Water Treatment Plant in a Refugee Settlement in Northern Uganda. *Water* **2019**, *11*, 647. [CrossRef]
36. EPA. "Current EPA Microbial and Disinfection Byproduct Regulations", Agencia de Protección Ambiental de los Estados Unidos. Available online: https://archive.epa.gov/enviro/html/icr/web/html/regulations.html (accessed on 20 November 2024).
37. WHO. *Guidelines for Drinking-Water Quality: Fourth Edition Incorporating the First Addendum*, 4th ed.; World Health Organization: Geneva, Switzerland, 2017. Available online: https://www.who.int/publications/i/item/9789241549950 (accessed on 20 November 2024).
38. EU. Directive (Eu) 2020/2184 of the European Parliament and of The Council of 16 December 2020 on the Quality of Water Intended for Human Consumption (Recast). The European Parliament and the Council of the European Union. 2020. Available online: https://eur-lex.europa.eu/legal-content/EN/TXT/PDF/?uri=CELEX:32020L2184&from=EN (accessed on 20 November 2024).
39. NTE INEN 1108. *Agua Potable. Requisitos*, 5th ed.; Norma Técnica Ecuatoriana: Quito, Ecuador, 2014. Available online: https://lc.cx/EEUYoT (accessed on 10 November 2024).
40. Salazar-Flores, C.A.; Kurbatova, A.I.; Mikhaylichenko, K.Y.; Milutka, A.C. Health risk assessment of drinking water: Case study of city of Latacunga and the canton of Pedro Vicente Maldonado (Ecuador). *Hyg. Sanit.* **2022**, *101*, 344–356. [CrossRef]
41. Cuenca, G.A. Plan de Desarrollo y Ordenamiento Territorial del Cantón Cuenca—Actualización 2022. Cuenca—Ecuador: Gobierno Autónomo Descentralizado del Cantón Cuenca. 2022. Available online: https://lc.cx/rBKHuI (accessed on 11 November 2024).
42. Arcentales-Ríos, R.; Carrión-Méndez, A.; Cipriani-Ávila, I.; Acosta, S.; Capparelli, M.; Moulatlet, G.M.; Pinos-Vélez, V. Assessment of metals, emerging contaminants, and physicochemical characteristics in the drinking water and wastewater of Cuenca, Ecuador. *J. Trace Elem. Miner.* **2022**, *2*, 100030. [CrossRef]
43. ETAPA. "Plantas de Potabilización", Empresa Pública Municipal de Telecomunicaciones, Agua Potable, Saneamiento y Gestión Ambiental del Cantón Cuenca. Available online: https://www.etapa.net.ec/agua-potable-y-saneamiento/operacion-y-mantenimiento-agua-potable-y-saneamiento/plantas-de-potabilizacion-agua-potable/ (accessed on 11 November 2024).
44. HACH. "THM PlusTM Method: Hach Method 10132—Total Trihalomethanes (THM) Reagent Set", HACH. Available online: https://ca.hach.com/product.detail-print.version.jsa?id=14533963759 (accessed on 11 November 2024).
45. HACH. "Trihalomethanes: Method 10132", HACH COMPANY. 2017. Available online: https://lc.cx/Sv_ZL6 (accessed on 11 November 2024).
46. Hung, Y.-C.; Waters, B.W.; Yemmireddy, V.K.; Huang, C.-H. pH effect on the formation of THM and HAA disinfection byproducts and potential control strategies for food processing. *J. Integr. Agric.* **2017**, *16*, 2914–2923. [CrossRef]
47. Sriboonnak, S.; Induvesa, P.; Wattanachira, S.; Rakruam, P.; Siyasukh, A.; Pumas, C.; Wongrueng, A.; Khan, E. Trihalomethanes in Water Supply System and Water Distribution Networks. *Int. J. Environ. Res. Public Health* **2021**, *18*, 9066. [CrossRef]
48. Valdivia-Garcia, M.; Weir, P.; Graham, D.W.; Werner, D. Predicted Impact of Climate Change on Trihalomethanes Formation in Drinking Water Treatment. *Sci. Rep.* **2019**, *9*, 9967. [CrossRef] [PubMed]
49. Masoud, M.S.; Ismail, A.M.; El-Hoshy, M.M. Kinetics and thermodynamics of the formation of trihalomethanes. *Appl. Water Sci.* **2019**, *9*, 99. [CrossRef]
50. Amarasooriya, A.A.G.D.; Weragoda, S.K.; Makehelwala, M.; Weerasooriya, R. Occurrence of trihalomethane in relation to treatment technologies and water quality under tropical conditions. *H2Open J.* **2018**, *1*, 69–83. [CrossRef]
51. Kalantary, R.R.; Oshidari, Y.; Amoohadi, V.; Niknejad, H.; Zeraatkar, R.; Arani, M.H. Investigating the relationship between free chlorine concentration and heterotrophs in water of swimming pool in Iran. *Heliyon* **2024**, *10*, e36804. [CrossRef] [PubMed]
52. Kwio-Tamale, J.C.; Onyutha, C. Influence of physical and water quality parameters on residual chlorine decay in water distribution network. *Heliyon* **2024**, *10*, e30892. [CrossRef] [PubMed]

53. Saldaña-González, I.; Ávila, H. Evaluación de la concentración de compuestos trihalometanos en el agua potable distribuida en la Ciudad David, Panamá y sus riesgos a la salud humana. *Rev. I+D Tecnológico* **2022**, *18*, 2022. Available online: http://portal.amelica.org/ameli/journal/339/3393183007/ (accessed on 19 November 2024). [CrossRef]
54. Sarmiento, A.; Rojas, M.; Medina, E.; Olivet, C.; Casanova, J. Investigación de trihalometanos en agua potable del Estado Carabobo, Venezuela. *Gac. Sanit.* **2003**, *17*, 137–143. [CrossRef] [PubMed]

MDPI AG
Grosspeteranlage 5
4052 Basel
Switzerland
Tel.: +41 61 683 77 34

Water Editorial Office
E-mail: water@mdpi.com
www.mdpi.com/journal/water

www.ingramcontent.com/pod-product-compliance
Lightning Source LLC
Chambersburg PA
CBHW062031220926
51850CB00010B/2512
* 9 7 8 3 7 2 5 8 5 1 3 7 9 *